Manifesto for
a New Medicine

Manifesto for a New Medicine ⌇

YOUR GUIDE TO HEALING PARTNERSHIPS AND THE WISE USE OF ALTERNATIVE THERAPIES

JAMES S. GORDON, M.D.

PERSEUS BOOKS
Reading, Massachusetts

The names of all those who have come to me for help as patients have been changed, as have a number of identifying characteristics. In every instance except one, I have drawn on the case history of a single patient. In one instance, I have combined elements from the experience of two patients.

Many of the designations used by manufacturers and sellers to distinguish their products are claimed as trademarks. Where those designations appear in this book and Perseus Books was aware of a trademark claim, the designations have been printed in initial capital letters.

Library of Congress Cataloging-in-Publication Data
Gordon, James S. (James Samuel)
   Manifesto for a new medicine : your guide to healing partnerships and the wise use of alternative therapies / James S. Gordon.
      p.   cm.
   Includes bibliographical references and index.
   ISBN 0-201-48383-1
   ISBN 0-201-89828-4 (pbk.)
   1. Self-care, Health.   2. Alternative medicine.   3. Physician and patient.   I. Title.
   [DNLM: 1. Alternative Medicine.   2. Holistic Health.   3. Self-Care. 4. Professional-Patient Relations.   WB   890   G663m   1996]
R733.G675   1996
613–dc20
DNLM/CLC
for Library of Congress   95-48962
                                                                      CIP

Perseus Books is a member of the Perseus Books Group

Cover design by Jean Seal
Text design by Robert G. Lowe
Set in 11-point Walbaum by Douglas & Gayle Limited

   5   6   7   8   9   10-DOH-03 02 01 00 99

To my mother and father, and my godchildren

Contents ∾

Acknowledgments 〜

My father died several years ago. I miss him, and I missed him particularly while I was writing this book. I think he would have enjoyed the process, and the book, and, of course, enjoyed pointing out ways I could have made it clearer and more complete.

I'm deeply appreciative of the people in the pages that follow and of countless others, not mentioned, who have helped to shape what I know and who I am. Three whose spirits are present throughout are William Alfred, Robert Coles, and Sharon Curtin. They were there during difficult times in medical school and after. Models of gentleness and generosity, they reminded me of why I was becoming, and being, a doctor. They also helped me to laugh and to cry, and even to laugh at myself.

At the National Institute of Mental Health, Bert Brown, Ira Lourie, Juan Ramos, Joy Schulterbrandt, and especially Steve Hersh made it possible for me to move more deeply into the new medicine.

Since 1991, when I started the Center for Mind-Body Medicine, I've had the support of my colleagues. David Wolfe and Jacqueline Mendelsohn were there at the beginning. Carole

O'Connor told me to "follow my dream" and helped me to do it. Carol Goldberg, Jane Kauffman, Susan Buell Gorner, Ann Patterson, Mary Lee Esty, and the Center's volunteers, donors, and Boards of Directors and Advisors have helped it to unfold.

Whenever other activities threatened to divert me, my agent, Beth Vesel, reminded me of the value of writing this book. Bill Patrick, the Editorial Director at Addison-Wesley, liked the idea as soon as he heard it, and I liked him and have enjoyed his guidance ever since.

Along the way, a number of students, residents, and practicing physicians have helped me gather the research on which this book is based. Among them are Joanne Bailey, Jeff Burns, Jeanne Chang, Brent Harris, Robert Heffron, Michael Joyner, Gary Kaplan, Langdon Lawrence, Jonathan Lee, Ted Leon, Jennifer McCord, Matthew Mintz, Andrea Perrone, Kevin Shilling, and Lisa Soldat.

Several good friends were kind enough to read and comment on all or part of the book and I'm very grateful to them. They include: George Blecher, Max Heirich, and Judi Jones, as well as my brother Jeff Gordon. Marshall Berman, Meme Black, Del Bryant, Brenda Dash, Carmen de Barrazza, Rick de Lone, Gerry Eitner, Jonathan Goldman, Carol Knowles, Lorna Malmberg, Jose Rosa, and Bob Schwartz offered wisdom and comfort. During all the days of this writing, my dear friends Alan Cheuse, Kris O'Shee, Victoria McCaleb, and Rudy Bauer were especially loving and supportive.

Finally, I want to thank two people who provided significant help in the final stages of writing and editing: Linda Copeland, who carefully gathered together the refer nces that I'd scattered over two offices and found those I'd lost; and Susan Lord, who line edited the manuscript and gently helped to focus my sometimes wandering authorial attention.

ONE

Time for a Change ⌖

THEIR VOICES have such urgency in them. "I have ovarian cancer," one woman begins, even before she tells me her name, "with metastases to my brain." "My arthritis is so bad," a man shouts into my ear, "it takes me an hour to get out of bed." "I'm depressed," intones another voice, as dark and deliberate as a funeral march. "They've given me every drug and nothing does any good." "My child has terrible asthma." "My blood pressure's off the charts." "I've got chronic fatigue syndrome." "My father has Parkinson's disease." They are like shipwrecked sailors shouting to a passing boat.

So-and-so said to call, they continue, offering me the name like an outstretched hand. Sometimes I recognize a referral from one of my patients, or a physician or psychotherapist I know. More often than not now, a friend of a friend of one of my patients has suggested it, or a few words of mine in a magazine, or a doctor, desperate for assistance, who has also heard or read "something." Why, I ask, into the rush of the appeal, against the tide of the story. "What have you heard? Do you know what you're getting into?"

Something, they say, about "alternative" medicine or a "holistic" approach, acupuncture or hypnosis, nutrition, herbs, or homeopathy; a story about someone who seemed hopeless but who is now well; some encouraging remark that rings an obscure bell. Glimmers of hope that beckon in the dense fog of depressing diagnoses and distressing procedures. They are sick and, it turns out, sick and tired too, of the way they've been treated as well as the treatments they've been receiving.

The "alternative" therapies they associate with me seem somehow more hopeful as well as different. They want a "holistic" approach, one which recognizes that they are whole people with feelings as well as fevers, with likes and dislikes in addition to lab values. And they, along with sixty million other Americans who each year use "unconventional" therapies, are ready to commit their minds, bodies, and money to what they hope will be a more effective, less toxic, less expensive, and altogether better way to receive care and care for themselves.

About once a week now, one of my callers mentions David Donne's name.

When David came to see me, he too was desperate. All his fingers angled like shanked iron shots toward his pinkies. They hurt from the moment he awoke to the moment he went to sleep, and they were capable of only the tiniest bend at their last joints. With a brow deeply furrowed from chronic pain and a belly grown soft from underactivity and overeating, he looked a decade older than his fifty-five years.

Like forty million other Americans, David had arthritis. He'd had the symptoms for more than ten years. He didn't have osteoarthritis, the bony erosion and overgrowth that accompanies aging and makes getting out of a chair an ordeal for tens of millions of older Americans. He had rheumatoid arthritis, the kind that comes to two million of us suddenly and early in our lives, swelling the supple joints of the young to heavy immobility and, after repeated "flares," hardening them to great knobby knots.

Because he was a well-to-do man, well insured by his Washington law firm and well connected, David had received the best medical care available. His internist, who was on the staff of one of D.C.'s medical schools, referred him to a respected rheumatologist. Both men continued to see David, the rheumatologist taking the lead in the treatment of his arthritis, the internist presiding at yearly physicals and available for other problems.

The rheumatologist had begun conservatively and confidently with aspirin, the time-honored anti-inflammatory drug. At doses high enough to afford David any relief, however, it irritated his stomach. The rheumatologist soon switched to "nonsteroidal anti-inflammatories," like Motrin but far stronger. He tried one after the other, each varying in chemical structure, all briefly useful but none effective for long. After a while he told David that arthritis is a chronic, life-long, and progressive condition with episodic exacerbations called flares. Indeed, every few months, in spite of the rheumatologist's best efforts, David's hands or knees, elbows or shoulders, grew large and hot with pain.

Sometimes David, who had spent six fruitful months talking with a psychotherapist, thought that these flares might be related to the stress of spousal quarrels. He tried to tell his rheumatologist about the war between himself and his wife. After eleven years of marriage they had separated. She was hurt and angry, he long-suffering and resentful, the children torn between them. David, a devout Catholic, explained to his doctor that divorce, which had once seemed beyond the pale, now looked like the promised land. The rheumatologist nodded politely. When David, discouraged by the pain and the increasing disability, wondered whether diet or maybe even prayer would help, his doctor responded by upping the pharmacological ante.

Relying on a still unproved theory that arthritis may be infectious in origin, the doctor ordered antibiotics. They did no good. On two occasions in the eighth and ninth years of David's suffering, his doctor put him on high doses of the synthetic steroids that resemble the body's own anti-inflammatory medicine, cortisone.

The pain and swelling in David's joints diminished, but his feet and face grew big with retained water. He lost his temper in the office, faltered in the courtroom, and grew teary at home. Finally the rheumatologist prescribed Plaquenil, a powerful antimalarial drug, which relieved his pain briefly but robbed David of his distant vision. Every day during the long years his doctor searched for the right anti-inflammatory regimen, David also had to take high doses of pain relievers—Tylenol with codeine and Percocet, a synthetic version of codeine.

By the time he came to see me, in the tenth year of his medical treatment, David was at his wits' end. His hands, unable to grip, were in constant pain. His left hand was all but useless. By two every afternoon he was exhausted. The anti-inflammatories and pain relievers ground away at his gut, damaged his liver, raised his cholesterol, and in any case were no longer effective. He'd all but lost interest in sex, was eating too much, and had put thirty pounds on his long but slight frame. The lost vision that the Plaquenil had caused had not returned when he stopped the drug.

David felt that each day he was deteriorating a little more. For months it had seemed that his mind was "going." He wasn't able to reason as closely as he needed, and vital details—the precise precedent he was searching for, or the right phrase to enlist the jury in his client's cause—seemed just beyond his reach. Golf, the joy of his youth and the enduring pleasure and balm of his adult life, had been out of the question for eight months. His rheumatologist, he told me, was even more despairing than he was. "I have," he told David grimly, "nothing left to offer."

David's situation is not unique. In fact, it is typical. The majority of American adults, and a significant minority of our children, suffer from one or more chronic, often debilitating, sometimes life-threatening illnesses.

Sixty million Americans have high blood pressure and are therefore particularly vulnerable to heart disease and stroke, the major killers of our population. Forty million of us have arthritis, and some ten million are afflicted with asthma. This year more than one million people will be diagnosed with cancer, and during our lifetimes as many as forty percent of us will develop one form or another of this feared and often deadly disease. It's been estimated that as many as thirty million people will have a clinical depression—one that includes physical as well as emotional signs and symptoms—at some point in their lives. Twenty-three million Americans suffer from the throbbing pain and nausea of migraine headaches, and up to 80 percent of our population will, at one time or another, have a "back problem." As many as one and a half million of us are HIV positive, and the number is increasing.

These illnesses are dangerous, debilitating, and enormously expensive: it has been estimated that *each year* back problems alone may cost our society as much as *$50 billion* in treatment and work time lost to pain and disability.

These conditions, many of which are unknown in aboriginal societies, have been called the "diseases of civilization." Some are rooted in significant genetic predispositions; others have specific causes. All, however, are shaped by the ways we think and feel, eat and exercise, work and play, by our environment, our economy, and our interpersonal world—by the stresses we experience and the way we respond to them.

Each year the incidence of these and other conditions increases. Almost 25 percent more people under sixty-five died of cancer in 1990 than in 1973. Since 1971 the overall incidence of cancer, according to the national Cancer Advisory Board, has increased by 18 percent, and the mortality rate has grown by 7 percent. The prevalence of asthma among children under eighteen increased by 39 percent between 1981 and 1988. A Mayo Clinic study indicated a 60 percent increase in people with multiple sclerosis between 1978 and 1985. The figures for migraine headache, back problems, Alzheimer's disease, depression, and eating disorders have all been following a similar pattern. Meanwhile new illnesses—fibromyalgia, chronic fatigue immune deficiency syndrome, Legionnaire's disease, and AIDS—are disabling, sometimes decimating, our population and frustrating conventional attempts at treatment.

Like David, those who suffer or may suffer from these problems are desperate for a fresh and more hopeful perspective. They are tired of being told they will "have to live with" illnesses that may cripple or kill them. They want to know more about the "alternative" treatments that, they have heard, can cure them or at least improve their sense of well-being. What about biofeedback and hypnosis for migraines, smoking cessation, and epilepsy? Are there really nutritional therapies that offer hope to people with cancer and arthritis? Is chiropractic the answer to back problems? Does acupuncture work for chronic pain, homeopathy for allergies and infections, and Chinese herbs for depression and AIDS? Can relaxation therapies, physical exercise, and meditation really change the course of heart disease, asthma, and anxiety? They want to find answers to these questions, and physicians and other practitioners to help them.

Large numbers of Americans have already decided to find the answers. A definitive survey of "Unconventional Medicine in the United States" published in the *New England Journal of Medicine* in 1993 indicated that more than one third of the adult population was, in 1990, making 425 million visits to practitioners of alternative therapies—a number of visits that exceeds those made to all primary care physicians. Equally impressively, these people were willing to pay for the services out of their own pockets: $10.3 billion out of a total of $13.7 billion spent. This latter figure, as the authors of the *Journal* article noted, was greater than the $12.8 billion spent out of pocket by all Americans on their hospitalizations.

Many of these people, like David, are fond of their physicians and impressed by their knowledge and technical skill. They regard the frequent and expensive tests they are given as hallmarks of professional thoroughness; appreciate their physicians' efforts to provide information about drugs and procedures; and do not balk at fees that are substantial if not outrageous.

But like David, they *are* troubled by the ineffectiveness of their treatment. They know and are pleased that it is "state-of-the-art." They just wish it were more helpful.

Others are discouraged not only with the treatment they have been getting but with the ways of those who have been treating them. They tell stories of doctors cruelly and casually breaking news about life-threatening diagnoses, then painting their bleak prospects with bland assurance. Their doctors, they say, seem to be oblivious of the side effects their words and their medicines cause, unequipped to deal with them as emotional beings, and unwilling to take seriously the alternative therapies their patients are so eager to learn about.

Rich patients recall famous physicians who hovered nervously at the door of their hospital rooms as if the cancer that ravaged their bodies were a flu that could be caught. Middle-class patients tell me about weeks of waiting lists in their health maintenance organizations, the impossibility of paying for a long-trusted physician not on the HMO's approved list, and care so cool and perfunctory they wish, once they finally arrive, that they'd never come. Meanwhile, the poor say they can't even get in the door—many doctors won't accept reduced fees or Medicaid—or that they must wait, groaning or bleeding for hours in the emergency room, for a few minutes with an intern who seems too tired to think straight.

In recent years caregivers have become almost as dissatisfied as their patients. They are accustomed to convincing successes, particularly in life-threatening emergencies, acute infections, and surgical interventions. Still, they know that they are able to offer only symptomatic stopgaps to the vast majority of their patients who suffer from chronic illnesses. They have also learned, to their dismay, that almost all of their treatments are fraught with debilitating side effects. Our overuse of antibiotics has produced a plague of antibiotic-resistant bacteria and deadly new infections. Anti-inflammatory drugs, like the ones David was taking, routinely wreak havoc on patients' guts. And surgical procedures, like prostatectomies, which once seemed rather benign, have been found to be not only overused but dangerous: a majority of men who have been operated on develop incontinence, impotence, or both.

These limitations distress physicians who are concerned about their patients' welfare. Many have become terminally *realistic,* a word that often doubles for *resigned* and may soon mutate to *cynical.* Whatever they're doing, they irritably tell their patients, is the "standard of care" for their specialty and this disease. It is all that can be done. So far as they are concerned, the alternative therapies that so many patients are eager to explore are by definition suspect. They aren't taught in medical school, aren't written about in the specialty journals, and aren't touted in glossy brochures produced by the drug companies. So how, the reasoning seems to go, can there be anything to them?

When patients ask about alternatives, some physicians are curious and encouraging. They are, as they should be, eager to learn if there are other, better ways to deal with conditions that they can't treat successfully. Many physicians, however, become self-righteous and defensive. They refuse to participate in the open-minded inquiry that is the basis of the scientific method or, indeed, in a simple courteous discussion. Instead, they retreat behind a wall of scornful but uninformed authority. "There's nothing to it," many of them sneer, without a shred of evidence to support their conviction. Not surprisingly, many patients refuse to tell their doctors about the alternatives they ultimately pursue—as many as 72 percent of them, according to the *New England Journal* survey.

Patients deserve better in other ways as well.

Physicians who should be bent in care and comfort are looking over their shoulders—at the insurance companies that continually call them to account, toward the threats of malpractice litigation that shadow every decision. When they turn to look at their patients, it is too often through the thick and expensive screen of diagnostic tests that they feel compelled to order—five hundred to two thousand dollars for a magnetic resonance scan (MRI) after a minor head injury, six hundred dollars for a "routine" stress test to assess cardiac functioning, and a hundred dollars for electronic fetal monitoring, which has never been shown to improve the health of low-risk newborns.

Good, kind, not greedy professionals also worry about the avalanche of initials that tumble toward them—HMOs and PPOs (preferred provider organizations) that threaten to scoop up their patients or their practices; DRGs—diagnostic related groups—that tell them, based on statistical averages, not individual health status, how soon their patients must leave the hospital.

Increasingly, physicians are becoming fearful of trusting their clinical judgment and disillusioned with the way they practice. Some wonder despairingly if they might not be replaced by intelligent clerks. In a 1993 American Medical Association poll, thirty-six percent of all those in practice said they would "definitely" or "probably" not go to medical school if they had it to do again. Even larger numbers are discouraging their own children and other young people from becoming doctors.

Medical students, sweet and hopeful in their first days, grow suspicious, and self-protectively cynical. Though more are now choosing family medicine and other "primary care" fields, disproportionate numbers still dream that when their time in training is up, they will enter high-paying, technologically sophisticated specialties and subspecialties—radiology and radiation oncology, invasive cardiology, anesthesiology, pathology, and orthopedic surgery. There they will be secure in their expertise, removed from the rich but often baffling complexity of day-to-day, lifelong contact with patients with chronic problems.

* * *

When I first spoke with David on the phone, he wondered aloud about the limitations of the treatment he'd been receiving. He didn't doubt his physicians' intelligence or sincerity, but he was troubled by their willingness to keep prescribing drugs that were both toxic and ineffective. He found it "curious and dismaying" that they had so little knowledge of or interest either in his emotional life or in the alternative therapies for arthritis that he was now reading about in popular magazines. Though he didn't want to criticize or offend the men who had loyally attended him for so many years, it was, he felt, time "to explore my options."

I asked him, as I do with all my prospective patients, if he was also willing to take a fresh look at his habits—of eating and drinking, exercising, thinking, feeling, and acting—at his job and his home life. He waited for a few moments before answering in measured lawyerly tones: "Yes, I think it's important that I do that." Then he began, in a great rush, to share the thoughts of a decade of pain.

David had long suspected that his troubles with his first wife had somehow precipitated his illness. And it was true that conflict—about the morality of divorce and the needs of his children and the demands of his job—did seem to make his condition worse. And he had always believed, in spite of what his doctors said, that certain kinds of food—maybe red meat, alcohol, and the sweets he craved—contributed to the pain and swelling.

I told him that he might be right on all counts and that we would explore these possibilities. Stress clearly can exacerbate rheumatoid arthritis, and food sensitivities have repeatedly been implicated in flares. I said that I would also work with acupuncture and Chinese herbs and manipulate his back and joints as osteopaths and chiropractors do. He was not surprised. "That's what Alice [his second wife] told me." When I said that he would have to do the lion's share of the work and that I might suggest long-term major changes in what he eats and how he exercises, he nodded and responded,

"Whatever it takes." And it was at least "okay" that he would have to wait a while to see me. "I've waited this long."

When, six weeks later, David enters my office, he moves with a quick lurching gait. He is wearing the Washington lawyer's workaday uniform—dark blue pinstripe suit, crisp white shirt, red-figured tie. He sits, slightly stooped, a careful man with iron gray hair and wire-rimmed glasses. "I need help," he says quietly.

Then, with precision born of years of careful courtroom preparation, he offers up the details of his history—long paragraphs on childhood and parochial school, college, his past sadness with the failure of his first marriage and present satisfaction with his second; thoughtful evaluations of each of his children; and crisp notations on the ten-year sequence of his symptoms, and on the drugs that have been prescribed, their effects and side effects.

He is determined to tell me everything that could be of use, willing to describe all the twists and turns that have brought him to my office. He wants to search for causes rather than suppress symptoms, to face and move through pain rather than turn from it.

David allows me to examine him, to touch, as kindly as I can, the tender red joints at his ankles, elbows, and knees. Hearing the soft pops as I reduce the dislocations in the small bones of his wrists, he grimaces. He watches with quiet but uneasy fascination as I put acupuncture needles in his hands and arms and legs. When I approach his belly, he looks at me with horror: "You're going to put needles down there?" He nods toward the lowest part of his abdomen and closes his eyes when I say yes. Twenty minutes later, when I take them out, he is calm, smiling, and obviously relieved. "I guess I made it."

I explain then that he will have to eat only watermelon for a week. He turns his head to the side slowly and looks at me out of the corner of his eye, over the bow of his glasses, as he might at a witness who has just stepped on his own best alibi. "Watermelon?" he queries. "Watermelon," I respond, explaining that it stimulates the kidneys' functioning and that in Chinese medicine the kidneys are connected with the bones and joints. For the two weeks following his watermelon fast, I would like him to eat only raw food, a diet that will stimulate his digestion while allowing his body to detoxify, to rid itself of all the chemicals he has consumed over the years. For three months afterward, 70 percent of his diet should be raw, and he should avoid all milk and milk products, sugar, red meat, wheat, caffeine, and food additives. People with arthritis are, I tell him, often sensitive to these foods. "Okay," he says, understandably incredulous but still game.

We go through the rest of the regimen: the regular acupuncture treatments to reduce the inflammation and keep the qi, the energy, moving and balanced in his body and yoga classes to recover long-lost flexibility and motion. I prescribe a combination of Chinese herbs to "warm" and dry his inflamed and frozen joints, relieve his pain, and enhance his immune functioning: clematis, siler, and cinnamon twig to "dispel the damp"; tang quei (Chinese angelica) to "tonify" his blood and astragalus, atractylodes, and licorice to "nurture the root" and raise his level of energy. I give him the name of a massage therapist and explain that her hands will encourage his blood flow and help mobilize his muscles. I recommend daily meditation to bring his mind and his nervous system into balance.

I am not sure what David makes of the brief explanations I offer or the profound changes this program implies, but he keeps nodding his head slowly, gravely.

"What about prayer?" he asks.

"Prayer," I say, a bit surprised at the words that arise to meet his need, "is a beautiful way to transform everything else you do, to help make this process of self-care a kind of sacrament. Besides," I add, more the medical professional now, "regular prayer seems to have a positive effect on our physiological functioning, including our immune system."

Before David goes, I teach him a meditation technique he can practice at home, a simple breathing exercise. He loosens the tie he has just knotted and, after I ask twice, risks closing his eyes.

"Slow breathing reduces the heart rate, lowers blood pressure, helps to synchronize the two halves of the brain, and quiets the mind," I explain, speaking to the concerns of his critical, rational mind, as I encourage him to loosen its control and to experience his body.

"Allow your belly to be soft," I say softly, allowing my belly to relax along with his. "Let it puff out as you breathe in, rising, and falling as you breathe out. I know it's a bit un-American," I tease him. "You can say to yourself 'soft belly,' as if it were a mantra." He cracks a smile. After a few minutes his breathing slows, and I can see his belly rise beneath his starched shirt.

"Now," I continue, "allow the softness to fill your thighs and knees, calves and ankles. Let it take the tension from your feet." His knees fall slightly apart, and his breathing slows. "Now let the softness move up into your chest, down into your arms, and let it fill your hands and soften the places that have been hard and bent." His poor crabbed hands begin to move with the breath. "Allow it now to move up into your neck and face and head. Let your eyelids lie gently on your cheeks," I suggest as I notice the effort he brings even to the closing of an eye. We breathe together this way for a few minutes.

"We're con-spiring," I say, stretching the Latinate word out to make the pun obvious. "We're breathing together." He nods and smiles. I explain to him that this meditation is one he can do at home, once or twice or several times a day, whenever he feels pain or tension. It will help ease the pain, help let him just be. When I ask him to open his eyes, he is still smiling.

He raises his hands, now a bit more mobile, as if to allow them to speak for themselves. "They don't hurt so much," he says.

Finally, before saying good-bye, we lay out a plan for which medications he should cut, and in what order, and by how much.

A week later David returns. He is barely able to suppress a grin as he watches me looking at him. "The watermelon certainly does work on the kidneys. It's had me peeing like crazy. I've lost eight pounds," he says, pulling the waistband of his pants away from his diminished belly, as proud as any schoolboy. "I cut the medication a little more than we agreed"—I nod—"and," he says, "the pain is no worse, maybe even a little better, and I can move these hands." He wiggles them now.

He's been doing the meditation at least twice a day and has had his first yoga lesson. "Alice is amazed," he says, grinning, looking at least five, maybe ten years younger than a week ago. "She can't believe what I've done. She wonders if she can go on watermelon too."

Two weeks afterward, on a diet of watermelon and other raw foods, David's lost a total of fourteen pounds. He's cut out all his medicine—six weeks ahead of our schedule. He's visited the ophthalmologist, who confirmed that his eyes were beginning to regain the ground lost to Plaquenil. David's thinking straighter, and his hands, unaided by any medication for the last week, are less painful and more mobile than they've been in years.

Three weeks later he is back again, positively beaming. "I'm really enjoying the yoga," he says, still not quite sure why or how such an alien practice would delight him, "and feeling better than I have in years." He is a total of twenty pounds lighter—"I've gotten a lot of compliments," he tells me proudly—and two inches less burdened in the waist. He weighs what he did when he played golf in college. He's begun to squeeze a ball to strengthen his hands and tentatively to pick up his golf clubs again.

He's also begun to pray regularly. As he defies conventional wisdom and his familiar doctors' directives, to find his own way to health, prayer seems a source of hope and a means for enlisting an ally. "All I really needed was your encouragement."

For years David had been a bit embarrassed about his desperate requests to God to relieve his pain. Now, putting his faith in a God whom he believes is wiser than any physician, provides a reassurance that David remembers from childhood. He feels connected to something larger than the sum of his symptoms and his thoughts. Each effort on his own behalf—he is a little uncomfortable saying this—really does feel like a sacred act, one done with God's support.

David's been back to see his rheumatologist as well. "Dr. Sanborn," David reports, "seemed a little nervous. He kept looking at me as if he couldn't believe what he was seeing," apparently shifting his gaze from David's slim body to his happy youthful face and his suddenly mobile hands. "He did tell me that medicine is 'not an exact science.'" The routine blood work the rheumatologist ordered shows an added bonus: David's cholesterol had plummeted from an excessive 285 to a respectable 195—in six weeks.

By the fifth month after we began treatment, David is hitting golf balls on a range, and soon after he's back on the course. He plays five rounds in seventeen days, and as if to celebrate his return, the gods—or saints—grant him two holes-in-one and scores to match the seven handicap he had had before arthritis overtook him. He is a very happy man, happy about other changes he is making in his life as well.

Though he felt weak and crippled, David hadn't realized that the passivity of patienthood had also been damaging. As a boy and young man, he had always been "good," inclined to obedience at times when rebellion might better have served him. He could see it in the way he had stuck out his marriage. He realizes now how his arthritis and its treatment repeated the pattern. He was as dutiful a patient as he had been a son, father, and husband. And his treatment had exacted a price that was reminiscent of the one he had paid in his childhood and first marriage. He had done what he was supposed to and felt worse, from the drugs he was taking as well as the disease, and from following well-meaning directives that had long since ceased to make sense to him.

Now he is striking out on his own. The acupuncture has had immediate positive effects—on the mobility of his joints and his mood. The herbs seem to increase his energy and relieve his swelling. But he is particularly delighted by what he has learned to do to help himself. He likes the way his new diet makes him feel and look, and he enjoys the discipline that enables him to follow it. Every day when he does his yoga, he can feel warmth and flexibility returning to his limbs and joints. And after he sits in meditation, he feels calmer about and more detached from the day's inevitable stresses.

David has addressed himself to the most intimate aspects of his physical functioning. He has learned to appreciate and care for a body that, in his rush to take care of professional or personal business or relieve pain, he usually ignored or silenced. To his amazement, he has discovered that he can effect changes that his physicians, with all their therapeutic tools, were powerless to bring about.

Over time, David's hard-won mastery has strengthened him emotionally as well as physically. Just as he has altered his habits of eating and exercise, so he has found that he is able to make positive changes in other areas of his life. Within a year, he left a job to which inertia had confined him and joined a new firm, where his work is more interesting and he is treated with greater respect. When his son goes through a time of crisis, he deals with the situation, and his ex-wife's fears, with a courage and forthrightness that amaze and delight him.

When David Donne first came to see me, he knew that after ten years he was at a dead end with conventional medical treatment. Though he couldn't say exactly what he was looking for, he knew he needed another approach, an alternative. He wanted clear answers to straightforward questions. Which alternative might be useful for him? Who might be knowledgeable enough to help him decide? Where could he find qualified practitioners?

But alternative therapies, and knowing when to use them, were not enough for David, and are not sufficient for any of us who are ill or hurting. We want and deserve someone who will listen respectfully to us, who will take seriously our point of view about the problems that are deforming our lives, who will help us help ourselves. And we are hoping, often after years of suffering and frustration, that somewhere there is a larger, more generous kind of medicine, one that combines conventional and alternative therapies, authoritative treatment with respectful care.

This is a book about the kind of care that David and so many of us want. It shows how patients and physicians can collaborate to transform medicine, and describes many of the approaches and techniques that we can effectively use.

The new medicine that we are creating together appreciates the great value of surgery and drugs but sees them as last resorts, not first choices. It makes use of the most sophisticated modern diagnostic techniques and research studies, but also puts value on the learning and experience that humans in all parts of the world have accumulated over millennia. It is a synthesis of modern technology and perennial wisdom, of powerful and definitive treatment and compassionate care, of Western and Eastern, high technology and indigenous and folk healing traditions.

This new medicine understands that each of us, like David, is unique, a whole person—biological, psychological, spiritual—in a total social and ecological environment. It acknowledges that each of these dimensions of our lives can be both a source of our distress and an arena for relieving it. This new medicine insists that healing be a fully collaborative partnership in which teaching is as important as treatment, and it regards self-care—particularly through self-awareness, relaxation, meditation, nutrition and exercise—as the true "primary care."

This new medicine is as concerned with enhancing wellness as it is with treating illness. It teaches us to mobilize our power to heal ourselves, and it makes full use of the extraordinary capacity of our minds to affect our bodies and of nondrug, physical approaches to enhance our mental and emotional functioning.

It draws on the perspectives and practices of the world's great healing traditions, including Chinese medicine and Indian Ayurveda, Native American, and African healing; and it gives a full and honorable place to popular European and American therapeutic practices that have been swept aside or scorned by our modern mainstream medicine—the use of spinal manipulation by chiropractors and osteopaths; such "natural" approaches as diet, herbalism, and massage; homeopathy and prayer.

It explores and encourages the great and largely untapped power that ordinary people have to understand and help one another—in support groups, therapeutic communities, churches, families, schools, and workplaces.

Finally, the new medicine, like the oldest healing that humans have known, recognizes that illness is a teacher on each of our spiritual journeys, as well as a physical misfortune and psychological challenge. It insists, as did the tribal shamans who were our first healers, that the work, the "profession" of those who "provide" health care, is itself a spiritual path.

This book is a guide to, and a manifesto for, that new medicine.

TWO

Biomedicine and Beyond ⤳

THE MEDICINE my father practiced seemed marvelous and terrifying to me but ordinary to him. In the bright light of his treatment room, gleaming scissors were lined up on white towels; scalpel blades, grainy glass syringes, and fierce needles emerged from the steaming sterilizer. I remember asking, at age three or four, how "instruments" that looked hurtful could also help. The scalpel, he explained, cuts away what doesn't belong. The needles inject medicine that makes sick people feel better. I nodded, dizzy at the thought of that power entering my body.

As a queasy high school senior, I watched my father operate for the first time. I held my breath against the possibility of error, while steel flashed, my father assuring me that surgery was only anatomy come alive.

In my father's office waiting room, men and women of all sizes and shapes were perched in their best clothes, reading magazines or staring at their good shoes. When I made rounds with him on the hospital wards, they lay neat and expectant under their covers.

My father was a large rough man whose arms moved a lot when he strode toward the hospital elevator. I remember once when he paused in his rounds for longer than usual. He sat on the bed of an elderly black woman. While he gently removed a bandage from her chest, he spoke to her in a voice far softer than any I had ever heard. As we walked down the corridor, my father told me that the woman had cancer and that she might not live much longer. At that moment I thought I might want to be a doctor. When I tried to explain how his kindness had moved me, he seemed not to understand.

When my father spoke of medicine, it was to dissect the steps in the diagnostic process, or to marvel at a colleague's careful research, or to remind me that I should learn the basic sciences well—"all of medicine is in pathology and physiology," he said. He was a general surgeon, at home in any part of the belly or limbs, willing to venture into the chest or head and neck. He worked from very early morning to late evening at five different hospitals. He operated, successfully, I like to add, on Joe DiMaggio's heel, as well as on the bodies of thousands of ordinary people. He was very good at what he did.

As time went on, my father seemed increasingly impressed by the men—they were virtually all men then—who had chosen to specialize in one or another aspect of surgery or medicine. He would show me their papers in the journals that piled up on his desk. He liked the thoroughness of their laboratory work, the improvements they had made in technique.

My father assured me that the papers they had written had gained them chairs at the great medical schools, the respect of their colleagues, and enormous fees for surgical procedures that he did for a fraction of the cost. We were, he told me thirty-five years ago, in the "Golden Age of Medicine."

I was impressed by their achievements but not moved to emulate them. The work of these researcher-specialists seemed to me more a matter of technical advance than great discovery. Besides, their lifelong concentration on a particular aspect of a single disease or treatment was uncongenial. I loved to listen to people tell the stories of their lives and wanted to become a psychiatrist. Freud, whose expertise ranged from speculating on the structure of the mind, to unraveling the complexities of case histories, to revealing the architecture of religion and politics, was my model—an explorer, not a land-holder. Science seemed a tool to me, a way of looking at the world and a means of understanding and helping, not an end in itself; specialization seemed too much like limitation.

Still, even if I questioned the specialization to which my father urged me and cast a youth's skeptical eye on the achievements he admired, I had a sense of what he meant by the Golden Age. Medicine seemed capable of almost unlim-ited invention. Science was penetrating every corner of its practice. The treatments these researchers were devising seemed equal to the task of addressing all ills. There was a balance between the precise, sometimes painful work that took place in the treatment rooms and ORs and the respect that patients and doctors extended to one another. Doctors were honored for their expertise, well loved and well paid.

The medicine my father practiced was based on a view of illness often called the biomedical model. This model is part and parcel of a way of looking at, analyzing, and acting on the world that characterizes modern Western civilization. It is variously called rational, scientific, or mechanical. It is grounded in a faith in the benefits of material progress, and in man's capacity to analyze and devise solutions for all the problems that confront him.

The biomedical model emphasizes the analysis of disease entities into their smallest, subcellular, biochemical, and molecular parts. It relies on treatments that address discrete abnormalities. It chooses its therapies based on a research that "controls for," or eliminates, other influences, other variables, in order to study the effectiveness of one particu-lar drug or procedure.

This biomedical model conceives of illness as a product of heredity, as the outcome of a string of predictable causative factors, or as an unfortunate aberration. It is considered a formidable enemy, and biomedicine uses a language of pathology and conflict that reflects this worldview. The physician is a detached scientist-strategist who rationally and objectively assesses the patient's symptoms; diagnoses the diseases from which he is suffering; and selects from and applies those therapies—"magic bullets," the great chemist Paul Ehrlich called them—that are most likely to subdue the invading bacterial pathogen or rectify the offending abnormality.

This model has shaped and catalyzed the great advances in pharmacology and surgery that we associate with twentieth-century medicine.

In the last thirty-five years, however, we have begun to realize biomedicine's shortcomings. It is inadequate to explain the origins or treat the consequences of the chronic illnesses, the disabilities, and the distresses that afflict more than 80 percent of those who seek medical attention. Its overuse and misuse has produced a deadly host of mutated bacterial and viral life-forms, and an epidemic of iatrogenic—physician-and-treatment-caused—illnesses. Its economic cost—almost one trillion dollars a year and close to 15 percent of our gross national product—has become insupportable. Even its metaphors of regulation and conquest, which once seemed fitting and hopeful, now strike increasing numbers of us as both grandiose and inappropriate.

We are not only *not* finding new magic bullets, but we are doing damage to ourselves with the old ones. We are losing the wars on cancer, hypertension, arthritis, depression, and AIDS, and we are taking civilian casualties at the same time.

We are in desperate need of a new medical model, new metaphors, and a new kind of medical practice, one adequate to the illnesses from which the vast majority of us suffer. But if we are going to create and make use of a new model, we must first understand why and how the old one grew and developed; appreciate its great intelligence, energy, and enthusiasm; and survey some of the problems it has so dramatically solved. It is precisely because biomedicine is so powerful and attractive—because it has grown so strong, explained so much, and helped so many—that it has been hard to see that it too is a stage in, and not the end point of, medical evolution.

* * *

Western medicine begins with Hippocrates, who lived on the Greek island of Cos in the fourth century B.C. In the works of Hippocrates there is a wonderful balance between respectful observation of, and experimentation on, nature and a deep appreciation for her mysteries. There is also breadth of vision. In addition to describing many distinct disease states, Hippocrates appreciated the social and ecological context in which illness occurs and the way physical manifestations of disease are shaped by psychological and spiritual forces.

During the European middle ages, Hippocrates' works were lost, and with them his experimental method and expansive spirit. Medieval monk-physicians were scholars, not experimentalists. They learned and parroted the Hippocratic concepts that were passed on to them by Galen of Pergamon. The words of this second century physician, Hippocrates' great, systematizing heir, were regarded as beyond dispute or question, like church dogma. So blinding was the light of Galen's authority, that medieval anatomists were unable to see the contours of the organs that lay before them. The liver, they asserted, against all the evidence of their senses, did indeed have the five lobes that Galen attributed to it.

The influx of Greek scholars and texts after the Turkish conquest of Constantinople in 1453 changed all this. For the first time, Western physicians had direct access to ancient Greek learning. During the Renaissance that followed, classical Hippocratic medicine, like classical art, was reborn.

The atmosphere of individualism, inventiveness, and exploration that pervaded Europe shaped Renaissance physicians' reading of the rediscovered texts. They were particulary impressed by Hippocrates' detailed attention to the origins, description, and treatment of illnesses. Inspired by him, they began to observe individual patients and particular disease phenomena at the bedside and the autopsy table, in the laboratory and the field. They wanted to know more so they could do more.

Within a hundred years, Renaissance physicians had planted the seeds for the sciences—anatomy, pharmacology, bacteriology, and physiology—that are still considered "basic" to biomedical practice and education.

By the early seventeenth century, European philosophers were developing a world view and a method which would foster these disciplines and serve Western medicine's inclination to objectivity and intervention. Francis Bacon, England's Lord Chancellor, was convinced that modern scientists would gain knowledge and power by aggressive experimentation, as well as observation. He urged them to "force" nature "out of her natural state and squeeze and mold" her.

Meanwhile, in France, René Descartes was maintaining that only rational thought was reliable. The mind, he said, was different from and of a higher order than the material world that it pondered. Some of the great Renaissance physicians still believed, as Hippocrates did, that matter and spirit were connected. For example, William Harvey, who discovered the circulation of the blood, was convinced that the heart was the site of vital energy, as well as a mechanical pump. So far as Descartes was concerned, however, there was a definitive separation between the mind and spirit and the body, between a disembodied intellect which observed and experimented, and a mechanical nature of which men were to be "lords and possessors."

For the next three centuries the scientific enterprise and the medical research it inspired, would be ruled by the descendants of Bacon and Descartes. These men would use their minds to explore and manipulate nature, including, most particularly, the human body.

This insistence on detached observation, analysis, and definitive treatment was facilitated by the reincorporation of surgery and anatomic dissection into medical practice, the creation of a university-trained class of physicians, and great technological progress. In the seventeenth century for example, the use of the microscope opened up a new window on nature: Leeuwenhoek, who developed this marvelous tool, was able to see "animalcules," bacteria that swam in drops of water.

With the invention of more powerful microscopes in the nineteenth century, the focus of medical attention shifted from the organ and tissue to the cell as the basic unit of functioning. At the same time the development of increasingly sophisticated diagnostic techniques made possible the delineation of clearer clinical pictures. Laennec's stethoscope enabled him to make elegant descriptions of pulmonary tuberculosis; Helmholtz's ophthalmoscope facilitated his explorations of the nerve tissue of the eye. By the end of the nineteenth century, Rudolf Virchow, the great Berlin pathologist, had laid the foundations for the distinctly modern understanding of the relationship between observable pathological changes in cells and particular disease entities.

At about the same time, discoveries in bacteriology and immunology were making possible a new understanding of the nature and treatment of some of our most devastating diseases.

Throughout history, humans had been vulnerable to outbreaks of baffling and terrifying illnesses. Some of these conditions were "endemic," that is, they were constantly present in a given population, their numbers and severity increasing and decreasing as environmental and economic conditions fluctuated. Others, called "epidemics," seemed to appear suddenly and without warning, in the midst of a population unaccustomed to them. Some physicians, following Hippocratic and Galenic precedent, attributed them to climactic conditions. Others, who were more influenced by the Church's perspective, located the cause in witchcraft or divine displeasure.

This began to change in the eighteenth century when Edward Jenner, an English country physician discovered that accidentally contracting a mild case of cowpox protected rural people against life-threating human smallpox. Soon Jenner was deliberately injecting humans with material from cows' pustules (pox). This procedure, which he called *vaccination* (from *vacca*, the Latin for "cow") succeeded in giving people immunity from smallpox.

In the mid-nineteenth century, the French chemist Louis Pasteur discovered that specific microorganisms were responsible for particular diseases, and developed vaccines against them. He found ways to attenuate, or weaken, the organisms that were responsible for chicken cholera, anthrax in sheep, and even rabies, and then injected them prophylactically.

The dramatic success of Pasteur's treatments in animals and people who might otherwise have died, made his name a household word in Europe. The germ theory of disease, with its concepts of clear and specific causes, predictable effects, and targeted therapeutics, became the model for medical understanding and rational treatment.

Over the next hundred years, biomedicine demonstrated its power in a dozen different domains. General anesthesia made lengthy surgery possible, while antiseptics protected surgical patients from the bacterial infections that had routinely killed them. Physicians and scientists developed anti-toxins to neutralize the bacterial toxins that produced deadly childhood diseases like diphtheria and tetanus.

In the early part of the twentieth century, Paul Ehrlich, who had helped develop antitoxins, provided a rallying cry for the new therapeutic enterprise. He coined the term "magic bullet" for the cures he was seeking. These magic bullets were chemical substances that would combat particular diseases without harming their human hosts. Ehrlich created Salvarsan, an arsenic containing compound that indeed destroyed the spirochetes that cause syphilis. Unfortunately, it proved too toxic for continued use.

Soon, however, scientists were discovering other, less dangerous, and more effective magic bullets. By the 1940s, the antibiotic penicillin and the antibacterial sulfa drugs were in wide use. They dramatically reduced the mortality from wartime wounds and the incidence of death, damage, and disability from a host of peacetime infections, including pneumonia, syphilis, gonorrhea, and meningitis.

Meanwhile, clinicians and researchers were looking for, and finding, magic bullets for a variety of other life-threatening conditions. By 1920, Frederick Banting and Charles Best had explored the role of the hormone insulin in regulating blood sugar, isolated it from the pancreas, and prepared it for injection into diabetics who were incapable of producing it themselves. Soon, scientists developed other forms of hormone replacement, as well as a host of drugs—some derived from plants, others synthesized—to combat cancer, lower blood pressure, remove unwanted accumulations of fluid, and stimulate and regulate the contractions of the heart.

By the time I entered Harvard Medical School in 1962, medical science was probing far deeper levels and more complex pathways of biological causation, and developing ever more precise pharmacological treatments. My classmates and I admired slides of the paired nucleotides that wound around the double helix of the DNA that makes up chromosomes. These simple amino acids, mixed and matched in almost infinite combinations, are, we learned, the matter of our genes, the blueprint for all our physical functioning.

In our biochemistry lab we did experiments that demonstrated the functions that DNA regulated. And, when the lights dimmed in amphitheater D, we saw, in the staggeringly intimate detail of electron micrographs, the organelles, the tiny factories within the cell where, under the guidance of DNA and its messenger RNA, the body's own building blocks are manufactured and do their work.

The next year, in pharmacology, we learned just how the latest drugs halt or reverse pathological functioning in these cells. We saw the actual receptors on the cell surface where the molecules we diagrammed dock and do their work. Soon, our professors suggested, we would be able to repair malfunctioning receptors, as well as do surgery on damaged genes, alter immune functioning, and replace diseased organs with healthy ones.

In my last two years, at Harvard's hospitals, I saw the great therapeutic benefits of the biomedical tradition. William Castle, tall and stooped, calm and kindly in tailored wool pants and a long white cotton coat, made rounds with us on the wards of Boston City Hospital. In 1926 Dr. Castle had discovered the intrinsic factor which is missing in the stomachs of people with "pernicious anemia." In 1966, he helped us to elucidate and name our patients' biochemical defects, and pathophysiological problems, and to make precise selections of the most appropriate drugs. Walking beside him, I marveled at how the science he had helped to create had moved on, and how gracefully he was keeping up.

Across town, in the Ether Dome of the Massachusetts General Hospital (MGH), where general anesthesia was first used in 1846, John Constable, the plastic surgeon, showed before and after pictures of horribly maimed children. Complex and delicate surgery had made them whole again. It was no wonder, I remember thinking, that my father and his colleagues were so gratified and impressed by the triumphal march of biomedicine, that they felt they were living in a Golden Age of limitless therapeutic possibilities.

Still, even as we learned to appreciate the immense power, range, and elegance of this medicine, I was feeling uneasy about it. The focus on the pathological processes in our patients, and the search for accurate diagnoses, identifiable causes, and precise remedies for their diseases often tended to overwhelm our concern for them as people.

Drs. Castle and Constable clearly respected and enjoyed the people we cared for. Too many attendings (staff physicians) and residents treated the men and women whose bodies we probed as if they were laboratory preparations. We were urged to observe people whose rare diseases or peculiar physical findings made them "interesting cases," as if they were exhibits in a museum. Patients were routinely referred to by their diagnostic labels, as "the gall bladder in 402" or "the lupus patient." Standing over them on rounds, we spoke as if the men and women whose treatments we were debating were absent, deaf, or already dead.

Discussion of the psychological dimensions of illness, and exploration of the patient's emotions were often neglected and sometimes discouraged. These were the domain of the psychiatric consultant. The effects of social and economic conditions, so obvious in the poor people who lay in their own feces in the corridors of Boston City, were footnotes in a few lectures on public health. A family's concerns about a sick member were the social worker's business, not ours. And spiritual matters—our patients' needs for faith, hope, and charity, or their concern with meaning and purpose in their lives—were best left to the priest, minister, or rabbi.

While I was trying to master the basics of the biomedical model, I was also struggling against the human indifference and narrowness of this approach. Wasn't it because of these patients, these people, that we were learning the details of pathology and perfecting our command of procedures? It seemed to me too, that once you got to know someone, pretty much anybody, regardless of diagnosis, was an "interesting case." Certainly it was the people who suffered, not the pathophysiology of their suffering, that most engaged and inspired me and made me want to be a doctor.

Often I felt terribly alone. I hoped to become a helper of the ill and a physician to the minds and souls of my patients as well as to their bodies. I was fascinated by people's stories, by what gave meaning and purpose to their lives. I certainly wanted to relieve their physical suffering, but I felt equally gratified when I helped my patients to take a fresh look at their lives or helped them off their bedpans or sat with them during a long night of fear and pain. But these concerns, which seemed to me to be central to the care of the people whose bodies we repaired, were considered peripheral to our medical education and the daily work we did.

Though I recognized and respected the great discoveries of biomedicine and their enormous utility, I decided to leave its practice to my classmates. I would specialize in psychiatry. There I would be able to focus on what moved and interested me most: the rich complexity of people's lives, and our relationships with one another and the world in which we lived.

Still, I enjoyed my medical internship. I thrived on being able to give suffering people immediate relief and on the energy and urgency of the medical wards and the ER. It felt good to be gentle with old people's bodies, to care for sick children, and to assist at the miracle of birth. But this seemed more a privileged interlude and a wonderful preparation than a final resting place. Once my psychiatric residency began, I knew I had come home. Now, at last, I could do the work that had inspired me to become a doctor.

Unfortunately, I found that the biomedical model was beginning to shape and narrow psychiatric, as well as medical, practice. Though the residency program at the Albert Einstein College of Medicine in New York was deservedly known for its emphasis on psychodynamic psychotherapy— on the thoughtful, respectful exploration, and resolution of the familial and interpersonal origins of people's emotional problems—there was, in the profession, a growing belief that this approach might be both a luxury and an anachronism. A significant number of my supervisors seemed to have decided that the problems of the more disturbed patients were *really* only diseases, neurobiological puzzles to be solved by the appropriate pharmacological answers.

This narrow, biological perspective didn't make sense to me. The men and women on the psychiatric wards—people diagnosed as schizophrenic, manic-depressive, and depressed— were different, even odd, but they certainly didn't seem sick in the same way as people with diabetes, gallbladder problems, or heart disease. My supervisors' explanations about why most were forced, like people hospitalized for surgery or heart attacks, to wear pajamas, and why virtually all of them were treated with medication, disturbed me. There was no certain abnormality in their brain chemistry, and even if there were, we had no way of knowing which came first, the troubled mind or the disordered brain.

The medications they were given sometimes *did* make them less anxious or less preoccupied with ideas that were strange to the rest of us, but they also made their minds sleepy and their bodies spastic and rigid. Often the patients protested, declaring that the medication was punishment for thoughts, words, and behaviors that were unacceptable to the staff. They said the drugs were a form of social control, not medical help, a way to keep them in line. If these protests were particularly loud or insistent, they were sometimes used as a justification for once again raising the dosage of medication—a classic catch-22.

The whole situation made me uneasy and angry. Disease seemed a misnomer for these people, and diagnosis too often a rationale for ignoring their humanity. Where was the respectful mutuality, the commitment to understanding that had always seemed the hallmark of psychiatry? It looked to me as if the biomedical model was being applied where it didn't belong, with results that were potentially dangerous as well as demeaning to our patients.

As a psychiatric resident, I found I could often make sense out of the idiosyncratic speech and unconventional behavior of even the strangest schizophrenics. Sure Mrs. Kucinski was carrying on a dialogue with ancient Egyptian deities, and Mr. Morris insisted on wearing five pairs of pants in the most brutally hot summer in memory. But they did have their reasons, reasons compounded of childhood trauma and particular life experiences, present stress, and desperate hopes. Their ways of speaking and behaving seemed to me to be their own attempt to adapt to, explain, and cope with life as they understood it.

As a chief resident in psychiatry I created, with my coworkers, a safe place for psychotic people, a largely "drug-free" therapeutic community in which they and their rights and needs were fully respected. On Ward 13 they could re-experience and reintegrate fragments of painful early experience and creative fantasy—just what those who were less obviously disturbed could do in psychotherapy. In the context of our therapeutic community, they could be appreciated for their sometimes desperate and confused but brave attempts to piece together their disordered lives.

Our job, so far as I was concerned, was to guide and guard and support them as they plunged into and moved through what Scottish psychiatrist R. D. Laing had described as "the natural healing process of madness." Some attendings thought we should give them drugs to help them "restore their premorbid personalities." I believed we should try to help them through the crisis of their disorder, perhaps to a greater wholeness than any they had previously experienced. Facilitating this process of transformation was, I believed, what psychiatry was all about.

By the time my residency was over, I knew that I wanted to bring this understanding into the larger world. I was going to the National Institute of Mental Health (NIMH) to be a research psychiatrist. There I wanted to explore alternatives to biomedical treatment, places where troubled and troubling people of all kinds could be guided through—and learn to navigate—the difficult passages in their lives. I wanted to reach out to people who rejected psychiatric help, to create with them new kinds of caring communities, and to share widely what we learned together.

THREE

A Healing Crisis ⌇

O NE SUMMER MORNING twenty-two years ago, three years after I came to the NIMH, I injured my back and set in motion a chain of events that would alter and enlarge my understanding of psychiatry and medicine. I was doing "the plow"—an upside-down yoga posture in which the weight is on the shoulders and the feet are extended over the head, toes touching the floor—when I felt a terrible pain in the lower part of my back. It shot from the slope of my lumbar curve, down to the left, sending fire into my left buttock and calf, and continuing on into the foot, where pins and needles sprouted. I wanted to stand but couldn't. Bent almost double, I cursed my attempt to go too far, too fast. And I tried— the legacy of years as a competitive athlete—to work it out and walk it off. I had an important meeting coming up.

The work I had been doing at NIMH was bearing serious fruit. For several years I had been spending my time with runaway and homeless young people and their counselors, in runaway houses, on hotlines, in free schools, and in group foster homes. These programs called themselves alternative services because they were alternatives—conceptually and practically—to police, social service, and conventional mental health agencies.

The counselors in these programs saw and treated the troubled and confused teenagers—as many as one million each year were running from or being kicked out of their homes—not as patients or clients or delinquents but as younger brothers and sisters, fellow refugees from confusing families and confining institutions, pilgrims in search of some better way to live with themselves and one another.

My work with runaway young people and their counselors seemed very much an extension of what I had done as a chief resident at Albert Einstein. I wanted to see if together the young people, counselors, and I could transform the experience of running away from a pathological process or a delinquent episode to a step on the path of personal growth.

Three years after I began my research and therapeutic consultation with runaway houses in the Washington, D.C., area, the NIMH was prepared to fund a number of these programs, and I was going to coordinate the national effort.

I was excited yet anxious too. It was important that these programs and the respectful way that they worked with young people get adequate recognition and funding. Perhaps, I thought, the anticipated stress of my new role as a program coordinator had somehow contributed to my haste during yoga and my back injury.

I made my way to and through our planning meeting in barely concealed agony. I explained to my bosses at the NIMH that the conventional ways of regarding and classifying these young people were wrongheaded and counterproductive. The medical model had been stretched and distorted to include the "runaway reaction of adolescence" as a diagnostic entity, a disease—and thousands of kids were being hospitalized to "treat" this supposed illness. Many other ruanaway and homeless young people—especially those whose families lacked money and status—were put, to the dismay of cops and judges who saw the inappropriateness and danger of this practice, in actual detention centers and juvenile jails.

The runaway house programs were a hopeful contrast. We refused to label or constrain these young people. We offered them what they felt they needed, not what we thought was best for them—a place to stay, some food, a sympathetic ear. We respected their point of view and their right to use their own intelligence to make their own choices. Treated this way, most runaways responded by acting as if they were just about as responsible as we assumed they were.

My bosses listened. They agreed to try to make our funding as responsive to these programs as the programs were to the kids. I was delighted—but my back was still outrageously painful.

The next morning I arrived at the Bethesda Naval Hospital where, as an officer in the U.S. Public Health Service, I was entitled to receive care. I was filled with a mixture of apprehension and hope. I was worried that one of the cartilaginous disks that ordinarily provide cushioning and facilitate movement of the bony vertebrae had slipped out of place. Perhaps it was compressing the nerves as they emerged from the lower part of my spine and causing the pain, the numbness, and the paresthesias—the tingling in my legs. I remembered patients on the orthopedic surgical wards at Harvard Medical School who had had such problems. I could still see their grim faces, years after surgeries that seldom seemed successful, and hear their bitter complaints—of inability to lift or run, of ongoing pain and disability. On the other hand, maybe I had just had a bad muscle strain.

The orthopedic surgeons—large competent types in crisp white uniforms with short hair and golden insignias on their shoulders—gathered around me that first day like linemen in a huddle. They watched me walk and had me stand on one foot, stroked my insteps, pricked my legs with pins, and nodded to one another. After a while, the one with the most brass turned to me. "It could be a disk," he intoned solemnly. They prescribed muscle relaxants and painkillers, two weeks of bed rest, and a heating pad and deferred their final diagnosis.

For two weeks I stayed in bed as much as I could, sometimes bemused by the drugs. I rose as infrequently as possible, hobbling to the bathroom or the porch. When I sat, I lowered myself gingerly, and once seated I moved unwillingly. I called my office often, and remembered longingly the time when I had driven so easily into and around town.

The pain abated when I was still, but it never really left me. For the first time I understood what the expression "having your teeth set on edge" means. A portion of my mind was held hostage. It and I were always uneasy, poised for more pain. My concentration and my patience were short. I had the sense that the body that had always served me willingly and well might betray me. I realized that my back, which I had never much noticed, was my very center. It had supported me, kept me upright, and made it possible for me to move. And now it was unreliable. Would it ever be well again? I began to worry about all the other parts of me that I took for granted. Could I depend on them?

When I arose after two weeks, I was little better. I made my way back to the NIMH and then again to the Naval Hospital.

This time there was more brass in the room. They repeated their examination. "What's your specialty?" an older physician asked. When I said I was a psychiatrist, they all nodded, as if this explained everything. They told me that even if I had a disk problem, I couldn't possibly have the array of signs and symptoms that I described—the numbness here, the pins and needles there, the weakness and ache in the front of my thighs.

I could feel myself getting defensive and angry. 'Who were these people—standing starched, upright, and pain-free—to tell me what I did or did not have? I told them that I was quite aware that my symptoms didn't fit the prescribed pattern—I'd been boning up on neuroanatomy—but I assured them that I really did have them. Their glances at one another were filled with meaning. They smiled and nodded again. I imagined the polite ones were speculating about a "psychosomatic component" to my illness, while the more blunt were assuming that I was a "head case" as well as a head shrinker. Meanwhile I was oscillating between rage at them and sympathy for all the patients who had described vague or hard-to-explain symptoms about whom I had harbored similar thoughts.

I went back to work. Staying in bed wasn't helping, and being unable to direct the program for runaway youth only made me feel more marginal and depressed. I did the prescribed back exercises, kept hoping against the odds of my experience that this condition was only temporary, and rested as much as I could.

Two months later I was only slightly better and exceedingly impatient. I was always worrying about where and how I would sit and how much energy I had and where to expend it—like an old man, I thought. My visits to the Naval Hospital were becoming progressively less cordial. I had begun to sense that my persistent illness and their inability to help were an affront to the doctors. Now they were speaking with increasing conviction and, I thought, a touch of glee, about a myelogram—an injection of dye into the spinal column—which I knew often produced blinding headaches and was, in any case, the prelude to back surgery.

I turned then from military medicine to what we called the private sector. Perhaps the chiefs of orthopedics and neurosurgery at one of the city's major teaching hospitals would have some better answers. They were cordial but equally discouraging. They reviewed the X rays, expressed concern, and recommended a myelogram.

By this time, I was desperate. Each day in the office was an ordeal. If I took muscle relaxants, I would grow sleepy during the meetings where we thrashed out the details of our program. If I didn't, I was in agony as I drove around the city to work with the kids and their counselors. My attention span was short. I couldn't write the papers I had promised journal editors. Ordinarily fairly even tempered, I was now poised on the edge of anger, ready to shout at anyone who crossed me. In constant pain, still stiff, and bent over, I felt three times my age.

Finally someone suggested that I see an osteopath. At the time, I didn't know what osteopaths were—nobody at Harvard Medical School had ever mentioned them—but it was clear from the name that they had something to do with bones. I was told that their training was essentially the same as that of M.D.'s, but that they also knew how to "manipulate" the back. The idea seemed to be that somehow—against all the warnings that I received during my own training—they might be able to move something, perhaps the errant vertebrae or disks, back into place.

I was exceedingly nervous about seeing an osteopath but, as I thought more about it, curious and vaguely hopeful. Over the years I had had some interest in exploring other medical systems and theories and talking to their practitioners. In the mid-1960s I had visited with George Ohsawa, the precise, supremely confident, cigarette-smoking founder of the Japanese dietary therapy called macrobiotics; and during my residency I had been intrigued by stories of the *curanderos*, the South Bronx healers whom my Puerto Rican patients swore by. Most recently I had become interested in the theory and practice of acupuncture and in an enigmatic Chinese-trained, London-based Indian acupuncturist named Shyam Singha.

It was, however, one thing to explore other medical systems, or even listen to charismatic fringe practitioners like Ohsawa and Dr. Singha, and quite another to submit my own body—a body used to the most sophisticated and scientific Western medicine—to the ministrations of such people. Still, I was desperate. I hurt all the time and could barely walk and anything seemed better than surgery.

The osteopath I consulted in Washington—I felt as if I were in the middle of a Dickens novel—was named Dr. Blood. A solid man with a crew cut, he pressed on my spine, pulled on my legs, turned my feet this way and that, and announced that I had a "lesion" in my back—the lumbar vertebrae were probably pressing on the nerve roots as they emerged from the spinal cord. He told me to lie on my right side and dangle my left leg from the examining table. He leaned on my lower back with his well-muscled right forearm, put his left hand on my left shoulder, and moved—swiftly and forcefully.

I heard a horrible crunching sound—my second thought was that I would be paralyzed, and my first that I would surely become impotent. A few moments later, however, I was standing—not bending over but actually standing up. The numbness and tingling were receding. I was ecstatic—until five minutes later the pain and paresthesias returned.

Still, *something*, however brief, had happened. I was eager for another appointment. Soon, however, I was disappointed. The relief after each treatment never lasted more than an hour or two.

Finally, I decided to call Dr. Singha in London. I did it because I was close to despair, almost ready to submit to a myelogram.

I had first heard about him a year before, during a phone call from an old friend in England. Richard, laconic and skeptical, had been unashamedly enthusiastic about this "mad Indian." Dr. Singha had put him on a grape fast for sixty days and stuck needles in him and changed his life. The most remarkable thing was the call itself: it was the first time I had ever spoken to Richard on the telephone. Until his treatment with Dr. Singha, he'd been so hard of hearing it was impossible.

At the end of our call, when Richard asked if I could arrange for Dr. Singha to come to Washington, I readily agreed. This was someone I definitely wanted to meet.

Dr. Singha in person had gleaming yellow eyes and flowing black hair. When he lectured, he wore impeccably tailored Savile Row suits and paced the front of the hall like a panther. He spoke gnomically of "energy" and "elements"—of wood, water, fire, earth, and metal—and cooked strange and delicious meals that seemed to alter my mood and heighten my level of awareness. Later he showed me different ways to cut vegetables and herbs and helped me smell and taste the varied odors and flavors that he could produce. His way of combining foods was, he explained, based on the same principles as the medicine he practiced.

An hour into his introductory workshop, Dr. Singha asked us all to stand. "We'll do some chaotic meditation," he announced. While I was trying to puzzle out how meditation, which I had thought to be quiet and still, could be chaotic, he showed us how to use our arms like a bellows. This, he assured us, would help us to pump the air in and out as fast and as deeply as possible.

"All right," he said. "Thank Nature for this opportunity—and begin."

After a minute or so, there was a pain in my side, and I was desperately wondering how long this would go on. I felt my breakfast rising in my mouth. Soon my head was light, my chest tight, and my arms tired. "Come on," I said half aloud, "it's enough."

"Keep going," Dr. Singha shouted over the moans and groans and sounds of retching. "Give one hundred percent."

When he finally told us to stop, after ten very long minutes, my shoulders ached and there was water in my eyes, but the world looked a little brighter. I noticed that my mind was both quieter and more alert, and that I was calm and smiling.

While we recovered, Dr. Singha stood at the front of the room, surveying the heaving bodies, nodding his head, and pursing his lips. He seemed to me then more like the indigenous healers, the feather-wearing, miracle-working shamans and medicine men I had read about in the pages of Mircea Eliade, Claude Lévi-Strauss, and Carlos Castaneda, than any physician I had ever come across. He fascinated me, and later, when I asked typical psychiatric questions about his background, he frustrated my attempts to figure him out.

Now, at the end of my therapeutic rope, I was reaching out to him for help over the telephone.

"Stop the medication," he said. "Take hot baths with Epsom salts and then cold showers. Eat three pineapples a day for a week and nothing else." I thought the transatlantic phone had gone bad. He repeated his prescription. I could hear what sounded like the roar of the ocean in the line, while I stood with my mouth open.

"Why?"

"It won't make sense to you."

"Why?" I demanded. (I'm a Harvard Medical School graduate, I thought, an NIMH researcher.)

"Remember what Hippocrates, the father of your medicine, said."

I could only say, "What?"

"'Let food be your medicine and medicine your food.'"

"Yes, yes. But pineapple?" I was getting impatient.

"Pineapple has malic acid."

"Yes, I understand that." I was even more impatient.

"Malic acid affects the lung and colon." He was fast losing credibility. "In Chinese medicine the lung and colon are the mother of the kidney and bladder." The mother? "And the bladder and kidney are connected to the back."

He was right—it made no sense to me. But I didn't want a myelogram, and I knew I didn't want surgery. Nothing else had worked, and none of my doctors even had anything else to offer. He had helped Richard. And something about Dr. Singha, an authority I did not understand, moved me. I decided to do what he said.

I took my baths and showers, and to my own continuing surprise, I ate the pineapples. I had them at room temperature, I froze them, and I heated them. I ate them with my fingers and a fork. I macerated them in a blender and drank them. And while my friends and colleagues stared and the homeless kids shook their heads in amazement, I kept on eating and drinking them.

After three days, I called Dr. Singha in London. "My mouth," I reported in a muffled and pained voice, "is full of sores. I have a 103-degree fever. My back hurts as badly, and the paresthesias are as strong as the first day I injured it."

"For the sores," he said, "coat your pineapple with honey." Why didn't he tell me that three days ago? "So far as the rest of it goes, it's very good. In Chinese medicine a chronic disease must become acute before it can be healed. In the East we call this a healing crisis."

At first I thought the fever had made me delirious and I had misunderstood. Then suddenly, for the first time, something about Dr. Singha's treatment made sense. In psychotherapy one often has to relive painful, traumatic experiences, to go through an emotional crisis as part of the process of recovery from a debilitating way of thinking or feeling. Depressed people may sometimes feel rage that has been bottled up, or they may face an even deeper despair. All my work with psychotic people had been to guide them through the center of their pain and confusion, not to avoid or to suppress it. Dr. Singha was saying that the body's pains and disability have to be navigated in a similar fashion, that the way out of physical illness is also through it. I felt like a character in a comic when the light bulb goes on over his head.

Maybe the body and the mind are far more intimately connected than I had ever realized. Maybe the principles that govern their functioning and healing are the same. Maybe the problem isn't, as I thought, that the conventional biomedical model is inaccurate for mental illness but that it is inappropriate even for physical illness. Maybe healing of all kinds is a journey through illness and a process of transformation. It sounded right, and it felt right.

Over the next few days my mouth began to heal, my temperature returned to normal, and the numbness and paresthesias diminished. The pain receded until there was only a small focus in the lower part of my lumbar spine. I felt good and different, not only physically light but somehow emotionally and mentally relieved as well. As I found I could move without pain, the world seemed more inviting. The obstacles to implementing the program for runaways seemed manageable, not overwhelming. I stopped grimacing and started smiling.

When, at the end of seven days, I called Dr. Singha, I told him that my back was 80 to 90 percent better. I was, I added, twelve pounds lighter and far clearer in my mind. "Good, good," he said, as if he'd known all along that it would be this way. "Now go back to the osteopath and let him adjust your back." I did. This time, after Dr. Blood's crunch, the adjustment held. I was well.

Neither my back, nor my medical practice, nor indeed my view of the world, has been the same since.

FOUR

Physician, Heal Thyself ∽

THE MARVEL of my recovery teased and excited me. I kept testing my back against small chores—driving for an hour to the NIMH without stopping to unkink myself, bending to weed in the garden, lofting forkfuls of wet hay out of the barn on the farm where I lived. My back ached, and when I stretched in the morning, I was still a bit stiff and vulnerable, but I was better. No question.

I had words for the way I'd become well—a description of the trajectory of a chronic condition to and through a crisis—but I couldn't get my mind around it. This law of healing, even if it resembled my psychiatric experience, was still antithetical to everything I'd been taught about the body; and the means had been even more outlandish and improbable than the man who'd made it happen.

I was fascinated. In medical school chemical reactions, disease states, and diagnoses had been dry things to me, watered only by contact with the humans in whose service we could put them. But something had come alive in me during this therapy, some direct full connection to my own biological processes, some inkling that there were, perhaps, secrets in the natural world that were not revealed by our texts of bio-chemistry and physiology. I was immensely eager to learn them. I felt again like a child discovering the limitless world of words and books.

Phrases of Dr. Singha's kept appearing on my mind's horizon: "the lung is the mother of the kidney"; "a chronic disease must become acute before it can be healed." Biology, it seemed, could be as personal and immediate, as subtle and rich with story as psychology. This new/old medicine that had so profoundly altered the condition of my back and the way I felt seemed to be inviting me to embark on a different kind of experiment. Instead of isolating and controlling variables, dissecting and measuring organs and outcomes, I would learn on myself. Instead of observing something or somone out there, like Bacon's ideal scientist, I would be both experimental subject and experimentor. I would befriend, not master, Nature and my own nature; come to know, not control her ways.

I wanted to learn about Chinese medicine, but the only two English texts I could find seemed relentlessly impenetrable. And no books had anything to say about chronic diseases becoming acute or about how eating pineapple could affect the structure and functioning of my back.

I sat with my dilemma for a while—until it occurred to me that the best place to begin my study was with myself, with those parts of me that were crying out for help, and those therapies that I could begin to learn about and easily use on my own. I took an inventory of my problems. I had bad allergies and frequent colds; unstable knees; and a wandering and doubt-plagued mind. The most pressing item got my attention. It was late summer, the height of the ragweed season. So I started there.

I didn't like having a stuffed nose and runny red eyes, let alone the asthmatic gasps and wheezes that sometimes overtook me. They made breathing an anxious chore, and sleep difficult. As I got to thinking about it, I realized that these symptoms also embarrassed me. Stuffed up and sniffling, I felt like a snotty-nosed kid, a sickly wimp.

Ever since childhood, when my pediatrician first prescribed them, I had been content to dose myself with secretion-drying antihistamines and sinus-shrinking decongestants. My medicine cabinet—and my suitcase—were filled with small bottles and paper packages of bright pills and two-colored capsules. For years, without ever really thinking about it, I had obliterated my discomfort and, not incidentally, erased the image of vulnerability and sickliness, by medicating myself.

The medicine gave me some relief and sometimes even a feeling of triumph, a sense that I had subdued my opponent. But it was short-lived, dependent on continual doses of drugs. And they certainly didn't lead to better health—four or twelve hours later the symptoms would be back, rebounding with, it seemed to me, even greater force than before.

I had always told myself that there was no harm in the medications. They weren't even prescription drugs. If the TV commercials and the display cases in drugstores were any indication, tens of millions of other Americans suffered as I did. Probably they took hundreds of millions of doses each year. I had never had what I would have called a "bad" reaction, but I began to think about it. I knew that antihistamines acted not only on my nose but everywhere in my body. They gave me relief by successfully competing at nasal receptor sites with the irritant histamine. But of course, they also had to interfere with the digestive role of histamine in the stomach. If they produced the desired drying in the nose by interfering with the neurotransmitter acetylcholine, they must have similar "anticholinergic" effects everywhere else in the body, including the brain.

I had, of course, learned this in pharmacology, but I had also learned to dismiss minor "side effects" as unimportant— what's a little drowsiness or dry mouth compared to the constant irritation of a stuffed and runny nose?—and major ones as ridiculously rare. Sure, one person in a hundred or a thousand might develop a serious side effect like urine retention, dizziness, or disturbed coordination. But I hadn't been one of them, and even if it did happen, then I could just discontinue the medicine and my body would quickly recover. I had never really wondered what long-term effects there might be on my stomach or urinary tract or brain—or on that of all those other people who were each taking hundreds or thousands of doses over many years.

All right, I thought, let's see if I can get rid of, or at least cut down on, the drugs. If I really get desperate, I can always go back on them. Living on a farm in rural Virginia, working in Washington, D.C., the allergy capital of the Western world, I couldn't get away from the offending pollens. I had to try to find something that would do the same thing as the drugs—with no side effects; maybe even something that would get at the cause as well as the symptoms of my allergies.

I looked in the only acupuncture book I'd been able to find, a dense and technical little volume that read as if it had been badly translated from the Chinese but that had actually been written in English. I located a couple of points on the face that seemed relevant—at the base of my nose, where the nostrils flare, and just above the nose, where the eyebrows approach each other. I didn't have needles and wouldn't have known how to use them if I did, but I pressed on these places—on both sides of my face—and rubbed the spots for a while. I thought I noticed a little relief, a slight opening of my nasal passages. I was impressed and tried again—a little more open. I kept on, but the effect was limited, and after a while the clogging resumed. I couldn't do it all day long.

What about food? I had noticed that my nose was clearer while I was eating pineapple, but I certainly couldn't face that for very long. What else? Within a year I would discover that milk and milk products, and indeed sugar, alcohol, food additives like monosodium glutamate, and preservatives, all increased my congestion. Now when I work with patients with allergies, I routinely suggest eliminating these and sometimes other foods for a while. But twenty years ago, I was unaware of these kinds of sensitivities—of how, for example, milk seems to produce excess mucus in so many people—or of how simple it is to eliminate and then reintroduce suspect foods, one by one, to see which, if any, has negative consequences.

Still, I remembered what Dr. Singha—and Hippocrates—had said about food being your medicine. Maybe there were foods that could not only achieve symptom relief but actually change my reactivity to the pollens and dusts—the allergens that caused me so much grief. Today it's possible to find hundreds of books on the therapeutic uses of foods, and as many more on European, North American, Chinese, African, and Indian herbs. Every health food store and many pharmacies have several lines of herbal products. In 1974, however, I could find only the naturalist's and hippie's bible, Jethro Kloss's *Back to Eden,* and a few raggedy copies of old herbals—compilations of herbs.

The herbs, arranged in alphabetical order and indexed by disease, were accompanied by line drawings or watercolors and Latin names. Some of the books, like *Mrs. Grieve's Herbal,* were both cozy and familiar, and rich with history and literature, myth and magic. I learned that Saint-John's-wort, Hypericum, which is used for lung and bladder problems and depression, was once believed to be "so obnoxious to evil spirits that a whiff of it would cause them to fly." And that parsley, which is a strong diuretic, was mentioned by Homer and held in high esteem by the Greeks. They believed it sprang from the blood of the hero Archemorus, and they used it to make wreaths to adorn the tombs of the dead as well as for medicinal purposes.

Mrs. Grieve and the other compilers seemed as assertive and innocent as the pungent herbs they described, and as eager to share their knowledge as Nature was to offer her bounty. Anyone could use their books, buy the plants, and prepare and take the herbs. No degrees or prescriptions were necessary. I was a bit skeptical of such folksy self-assurance. But I was willing to give it a try.

I looked up allergies and stuffed noses, colds and sinusitis, and pieced together a program that seemed to make some sense. At meals I ate as much garlic and onions as possible.

They were said to dissolve mucus, improve the lungs' capacity to clear secretions, and forestall infections. In between, I drank herbal teas: elder flowers—to help break up the mucus that made me so miserable; mullein, goldenseal, and borage to tone the membranes of the nose and sinuses and to reduce inflammation; and echinacea to repel possible viral and bacterial invaders. I brewed these plants in various combinations—boiling them in water—added honey and lemon, and on occasion black pepper (also good for dispersing mucus) to make the mixture—the decoction, the herbalists called it—more palatable.

I got better—not all better but enough so that I could endure my residual nighttime nasal stuffiness and wake without my eyes cemented together. This was progress, and it was fun too. In times of real trouble I had been grateful for the potency of pills, but they had never really pleased me. Whole plants were different. There was a sense of adventure and satisfaction in finding and holding, preparing and using these remedies. I felt Nature was my ally, not my enemy, and that I was engaged with, not overwhelming my body. I was almost sorry when allergy season ended.

That winter, in time away from my work with runaway kids, I began to read in earnest.

Initially, I wanted to find out more about the approaches I had already experienced. I started with herbalism, which is generally believed to be the oldest form of medicine on the planet. Some animals, I read, were known to use herbs, and traces of medicinal plants had been recovered from some of the earliest archaeological digs. Herbalism had also, it turned out, been a powerful force in American medicine until the late nineteenth century, when the effectiveness of some pharmaceuticals, and the opposition of organized medicine, had cast a shadow on it.

We had learned in medical school that drugs derived from plants are more potent and more easily quantifiable than the plants from which they have been isolated. This is true, but it is also true, according to the herbalists I read, that by extracting them, we lose as much as we gain. Whole plants contain many "active ingredients," not just the single one that chemists isolate. When we use whole plants as medicines, these substances act in concert, contributing to one another's effectiveness, counteracting each other's toxic properties, and decreasing the side effects that the single, isolated active ingredient produces.

As I read on in books of "natural medicine," I learned that I could further diminish my allergies by making use of a folk remedy well known in Europe and North America. Three times each day, for three months, I was to chew a cubic inch of locally produced honeycomb. The pollens deposited there would confer a kind of immunity on me. I chewed devotedly and, in the spring, discovered that my allergies had all but disappeared.

I read cookbooks and started cooking Indian meals, hoping to understand some of the ways in which Dr. Singha had combined foods, spices, and herbs; struggled to penetrate the unfamiliar concepts of Ilza Veith's translation of *The Yellow Emperor's Classic of Internal Medicine,* the fundamental text of Chinese medicine; and planted an herb garden.

I also began to realize that my personal quest for new and more effective remedies was part of a larger process of questioning. Many people were discovering the limits of biomedicine and putting its history into a broader perspective.

My first tutor was the great microbiologist René Dubos. In 1959, in *Mirage of Health,* he had disputed the prevailing belief that medical progress had been, and would be, responsible for the defeat of disease. Dubos was well aware of biomedicine's great triumphs, but he maintained that the advances that he and others had made had been vastly overrated. Antibiotics and other drugs were certainly useful, even life-saving. But from his reading of the evidence, they had far less to do with the improved health and life span in industrialized countries than economic, social, nutritional, and behavioral factors—better sanitation, housing, nutrition, and

birth control. In the future, he believed, the way we inter-
acted with each other and the environment would influence
our health far more than any discoveries we might make in
the laboratory.

Over the next few years a chorus of other critics would
take biomedicine to task for its excesses and shortcomings,
as well as for its self-importance. In 1973 *Consumer Reports*
documented our grotesque overuse of prescripion and over-
the-counter drugs—five to seven billion of the tranquilizers
Valium and Librium, 20,000 tons or 225 aspirin per American adult per year. In 1976 Ivan Illich published *Medical Nemesis,* an unrelenting critique of the promiscuous and mindless
use of drugs and surgery and of the "medicalization" of
everyday life.

That same year the House of Representatives issued a
report documenting some 2.4 million *unnecessary* surgeries,
which cost patients $3.9 billion per year and resulted in the
loss of 11,900 lives. Meanwhile, the Rockefeller Institute was
convening a conference on the limits of medicine, whose proceedings were titled *Doing Better and Feeling Worse.*

At the same time other critical perspectives were being
brought to bear on the biomedical model. Anthropologists
were publishing data that suggested that biomedicine might
not represent, as we had always assumed, a clear evolutionary
advance on the healing sytems of other cultures. Physicists
were suggesting that even medicine's claim to scientific
objectivity might be illusory, arguing that the perspective of
the observer influences what he observes. Feminists began
to seriously question doctors' attitudes and judgment. Why
were they treating patients with condescension and rushing
to perform such large numbers of cesarean sections? Were
they making women's health and welfare secondary to their
own convenience and economic gain?

At the conferences where I heard these critiques, I met
other people who were exploring other medicines. Some were
health professionals who, like me, had run up against the
limits of biomedicine. Others were people from non-Western

cultures who were rediscovering the power of their traditional practices. A number were chronically sick and troubled people, "consumers" hoping for help.

A year after I recovered from my back problem, Dr. Singha came to the United States again—for another workshop, and to do acupuncture and osteopathic manipulation with me and a few other brave or desperate souls. I had a sense by then that my questions were part of a much larger intellectual reevaluation of biomedicine, and that my own search for more effective remedies would be far more important to me than I had first suspected.

Listening to Dr. Singha speak about the ancient laws of Chinese and Indian healing, I could feel his words, like some living force, working and surging in me. Later, when he treated me, I felt a power I had never imagined.

The first time he put acupuncture needles in my body, waves of pleasure swept from my feet toward my head. On the same table, three days later, without warning, my arms and legs began to shake so hard that the trays of instruments across the room clattered. He looked in on me, impassive, and nodded: "Good, good." Meanwhile my head was vibrating and my teeth chattering. Would I, I wondered with surprising detachment, go unconscious like an epileptic, lose my urine, or bite my tongue?

"That is what the Chinese call *qi*," Dr. Singha explained half an hour later, when I managed finally to open my trembling mouth to ask. "The Indians called it *prana*, Henri Bergson said it was *élan vital*, and Wilhelm Reich, your Western psychoanalyst, named it *orgone energy*. It is the life force. The acupuncturist's job is to move and balance the qi. Everything else—bliss, shaking, tears—arises as the being moves toward balance."

"Yes," I said, eager as any eight-year-old, "but how does it happen? What can it do? How can I learn more?"

He laughed. "In the East we say that when the disciple is ready, the teacher arrives."

"Well," I said, "you've arrived, and I'm ready."

"Good, good," he said. "First you were angry. Who was I— some impudent wog—to tell you, an important M.D., that you couldn't understand how pineapple works." (How does he know that? I'm wondering.) "Then you ate the pineapple and were confused. You got better and were curious. Now you've experienced energy, and you're eager."

I dropped my irritation at being found out. "You're right," I said. "I'm very eager. I have all these kids I work with whom we might be able to help. Some of them have been on tran- quilizers for years—"

"Forget about those kids," he interrupted. "Look to your- self. It's your medicine, the medicine you are now questioning, that says treatments can be learned like recipes, that doc- tors are no more than second-rate cooks or plumbers. That is not what I do nor what I teach. Treatments and techniques are available, and they do work, but first the being who uses them has to change."

"So what do I do?" I asked.

"Your medicine," he began, "was not always so. Hippocrates, the father of your medicine, said 'Physician—heal thyself,' and I say the same." He paused as if this were sufficient instruction.

I urged the conversation on, and it wound its way among stories and more uncanny sensing of my thoughts. I politely challenged his facts, and he not-so-politely challenged my ways of thinking. Meditation and medicine, he explained, have the same linguistic root. In the East meditation is an integral part of the training of all physicians. The mind, he assured me, has to be used as a servant not worshipped as a master. One has to free oneself from the limitations of rational thought, as well as its endless doubts and pointless disputes, in order to use any technique or treatment appropriately. To become open to the limitless wisdom and inventiveness that is avail- able to each of us, we have to abolish the mind's incessant chatter and enter the silence from which it originates. The path to this silence is meditation.

At this point he paused—and I leaped into the gap or, as I later thought, the trap: "What kind of meditation should I do?"

"Forty minutes of chaotic breathing," he answered, springing it shut. Then he added, as if this were a harmless afterthought, "each morning for at least six months."

Dr. Singha left for London, and the next day I began. In the workshops ten minutes of this mad exertion had made me weak and light-headed. Forty seemed impossible. I couldn't imagine it, but I couldn't imagine not doing it either. Entering psychoanalysis during my residency, coming to understand more about who I was and how I got that way, had been crucial to my becoming a psychiatrist and helping others to understand themselves. This process seemed analogous: I had to move and feel my own energy before I could work with others; free myself from my preconceptions so that I could have a direct experience of what Nature and my own nature had to teach me.

The next morning, alone in the city where Dr. Singha had led his workshop, I awoke early and apprehensive. I set a kitchen timer, took a few slow deep breaths, thanked Nature as Dr. Singha had advised, closed my eyes, and started.

I breathed as fast and as deep as I could, in and out through my nose, my knees bent to brace and sustain me, my hands clenched in tight desperate fists, my shoulders rising humped toward my ears, my arms pumping. I must, I thought, look like a crazed chicken.

Within five minutes my mouth tasted of metal and my head ached. I could think of nothing but the impossibility of keeping this up. The prospect of forty minutes lay on my chest and shoulders like a leaden blanket. I tried to slow down, to pace myself, and Dr. Singha's face appeared, disgusted. "Give a hundred percent," I heard him shout. I picked up speed again, dragging my arms up. I felt a wire band tightening across my diaphragm; I coughed and sputtered.

This can't be good for you, my mind—whose mind, my physician father's or my anxious mother's or mine?—warned me; you're going to dislocate your shoulder, hyperventilate, faint, and smash your head. I started laughing at myself, knowing that these voices were also evasions and, against all doubt and fear, picked up the pace again.

How much longer? The wire band was tightening again, but this time, more determined than I could have imagined myself to be, I kept breathing, faster, deeper. And then, without warning, it all changed. My arms were moving on their own, my head sat light on my shoulders, the air was cool on my face and sweet in my lungs.

I smiled. I thanked God or Nature, and thought that this must be what grace is—and then, just as suddenly, I found myself pounding away again, returned to earth by thought and self-congratulation. Okay, I said, let me pound and breathe, pound and breathe, fall into the rhythm, do this because, without knowing exactly why, it is what I asked for. My own stubborn dumb desire made me smile and breathe harder and faster, and smile and breathe, and then the timer sounded.

I did this meditation for more than six months. It was never easy to begin or finish. I watched my mind wander during my morning meditation, until, reluctantly, I brought it back to the task at hand. Each day, along with physical exertion, I met whatever the breath churned up from my mind. I saw how fearful I could be—of injury to my body, of looking foolish and being wrong, of a dozen other ogres of childhood and adolescence.

Years of psychotherapy and psychoanalysis had helped me to see what troubled me and why. Months of meditation now helped me to relax in the presence of my fears. Slowly and gently, they seemed to loosen their hold on me. My mind became clearer. I seemed more aware of my own reactions, more intuitive about other people's feelings.

Sometimes I laughed as I breathed, more often tears streamed down my cheeks. I learned I could do what hadn't seemed possible. And I learned that if I put out total effort, without expectations, that sometimes something else, something utterly beyond me, would take over. Then everything hard would become easy, and I would watch with delight as the breath breathed me.

FIVE

We Are All Unique ∽

S IX MONTHS LATER, when I saw Dr. Singha again, I felt more at home in my body, looser in my injury-jammed knees, lighter on my feet, more responsive to the taste and texture of foods, a bit more sure and loving in the way I touched others. My nose was definitely clearer, and my back wasn't bothering me. "Good, good," he said, pursing his lips and looking me up and down. "Something has happened.

"Nature serves," he went on, "but we don't know how to receive. Every moment she is showering grace on us, but we put up a parasol. It is so simple, but we don't want to know. We want to accumulate, to pretend that we can control. We want rules and recipes. Then we can put it all down and chalk it up and say, 'Yes, I've read that and done this.' But no one can tell you.

"The Western mind makes up the story that the Chinese learned acupuncture by trial and error, that once upon a time a warrior was wounded with an arrow here"—pointing to his ankle—"and a physical illness disappeared there"—indicating his abdomen. "Then there was another injury and another correlation. Bullshit. The doctors, the acupuncturists were monks. They meditated six, eight hours a day. In meditation they felt the points from the inside and knew which was connected where.

"Knowing arises within. And knowing also knows that at each moment truth is different. Heraclitus, your Greek philosopher, said you cannot step into the same river twice. I say you cannot step into the same river even once. It is already changed."

I didn't always know exactly what Dr. Singha meant. Sometimes I asked, questions tumbling after answers, pursuing him, he would later tell others, "everywhere, even into the bloody loo," until finally I came to some resting place of acceptable comprehension. When I was really trying to be a good student—he had once told me a story about three monks who lived together in silence, and the annoyance of two at the third who insisted on a yearly greeting—I'd just be quiet and wait till, sometime, maybe minutes or months later, when understanding would arise on its own.

This time, though the implications were pretty astonishing, I didn't need to ask. Maybe by going within, we really can know everything we need to—perhaps not in the special language of our science but in some way that is quite real and useful. Each of us comes to our knowledge differently and uses it differently.

A few months into my daily meditation, I'd had some inklings of intuition that were, to say the least, surprising. I became aware of the foods and emotions that made my allergies worse on one day than on another. I discovered that I knew which herb to use for what condition, and I somehow "guessed" that rubbing a certain point, far removed from an offending ache, could indeed relieve it. I wasn't sure what to make of all this and couldn't absolutely rule out prior but forgotten knowledge, but something else, some other kind of knowing, seemed to be at work. As unsettling as it was to my rational mind, it was certainly suggestive and inviting.

Secondly, if I was understanding Dr. Singha correctly—and I was pretty sure I was—every person really *is* different from every other. And different from moment to moment.

I had a sense of what this meant in my personal life. Clearly, my moods could dive and soar, and with them my opinion about my intelligence, my looks, and my prospect of ever feeling any different. I knew as a psychiatrist that patients who seem quite crazy enough to be committed can a few minutes later be saner than the doctors or judge who are deciding their fate. Have they stopped being schizophrenic, or is diagnosis itself far more mutable than most anyone cares to believe?

I wondered what this meant for our understanding of physical illness. I already knew that one person's character may help him deal with an overwhelming situation in a different and healthier way, and that another's "good constitution" may fortify her against physical illness; and that some people, for no obvious reason, recover from conditions—from cancer to car accidents—that customarily kill others. Surely there are powerful individual differences at work.

Maybe every person's illness is different from everyone else's. Perhaps my gallbladder problems, even my pneumonia, are different from yours. Not in the sense simply that my interpretation of my condition or my reaction to it is different, but that in some radical, deeply biological way, it is different enough to make a real difference. Not only that, it can be different from one hour to the next, and different depending on who assesses it.

This perspective is quite—no other word comes to mind—"different" from any we adopted in medical school. There the focus was on defining discrete disease entities and matching particular treatments to them. We took cultures from the throat and blood and tested the bacteria that grew from them against a variety of antibiotics, looking for the one that most effectively inhibited growth. We chose, in a particular order and from a small menu, drugs to prompt the kidneys to excrete the excess fluid that was burdening the heart. The rich and complex individuality of the person who was being treated faded into the background.

Here, in this world of "other medicines," we were considering the disease as one element of the larger picture that is the whole person. In Chinese or Indian Ayurvedic medicine, there might, Dr. Singha said, be half a dozen, or twenty, or more, very different treatments for people with exactly the same Western medical diagnosis. For example, a person's age and sex, sensitivity to heat or cold, predominance of one or another emotional factor, the shape of the pulses at the radial arteries—there are twelve in Chinese medicine, he assured me—and even the time of day at which the treatment is given, are all taken into account. There is no standard treatment for congestive heart failure or even pneumococcal pneumonia, but many different ones, different combinations of herbs and acupuncture points, physical exercises, and psychological advice, each designed for that particular person.

"Nature is so generous," Dr. Singha confided to me on the way to the airport. "In India we say there is not one god but six hundred million. Each person is a god. When a child is born, we say, not even that it is a gift of god, but that the god has come. We are all unique like gods, each with a different fingerprint"—waggling his fingers at me. "Walk in the woods. Take the leaves from one branch of a single tree, and look at them carefully. The same genes, the same DNA, but they will all be different—a sharper angle here, a vein crossing a bit to the left there. Take a magnifying glass to the beach, and sit for a few hours. Look at each grain in a pinch of sand. All different."

It took many months, but I did as he advised. And once I'd done it, spent an afternoon with the leaves and one with the sand, I never forgot. Yes, I thought, if even such simple forms—of minerals and of plant life, can be so obviously, morphologically, grossly physically different, then how much more so each of us large complex and complexly grown humans, with our unique DNA and our particular parents and daily lives and our long many-branched histories?

What Dr. Singha was saying was true. And when I reflected on it, I realized that this perspective had always shaped my interactions with people. Still, I wondered how deeply it went, and what its implications for physical illness might be.

At about this time, in one of those coincidences that really seem like more than coincidences—the psychiatrist Carl Jung called them synchronicities, events connected not by cause and effect but by their occurrence at the same time and their relevance to one another—I came across the work of Dr. Roger Williams.

Williams was a professor of chemistry and director of the Biochemical Institute at the University of Texas, a man who in the mid-1970s was already in his seventies. He had isolated and synthesized vitamin B5, pantothenic acid, and had written many papers on biological chemistry and nutrition for scientific journals. In recent years he had become particularly interested in what he called "biochemical individuality," and it was his papers and books in this area that drew my attention.

Williams had studied individual differences in nutritional requirements and had begun to pull together the literature on the subject. His findings were eye-opening. It turned out that among normal populations the need for specific nutrients—for example, vitamins, minerals, and the amino acids that are the building blocks of proteins—varies enormously. One "normal" thirty-year-old man might require two or ten times as much vitamin A as another or twenty times as much zinc for ordinary functioning. Williams postulated that these differences might be the result of genetic variation or previous life experience and illnesses. These variations, in turn, might produce different kinds and amounts of bacteria in the gastrointestinal tract, different speeds of absorption into the bloodstream, and different metabolic rates and requirements.

Whatever the cause, the implications were great. First of all—and Williams made this point repeatedly—these individual variations call into question the customary way that the Department of Agriculture calculates the Recommended Daily Allowances of nutrients. If I need twenty times as much of a particular nutrient as the statistical average on which the

RDA is calculated, then I am ill served by getting only that amount. Secondly, his findings showed that the so-called "normal" blood levels of these nutrients may also be poor indicators of someone's actual nutritional status. If, because of a difficulty in metabolizing the amino acid arginine or vitamin C, I need twice or ten times as much as my neighbor, then a "normal" blood level in fact reflects a deficiency *for me.* Finally, his studies made clear that the levels of nutrients, and our need for them, may fluctuate considerably even in one person at different times of the year or indeed the day.

Since these nutrients are crucial to biological reactions throughout the body, a lack of one or another may have significant consequences. It may be responsible for a deficiency disease or for a vulnerability to either infectious or noninfectious illnesses. And since it is statistically quite likely that a given individual may have greater-than-average requirements for more than one nutrient, there is a significant possibility that many of us—with average intakes and normal blood levels—have an undetected nutritional vulnerability to a number of disease states.

Williams pointed out that there are also significant differences in normal people's sensitivity to, and rates of metabolism of, the pharmaceutical agents that we prescribe and use. It was well known that some people have a "hypersensitivity" to certain drugs—an exaggerated rise in blood pressure to a decongestant—or indeed a paradoxical reaction to them—growing agitated, for example, rather than quiet, after an injection of morphine. It was less well known but equally important that blood levels of drugs (given to people in equal dosages) and sensitivity to them vary enormously from person to person and sometimes even within a given person at different times of day.

As I read Williams's work, I knew that I had come upon a Western biochemical perspective that was analogous to the one Dr. Singha had been urging on me, a modern validation of ancient observations. The diagnostic entities and statistical norms that dominated my medical education were indeed only relative truths based on statistical averages. The excessive reliance on tests and lab values might be subversive not only of a close doctor-patient relationship and of clinical judgment, as I had suspected, but also of a precise scientific understanding of the person a doctor is supposed to help.

It was becoming clearer that conventional medical wisdom was not necessarily the final arbiter of how we should help ourselves. Williams's work suggested that we all needed to be far more sensitive to the way we felt, and far more assertive in investigating and meeting our own needs, than we had been led to believe. For example, even if my diet seemed adequate, and my doctor told me my lab tests were within normal limits, I might still need nutritional supplements. And the only way I would be likely to find out if this were the case would be to experiment for and on myself. Similarly, even though the blood levels of medications I might be taking were "within the therapeutic range," the dosage might be inappropriate for me. The therapeutic range, Williams was telling us, is only an average. It may be therapeutic for one person but toxic for another and entirely inadequate for a third.

In the years since Williams first made these points, the basic tenets of his theory of biochemical individuality have been borne out. For example, recent studies on several of the B vitamins have shown that people who have both normal intake and normal blood levels of B12, B6, and folate are, in fact, suffering from functional deficiencies of these vitamins. In one recent and careful study, five percent of people suffering from neurological symptoms clearly attributable to B12 deficiency had *normal* levels of B12.

Williams's findings, and the studies that have subsequently appeared, confirmed my sense of the importance of understanding and treating each person as unique. What had originally seemed to be common sense, an ordinary courtesy to troubled and ill people, what Dr. Singha had declared to be a reflection of Nature's ways and a metaphysical truth, now was taking on the force of a biological imperative and the sharpness of a scientific fact.

SIX

Whole People in
Their Total Environments ❧

W E ARE WHOLE AS WELL AS UNIQUE, and each
aspect of our lives—the emotional, mental, and spiritual as well as the physical—is rich and complex
and deeply connected to the others. Each of us is brought up
in a particular family at a given time and in a specific place.
Each of us is a member of a socioeconomic and ethnic group.

These are not merely sociological platitudes or items to
include in an inventory. Understanding all the dimensions
of a life is crucial to understanding each person and his or
her illnesses. Addressing them may make possible a successful treatment that a more narrow approach would dismiss or ignore.

Working as a psychiatrist, and being a patient in psychotherapy and psychoanalysis, had sensitized me to the
importance of family and social circumstances in shaping our
emotional reactions and our ways of looking at the world. It
seemed no accident that my two brothers and I all share a certain level of self-flagellating perfectionism and recalcitrant
self-doubt with my father; nor that each of us is as comfortable and curious in unfamiliar situations as both our parents

seemed to be. Nor did it seem odd that my paranoid patients often had grown up in homes where they were teased with secrets or unpredictably abused, beaten, or berated. These were the commonplaces of self-examination and psychotherapy. My work was to explore the origins of these thoughts, feelings, and behaviors and to free myself, and help my patients to free themselves, from those that limited or damaged us.

I also believed that mental and emotional states can affect the course and outcome of physical illnesses. I had seen it as a child in my family: my father's blood pressure hitting the ceiling after a fight with my mother; high levels of tension making one of my brothers wheeze with asthma; my own skin showing the effects of prolonged worry. Two months into my internship, I was sure of this connection between family relationships and physical illness.

I was on pediatrics one Saturday, running back and forth from the ward and nursery to the ER, when Mrs. Tyson, a thirtyish black woman, brought in Jerome and Jermayne, her two well-dressed young boys. The boys were wheezing so loud, I could hear them before I rounded the corner and saw them. I was struck by the mother because her mouth was tight and her posture rigid; and by the gasping boys, because they looked and sounded so bad and reminded me of my own brother. It was the second straight Saturday that they'd appeared in this condition.

While I was drawing up a syringe of adrenaline to break their asthma attacks, their mother left the examining room to go to the bathroom. I started talking to the boys then, telling them they'd be fine and saying how my brother had had asthma and he'd gotten over it. Within a minute, before I'd even filled the syringes, the pace of their breathing had slowed, and the volume of the sound was down. I waited a while longer, still talking, telling them how great they were doing. Ten minutes later they were giggling and playing with my stethoscope, and telling me about their grades in reading and spelling, and who the best ballplayers in the neighborhood were. I hadn't given either of them a drop of adrenaline.

When their mother came back—she'd gotten lost on the way to the bathroom—I asked her if the boys had attacks during the week. It turned out they didn't. What was special about Saturday? I wondered. She thought about it for a moment and told me that it was the only day she had off. She worked three jobs, more or less around the clock, and Saturday was the only time she had with her sons. Maybe it wasn't all that good a time, she thought, because she was always so nervous about squeezing a week's worth of love and caring into one day, and so guilty about not supervising their schoolwork at other times, or talking to their teachers or cooking their meals. She found herself fussing over every detail of their Saturday diet and dress, and squeezing their hands too tight, even when they were walking on familiar streets.

It seemed so clear as she spoke that the terrible pressure of time and money, the anxiety and guilt of living the way she had to, was being transmitted to them and transformed in them, for reasons of biology and heredity that I could only guess at, into spasms in their bronchi: the vulnerability of her life triggering the vulnerability in their biology.

I told her what nice kids they were, how bright and friendly, and said that I understood, or thought I did, how hard it is to have to work such long hours and not be where you feel you should be, to do everything you feel you should do. But I said that it seemed to me that even if it was very hard and not fair, still it was all right. She was doing such a good job.

I felt like I was blundering on, and I was on the edge of tears myself, feeling the sadness of her trying so hard and just making things worse. I'm not even sure that she heard everything I was saying, but it seemed to make her shoulders relax. She was smiling, and the boys were breathing easy when she left. They didn't come back on any of the other Saturdays that I worked on pediatrics. And when I asked a few months after I finished peds, none of the other interns had seen them.

Years later, when I began to read over the literature on how familial and social factors may affect health and illness,

I remembered these boys and their mother. So much that is so important, so much that we have since then systematically examined, was there in that half hour in the ER—so much that is still, to all of our detriment, too often ignored.

While I was still working as an intern in San Francisco, Salvador Minuchin, the psychiatrist and pioneering family therapist who directed the Philadelphia Child Guidance Center, began a series of simple but elegant studies on children and adolescents with serious physical illnesses, including asthma, rheumatoid arthritis, anorexia nervosa, and juvenile diabetes. Minuchin's hypothesis was that these were emotional as well as physical conditions, and that family interactions could profoundly affect their course and outcome.

I was particularly struck, years later when I read it, by Minuchin's description of his work with families whose children had juvenile or insulin-dependent diabetes. Minuchin found that some of these kids had what he called "psychosomatic" diabetes. They were normally indistinguishable from other juvenile diabetics, but in the context of certain kinds of family stress, their physiological responsiveness changed dramatically. Then their free-fatty-acid levels (the indicators of emotional arousal that Minuchin measured) would rise rapidly, and their blood sugar would go wildly out of control; sometimes no amount of insulin could bring it down.

When Minuchin looked closely at these families, he found that the children were either the objects of their parents' overwhelming attention or served as "mediators" of parental conflict. When he interviewed the parents by themelves and pushed them to deal with conflicts between them, the free-fatty-acid levels of one or both rose. When the diabetic child was brought into the situation, she became a lightning rod for family stress. While the parents' free-fatty-acid levels remained constant, hers escalated precipitously, setting in motion a whole chain of events that sometimes led to a diabetic crisis.

Minuchin concluded that sometimes juvenile diabetes, one of the most clearly delineated of biomedical disease states, is in fact a family illness as well as an individual one; its proper treatment requires not only dietary management and injectible insulin but family therapy.

And it's not just children whose illnesses are entwined with family functioning. At about the same time Minuchin was doing his work, a Ph.D. candidate named Fred Hoebel was taking a look at a group of men with coronary artery disease. These men were considered by their exasperated physicians to be particularly "difficult to manage" and therefore at high risk of dying from their heart disease. Nothing the doctors said or did could convince them to take their medicines, lose weight, exercise regularly, or eat properly.

Instead of trying to find better arguments to convince the men to change their behavior, Hoebel took another tack. Believing that heart disease is as much a family affair as a matter of pathology in the men's chests, he decided to try instead to alter the patterns of their relationships with their wives. These patterns, he believed, were helping to sustain the men's self-destructive behavior. Hoebel decided to ignore the men and meet with their wives for a maximum of five hours each.

Hoebel tells us, in his account of his work, that he convinced one wife *not* to encourage her depressed, sedentary, overweight, out-of-work husband to take better care of himself. Over the years all her attempts to be encouraging, consoling, and helpful had come to naught; her husband just seemed to get heavier, more inert, and more depressed.

When, with Hoebel's insistent tutoring, she was able to tell her husband not to bother to do anything, that he was clearly incapable of changing his behavior, everything did in fact change. He began to exercise, lose weight, be more cheerful and hopeful, and even look for and find a job. Altering the family pattern, springing him from his role as the pampered and nagged but hopeless patient, had made it possible for him to change health-destroying individual patterns that had seemed unalterable.

The literature on the effects of social and economic forces on health and illness is, if anything, even more dramatic.

Poverty and racism, all but ignored in medical education, diagnosis, and prescription, are of particularly great importance.

People of color and poor people generally have a far higher incidence of chronic illnesses and of morbidity (disability) and mortality from these conditions. Asthma, for example, has been increasing steadily in the last two decades, its incidence probably elevated by environmental pollution, adulterated food, and stress. Between 1981 and 1988 it climbed by 39 percent for all children under eighteen. During this same period the incidence and hospitalization rates for asthma were 300 to 400 percent greater for black children, like Jermayne and Jerome, than for white children. The mortality rate from this condition was five times higher for black males than for white males.

The discrepancies between blacks and whites are also striking for cardiovascular disease, cancer, and blindness, as well as for AIDS, depression, drug abuse, and death from violence. Writing in the *New England Journal of Medicine* in 1990, Drs. Colin McCord and Harold Freeman observed that "black men in Harlem were less likely to reach the age of 65 than men in Bangladesh," a country synonymous with natural and man-contrived disasters, abject poverty, and malnutrition.

Social dislocation, and alienation at work and in the world, are less dramatic but equally important and pervasive contributors to ill health. Over the last thirty years the increased incidence of a variety of disorders has been closely linked with removal from familiar settings and supportive communities. One famous study was done on Italian-Americans in Roseto, Pennsylvania. The children of immigrants who remained in this small cohesive town enjoyed the same good he.lth, good spirits, and longevity as their parents. Those who left to seek their fortune elsewhere tended to become as ill as the people who lived in the towns and cities to which they migrated.

The same findings hold true for other ethnic groups. In Japan, for example, the rates of heart disease in the 1960s and 1970s were extremely low, as were the incidence of and death rate from other chronic illnesses. However, Japanese who migrated to the United States and adopted the ways of their new country soon came to have morbidity and mortality rates comparable to other Americans.

On the other hand, those who kept close ties to the Japanese community and observed traditional customs maintained the same good health as those they left behind in Japan — *even if they ate the conventional high-fat American diet*. It would seem that deprivation of membership in a close-knit and supportive group is dangerous to our health, while integration into such a group is therapeutic.

Work satisfaction and employment status also have definite effects on health and illness. The data is particularly striking for cardiovascular disease but may well apply to other conditions too. In 1973 a Department of Health, Education and Welfare survey in Massachusetts revealed that the best predictor for a heart attack was not high blood pressure or cholesterol level or smoking but job dissatisfaction.

More recently, Robert Karasek of the University of Massachusetts has shown that people who work at jobs characterized by "high strain" — a great demand for productivity and little room for freedom to determine how that demand will be met — have an increased risk for developing cardiovascular disease and indeed, a significantly higher death rate from all causes. This is true, for example, of assembly-line workers, waiters in busy restaurants, and gas station attendants.

Interestingly, heart attacks in the United States, as well as in other Western countries come with significantly greater frequency on Monday mornings between eight and nine o'clock, at the beginning of the conventional work week.

Family feelings, social and economic forces, work status, ethnic identity, and individual biological differences all come together in each of us. And each of us, as the South African biologist Jan Christian Smuts pointed out seventy years ago, is also more than the sum of these vital parts. Smuts said we were whole organisms, whole people, and he named his way of looking at us *holistic*, from *holos*, the Greek word for "whole."

When I first heard the word *holism*—some people spell it *wholism*—in the early 1970s, I was impressed and even moved by it. *Holistic medicine* seemed exactly to fit what I was trying to learn about and practice and live. *Psychosomatic medicine* and *behavioral medicine* both seemed too narrow and too stiff; *humanistic* emphasized the kind of care I wanted to give, but not the means I wanted to use; *alternative* covered part of what I was doing but didn't take into account the richness and utility of conventional biomedicine.

Holism is inclusive and generous, comprehensive and integrative. Holistic medicine widens its lens to observe and describe the familial, social, economic, environmental, and ethnic dimensions of each of our lives. It includes conventional as well as alternative therapies.

Holism is also deeply psychological and spiritual. The word even has the same root as *healing* and *holy*. It implies that healing comes through wholeness, through recovering and reintegrating all those parts of ourselves that we have denied, ignored, or repressed; and it implies that our spiritual life is not separable from our physical and emotional life.

The word *holism* and the concept seemed right. Still, at times the *adjective* holistic felt both redundant and confining. I wanted all of medicine to be holistic, not for a small group of believers to lay claim to the title. My real work, I felt, was to bring the philosophy and practice of holism to all physicians, medical students, and patients, whether or not they ever chose to use or even recognize the name.

Now, when someone calls my practice holistic, I agree, but I also nod when asked if I work with alternative medicine or complementary medicine. And when the time came for me to create a nonprofit institution, I called it the Center for Mind-Body Medicine.

Yes, I say, I primarily use alternatives, techniques that are other than those I learned in medical school, ones that may work where more conventional practices have fallen short. And yes, I feel comfortable with the Europeans who speak of complementary medicine, of therapies that fit with and "complement" conventional practice. I call my center Mind-Body because so much of what we do is concerned with bringing mind and body into harmony and helping each to transform the other. But what I'm really interested in is helping to create a new *medicine*, a more respectful and responsive health care, a larger synthesis that transcends categories and any attempts to categorize it.

Everyone who has embraced the comprehensive, integrative, holistic approach of the new medicine has done so in his or her own way. Each person's practice is shaped by the particularities and peculiarities of his or her life history, aptitudes, and interests. For example, I was drawn more to Chinese medicine than to Indian Ayurveda, or to American Indian or African healing, though I recognize their power and utility. Some of my colleagues have devoted themselves to one alternative technique or system: for example, nutrition, Chinese medicine, or homeopathy. Others, like me, have worked with a number of different approaches. All of us use and combine them in different ways.

Still, even though its practice is highly individual, the new medicine does have certain consistent and recognizable features. All of us who practice it take seriously Hippocrates' injunction, "First do no harm." This means we use what is least harmful first. Only when the situation absolutely demands it do we use those therapies that are potent but potentially damaging.

The heart of our healing practice is those approaches that each person can undertake for himself or herself: self-awareness, relaxation, meditation, diet, and exercise. Next in line are methods and techniques that usually require professional assistance—manipulation, massage, acupuncture, hypnosis, and homeopathic and herbal prescribing among them. These modalities promote the balance that disease has disrupted and restore the body's own potential for healing. Finally, reserved for special and specially demanding or threatening situations—and for people whose defenses are overwhelmed—are potent pharmacological remedies and powerful surgical interventions.

Those of us who practice this way spend a great deal of time taking a history. We don't, as too many physicians do, touch only lightly on "family history," simply record a patient's job title or ignore her spiritual life. We regard all of these aspects of life as of fundamental importance. We ask not just what our patients' parents died from or what their health is like but what are, or were, *they* like? What hopes and fears, expectations and disappointments did they surround their children with and project onto them?

We want to know where each of our patients lives and with whom; whom they love; and what the joys and tensions of those relationships are. We are interested in how they eat and exercise and, most especially, what gives their lives meaning. How do you like your work, and what do you get out of it, and why did you choose it, are all important questions. And what makes it worthwhile to get out of bed in the morning, and why do you think you're here on this planet?

This same breadth of understanding informs and shapes our therapeutic approach. Because an illness manifests in a physical way doesn't mean that its origin is or its treatment ought to be exclusively or even predominantly physical. Virtually every chronic illness has a powerful psychological component, and almost always, the work of untangling the fears, resentments, and misconceptions that prevent emotional and intellectual change is a necessary precondition for physical healing. Similarly, the best approach to conditions described as psychiatric disorders is not necessarily psychotherapy or medication. I've found, for example, that physical exercise is often the single best therapy for mild to moderate anxiety and depression.

Always, whether a disorder produces physical or emotional symptoms, I am concerned with the spiritual dimension of my patient's life. What meaning does a particular illness have for the person? Does it signal the inadequacy of an old way of living, a need for a new direction and a deeper sense of meaning and purpose?

a workaholic. That wasn't the problem. The problem, she reminded me, glancing at her watch, was that she had multiple sclerosis, and it was getting worse. Twice this month, four times in the last five months, she'd had exacerbations, periods of many days, even weeks, when there was serious numbness and tingling in both her legs, and weakness in her right arm. Then she'd had trouble taking notes, and several times co-workers had wondered why she wasn't walking as quickly as they. Once she'd even thought that the horrible near blindness, the inflammation of the optic nerve that had heralded her first attack nine years before, was returning.

Leslie had heard from a friend whom I'd treated for ankylosing spondylitis, a severe rheumatoidlike arthritis of the spine, that I had helped her with diets, acupuncture needles, and Chinese herbs. Ankylosing spondylitis is an autoimmune disease, Leslie knew, a condition in which a person's immune system—designed to repel bacterial invaders and to destroy abnormal cells—seems to go out of control and attack normal tissue. Multiple sclerosis is now also presumed to be an autoimmune illness, and Leslie reasoned that I might be able to help her with it as well.

When she'd called, we talked about her MS. She'd told me that her attacks were becoming more frequent, and that scans of her brain had shown a number of large bright "plaques." These were areas where the immune cells were presumed to have attacked and destroyed the fatty myelin sheaths that protect and nourish the nerve cells. Leslie could see on the scans that her brain was damaged and could feel that her body was becoming ever more vulnerable and feeble. This was "exceedingly distressing" to her. Had I ever treated someone with MS?

I told her I was currently treating several people with MS, that two were doing very well and one was holding his own. I explained what my approach was and asked if she was willing to look at her life and lifestyle, at all the possible influences on her illness. "Yes, of course," she said, in what I knew was actually a form of dismissal, "but what about the acupuncture and the herbs?"

I said they would probably be helpful and once again began to explain—patiently and pleasantly, I thought—how powerful emotional and mental factors can be in the onset, course, and successful treatment of MS and other chronic illnesses. She cut me off: "When can I have an appointment?"

I found myself getting irritated. This woman wasn't interested in the kind of work I did or the way I saw things. She didn't want a healing partnership. She wanted me to do something to or for her, and she was, by God, going to tell me what it was and when she wanted it done. She wasn't interested in doing anything for herself except ordering me around. I thought about commenting on her behavior, or trying once again to explain the need for looking at herself and possibly for deep change as well, but it was clear that it wasn't going to get us anywhere.

Our first session was, if anything, even less promising. She arrived half an hour late, having confused my address with another. She dropped angrily into her chair, a dark-haired, pudgy, sullen-faced young woman in a shapeless gray pantsuit. When I told her we wouldn't have as much time as I liked, she wanted me to do acupuncture that day and continue with the history the next time we met.

I explained that I needed to know who she was before I began to treat her. While she sat smoldering, I began to ask questions that yielded information about her early life and her work. It was like pulling teeth. She was the long-suffering striver; everyone else, she intimated, from her parents to her co-workers, was either exploitative, inefficient, or neglectful. When I asked whom she lived with, she became indignant. What kind of a question was that?

At about this time, I started wondering who else I could refer this woman to, but even aside from the obvious difficulty of finding anyone who would be willing to see her, something stopped me. She *was* suffering and terrified, and if she was being controlling and rude, so what? Why was *I* getting so irritated? What buttons was she pushing in me?

It was clear to me that Leslie was one of those "difficult patients" that other doctors claim fill their practices, one of those people who, they are sure, will never be interested in the kind of approach I offer. These people, I had often been told, insist on the magic bullet and will steadfastly refuse to help themselves. She was also, I realized, a living, breathing, suffering caricature of all of us, or at least of the part of us that desperately wants someone else to take care of us, and of all the attitudes and expectations that our biomedical approach has helped to create.

Leslie didn't believe that her illness had anything to do with her mental or emotional life or, indeed, with her as a person. She had a problem in her nervous system, and I was the expert who could find its solution. She wanted me to use techniques associated with the new medicine, but to use them as if they were drugs and surgical procedures. She was challenging me in a very deep way. I had a feeling that if I could relax and keep my cool, I could learn a lot.

Coming to see the intimate connection between the mind and the body, and to realize the power each of us has to affect not only how we feel but indeed the course and outcome of our illnesses, has been a long and difficult struggle. It has been particularly long and difficult, I think, because it has required us not only to overcome 350 years of intellectual conditioning but because it has forced us to reclaim truths that many of the best minds of biomedicine have dismissed as unsubstantiated or trivial.

Thirty years ago, when I was in medical school, the connection between mind and body that was the cornerstone of Hippocratic medicine was for all practical purposes ignored or sundered. Everyone knew from personal experience that embarrassment can produce a blush, fear a fast heart rate, and anxiety a need to urinate. The information to substantiate the connection was available in our physiology courses. Still, our eyes seemed to slide over the forest of its meaning as we rushed to identify and master the trees of cardiovascular dynamics, pulmonary gas exchange, and kidney filtration.

We read about Claude Bernard, the nineteenth-century University of Paris professor and "father of modern physiology," who had observed that the organism has a *milieu interieur*, an "internal environment," that it strives to maintain in a constant state, despite changes in its external environment.

We also studied the work of Walter Bradford Cannon, who had been a professor of physiology at Harvard. Cannon had described the dynamic equilibrium or balance of forces within an organism as *homeostasis* (from the Greek *homoios*, meaning "similar," and *stasis*, meaning "position") and had named the "fight-or-flight" syndrome that threatened animals' experience.

We even paused for a moment to note the Canadian Hans Selye's definition of stress—"the nonspecific response of the body to any demand"—and his description of the general adaptation syndrome, the way the body mobilizes itself to meet the demands of any physical or emotional stress.

Unfortunately, we never considered the implications of this work—the unified picture of mind and body, and the power of the mind to affect the body—which their concepts offered us. Even in psychiatry the mind and body seemed to go their separate ways. Heinroth had first used the phrase *psychosomatic medicine* in 1818, and the American psychiatrists Helen Flanders Dunbar and Franz Alexander had, over a century later, made heroic efforts to correlate specific disease entities with particular psychological states. (Patients with rheumatoid arthritis, for example, were said to be rigid and filled with suppressed anger.) But this field and their work were presented as quaint, impractical, and largely of historical interest. It didn't matter that common sense appreciates, and ordinary language preserves, these connections between the emotions and physical functioning: people have "gut feelings," experience others as "a pain in the neck," and carry "back-breaking" emotional burdens.

Perhaps years of lying on an analyst's couch "free associating," letting thoughts emerge spontaneously, would establish links between the emotional states and disease processes. But who could be sure? We were sometimes encouraged to combine psychotherapy and psychopharmacology in the treatment of "mental illnesses." When it came to physical illnesses, we were advised to reach for the prescription pad.

This perspective began to change, at least in some quarters, in the late 1960s. A new generation of researchers, grappling with the prevalence and recalcitrance of chronic illness, rediscovered the power and intimacy of the mind-body connection. Researchers on cardiovascular disease reviewed the details of Cannon's fight-or-flight response, while those who were studying cancer, autoimmune disorders, and infectious disease began to ponder Selye's studies on stress.

Cannon had observed that during the fight-or-flight response, animals have an increase in heart and respiratory rate; greater muscular tension; coldness and sweatiness; a decrease in intestinal activity; and a dilation, or increase in size, of the pupils of their eyes. All these are manifestations of activity on the part of the sympathetic nervous system, one of two branches of the autonomic ("beyond our control," as opposed to voluntary) nervous system.

The sympathetic nervous system, like its complement, the parasympathetic nervous system, is regulated in the brain by the hypothalamus. It communicates not only with centers in the lungs, heart, and arteries but with the medulla or inner portion of the adrenal gland. There it provokes the release of epinephrine and norepinephrine, which further stimulate heart and respiratory rate. All of this sympathetic activity primes animals—and humans—to flee from a predator or, if necessary, to fight.

Where Cannon's work focused on the effect of emotions on the autonomic nervous system, Selye's was concerned primarily with alterations in the endocrine and immune systems. As a medical student in the 1920s, Selye had observed that people in the hospital all had a certain "sick" look about them, regardless of their diagnosis. As a researcher, he set himself the task of discovering whether there were consistent anatomical and physiological changes in all these sick people, regardless of the cause of the disturbance.

Selye pinched and poked, heated and froze animals. He subjected them to loud noises and electrical shocks and overcrowding. What he learned was that all animals, regardless of the nature of the "noxious stimulus" and in addition to such local manifestations as bruises or burns, showed certain consistent findings. These included, most importantly, an enlargement of the outer part of the adrenal gland, the cortex, which secretes steroid hormones that accelerate physiological functioning and decrease inflammation; and shrinkage of the thymus, spleen, and lymph nodes, major organs of the immune system. Selye called the body's consistent response to these stresses the "general adaptation syndrome," to differentiate it from the local adaptation that varies from stimulus to stimulus.

Selye hypothesized that the first stages of the general adaptation syndrome—the periods of "alarm" and "resistance"—represent a creative response, a mobilization of the body to deal with stress. If the stress is prolonged, a phase of "exhaustion," in which the body's remaining defenses are called into play, will supervene. Either these defenses are effective, or else the defenses in one vulnerable part of the body collapse and illness occurs. If the stress continues unabated, the organism, animal or human, may be completely overwhelmed and die.

The stress response is registered in the conscious and unconscious portions of the brain, Selye continued; it can be amplified and modified by the parts of the brain that control and register emotional responses and sensory imagery. It is then communicated to the hypothalamus, the same part of the brain that mediates the fight-or-flight response. The hypothalamus, in turn, transmits signals to the nearby pituitary or master endocrine gland. The pituitary sends messages to the adrenal cortex, calling on that gland to secre'e the hormones that produce the "stress response" that characterizes the general adaptation syndrome.

By the early 1970s, researchers were beginning to suggest that the fight-or-flight and stress responses might account for a variety of human disease states. According to Cannon's observations, endangered animals quickly flee and quickly recover or else die fighting; some civilized humans, however, seemed to exist in a perpetual state of fight-or-flight. The angry, time-obsessed, hypertension-and-heart-attack-prone type A executive, described by cardiologists Meyer Friedman and Ray Rosenman, was the prime example. Feeling unable either to fight or flee—he might lose his job or his status either way—hoping things would get better, toughing it out, he was in a chronic state of anxious readiness. In time, Friedman and Rosenman hypothesized, this produced a steady state of hypertension and physical damage, most significantly in the arteries and heart.

Selye's work, on the other hand, suggested a physiological basis for correlations that were being observed between early or ongoing emotional trauma—the loss of a parent, for example, or the death of a spouse or chronic tension at home—and an increased incidence of cancer, depression, and other chronic illnesses. Perhaps people whose immune functioning was compromised by high levels of stress and prolonged secretion of steroids were more likely to exhibit both the deficient immune response observed in cancer and the disordered immune functioning of the autoimmune diseases, as well as a vulnerability to chronic infections.

At about the same time, other lines of research, initiated by George Solomon at Stanford, Robert Ader at the University of Rochester, and Candace Pert at Johns Hopkins, suggested a third pathway by which mental attitudes and emotional responses could affect physical functioning and produce illness.

In the 1960s, Solomon, a psychiatrist, followed up on a little-known Soviet study that suggested that the hypothalamus is the "headquarters" of immune regulation. He found that when he destroyed the hypothalamus in rats, they had a marked decline in immune functioning. Ten years later, Ader discovered that the cells of the immune system, which had always been regarded as an autonomous defense network, can in fact be "conditioned" in much the same way that Pavlov had conditioned dogs to salivate at the sound of a bell. Meanwhile, Pert was revealing that similar receptors for the short-chain proteins called peptides exist on cell walls in both the brain and the immune system.

Solomon pinpointed the central role of the hypothalamus in immunity. Ader showed that the mind, presumably acting once again through the hypothalamus, can affect immune activity. And Pert was suggesting that peptides are the agents of communication between brain cells and those of the immune system. Ader named the new field they were mapping *psychoneuroimmunology*, to emphasize the interconnections among mind, brain, and immune system.

As this work accumulated, a panoramic picture of the links among social stress and thoughts, feelings, and physical functioning began to emerge. The connections between the mind and the emotions it produces, and three of the body's most important regulatory systems—the autonomic nervous, endocrine, and immune systems—became ever more clear. It looked as if the kind of stress we experience, and the way we interpret and deal with it, may be significant factors in the production of many of the diseases from which we suffer.

I knew my second, crucial task with Leslie would be to help her understand that her mind—the way she looked at the world and how she felt about it and herself—could indeed affect her brain and her body. My first task, which I had to address before I could expect her to focus on the second, was to relieve some of her suffering and meet some of her expectations. But before I addressed any tasks that had to do with Leslie, I had to take on one of my own: I had to get over my own self-righteous resistance to her rudeness and lateness.

I took a couple of deep breaths and told Leslie that I understood that she was afraid and that her fear probably made her impatient and demanding. But, I told her, she was also making me irritated. I had an idea, I said, to help us both get back on track. Would she be willing to try it? Grudgingly, she said she would.

"Okay," I said. "There's a beginning Zen meditation in which you count your breaths from one to ten and then from ten back to one. The full breath, inhalation and exhalation, is one, and so on. If thoughts come up, you notice them, then go back to your counting. It's very good because it gives your mind something to work with, to focus on."

Leslie looked at me as if I'd lost *my* mind. Then she started laughing. "You mean," she said, "like you count to ten when you're ready to punch someone in the nose and would rather not?"

"I guess so," I said, realizing my own unconscious had been working overtime.

"Why not?" she said.

After ten minutes of silent counting together, Leslie and I both felt different, quieter, even content to be in the same room with each other. "That's better," she said, and while I was still nodding my agreement, she began to tell me whatever came to her mind, first volunteering information about her "miserable junk food diet." She was looking straight at me now, smiling as she described "orgies of donuts and diet sodas." Then she began to apologize for her "bad attitude."

"I've had a terrible day at work," she went on, "and I started feeling that tingling and weakness again. For nine years the doctors have all been—you'll pardon my French—such assholes. The first two years, they didn't have a clue what was going on, and they acted like *I* was crazy. And then when they *finally* decided I had MS, they started acting like they were God Almighty and had known it all the time. And they began to talk at me—yes, *at* me, not *to* me—with these puffed-up voices, telling me all the things I couldn't do and how I was going to surely wind up in a wheelchair. They even sent me to a 'support group' where they handed out a magazine with beaucoup advertisements for wheelchairs.

"I guess I was just waiting for you to act the same way. Then when you asked me, who I live with, that was the last straw. You see, I'm a lesbian, and I'm not 'out,' and when I once told a neurologist, he got this weird look, and I felt like he was thinking, 'Well, what can you expect?'"

I wrote a prescription for Leslie. I asked her to eat only raw food for three weeks. No coffee or sugar. This, I explained, would help clean out her system and help her gut work more efficiently. It would remove the biological stress produced by diets high in fat, sugar, and food additives. I asked her to begin yoga lessons and to walk half an hour every day. I prescribed some Chinese herbs designed to balance her immune system and to help her deal with the tension she always felt, in her mind and in her gut.

A week later she came back, a bit shell-shocked after the withdrawal from caffeine and sugar—"my God, I felt like some street junkie, scratching and whining and snapping at Kate, my partner"—but less harried, more upright, slimmer, more cheerful, and on time. She allowed as how the walking had relieved some of her stress—"who would have thought it, such a simple thing"—and the yoga was helping her to feel more confident in the body in which she had lost faith. She looked more like a person, and less like a drudge, and when I said so, she laughed and shook her head.

Leslie began to tell me about her life at work. The efficiency on which she prided herself was won at the price of too long hours and enormous strain. She had become, she realized, a kind of machine, taking in huge amounts of data, processing it, and grinding out complex solutions. Sometimes, even before she developed the MS symptoms, she had felt as if her whole body, from her neck down, had gone numb or was missing. "I was a walking brain—wind me up and set me down in front of a problem." She hadn't been able to imagine leaving her high-paying job and couldn't imagine not feeling overwhelmed and numb while she did it.

It seemed the right time to explain to Leslie that prolonged stress can contribute in very significant ways to the onset of illness. I told her about the research that George Engel, a professor of medicine, had done at the University of Rochester. Over a period of twenty years, Engel and his colleagues had taken detailed histories from hundreds of patients with a variety of chronic illness. Prior to the onset of their illnesses, 70 to 80 percent of them had experienced extended periods of "helplessness," times when they had felt like "giving up." This was true of people with heart attacks, cancer, stomach ulcers, ulcerative colitis, and a number of other conditions, including multiple sclerosis. Exacerbations of these conditions were preceded by similar feelings.

In order to make sure that these people weren't being influenced by their reaction to their illness—feeling helpless *because* they were sick and projecting that feeling onto the time before the onset of the illness—Engel took detailed histories from their family members. In virtually every case, family members had observed the same state of "giving up" and "given up" that the patients had reported.

I told Leslie that my own experience matched Engel's: most of the people with chronic illness whom I had treated had begun to develop symptoms after a period of prolonged and intense stress. They felt overwhelmed and frustrated and often despaired of ever finding a way out—just like her.

Each of us, I went on, is biologically unique. Because of this, it isn't surprising that we have particular and different areas of vulnerability. In some illnesses there are clear anatomical and physiological pathways from emotional stress to symptoms in particular organs: the repetitive evocation of the fight-or-flight response gives rise to hypertension and heart disease in some people. In other cases, the target organ and the illness seem to be determined by the person's genetic makeup—diabetes, breast cancer, and asthma were the examples I gave.

Other illnesses may be occupationally determined—like carpal tunnel syndrome, or the compression of the median nerve at the wrist, in the hands of some typists and toll collectors. In still other cases, the site of vulnerability may be shaped by its personal symbolic meaning. I told her about my own bad back and how it had collapsed when I felt burdened by the responsibility of developing the national program for runaway and homeless youth.

I went on, knowing, I suppose, that smart and thorough Leslie would enjoy this kind of explanation. In any case, I said, whether or not I or anyone can be sure of why a particular illness or symptom occurs, there seems little doubt that what is going on in our lives and our minds may well have something to do with the onset of our illnesses. We have, I assured her, everything to gain and nothing to lose from assuming we can understand the origins of our stress and do something about them. The worst that will happen is that we learn something about ourselves. At best, we may discover psychological states, social situations, and biological pathways that we can address and alter.

The first step is to become aware of what may be affecting us. Most of us don't feel the need to be aware when all is going well. Life is on a kind of automatic pilot. But when illness or unhappiness comes and we feel overwhelmed, awash in an undifferentiated sea of events and emotions, awareness can be a lifeline. There are many routes to awareness, I said, each appropriate for different people or for the same person at different times.

I told her that when I was in medical school and many times since, I'd kept a journal. Writing, not for grades or publication, but only for myself, is a way for me to see what I am thinking and feeling. There it is, uncensored on the page. Writing also helps me to take some distance from what is otherwise unbearable. In the act of putting words on paper, I am meeting my pain and fear as an equal, not, at least for those moments, as a victim. Other people use drawings to do the same thing. Many, including me, have also been turning to meditation, like the counting Leslie and I did that first day.

Leslie, who until that moment was attentive and receptive, visibly flinched. When I asked about it, she told me that counting one time was okay—"Hey, we might have killed each other"—but that the thought of regular meditation made her nervous. She couldn't possibly "sit still and think of nothing." Besides, it had "overtones of something pagan, of giving up your free will to some guru. I know I'm a dyke," she went on, "but I'm still a Catholic."

I explained to Leslie that meditation is a physiological phenomenon as well as a spiritual practice. Years before, Herbert Benson, a Harvard cardiologist, had done studies that showed that a variety of different kinds of meditation and prayer all produced what he called a "relaxation response." Relaxation is a kind of antidote to the fight-or-flight response, I explained. It restores the balance between the hyperactive sympathetic nervous system and the quieting, or parasympathetic, half of the autonomic nervous system.

When you're relaxed, I went on, your heart beats more slowly, your respiratory rate decreases, and tight muscles ease up. Blood pressure falls, and brain waves become slower and more synchronized. More recently, Benson and others had found that regular relaxation also can decrease levels of stress hormones, improve immune functioning, diminish chronic pain, improve mood, and even enhance fertility.

"Yeah?" Leslie said, warming to the topic. "Does it improve your sex life too?"

"Could be," I said, laughing, and went on. Meditation isn't one particular kind of practice, I told her. She didn't have to take vows or belong to a group or even pay money to do it. It's available to everyone, and if one kind didn't suit her, there are hundreds of others. Saying the rosary is a form of meditation, one of many kinds that depend on concentration. Repeating a Hindu mantra, a Sanskrit sound, to oneself is another, as is gazing at a candle.

There are also "awareness" or "mindfulness" meditations, such as the ones taught in the Southeast Asian Vipassana tradition. Here practitioners are asked simply to be aware of whatever thoughts, feelings, and sensations arise and to let them come and go. Finally, there are meditations of surrender and self-expression, like my chaotic breathing. Each is different, but ultimately all help us to live more in the present moment, to find a calm observing center in ourselves, to be more aware.

The word *meditation,* I explained, seems to come from the same Greek and Latin roots as *medicine.* Both are derived from words meaning "to take one's measure." In traditional societies, where the physician was a spiritual guide as well as a temporal healer, it was customary for him or her to prescribe meditative techniques for his or her patients. Over the years it has become a vital and integral part of my practice. It provides a physiological and psychological "time out." It is also, I believe, something more: a direct route to the awareness that helps us make deep changes.

The idea that there is only one way to meditate is a misconception as well. It's true that some groups insist that only their form is useful, that all others are inferior, or that you have to be serious or holy to do it. But this is both arrogant and ignorant.

The practices that most of us associate with the word *meditation,* the silent sitting, the focusing on the sound or breath, the emptying of the mind, are wonderful and wonderfully useful. But they were developed in ancient agricultural societies, in a time without machines, in monasteries, schools, and ashrams that were separated and protected even from that pastoral world. They may be perfectly appropriate for some people two or three millennia later, but not for others.

Meditation, like any other healing practice, has to be individualized. The ancient masters knew this. One of the early systematic guides to meditation, the Indian *Vignana Bhairava Tantra,* a dialogue between the god Shiva and his consort Parvati, describes one hundred and eight different kinds — meditations on the breath and sounds, moving meditations, lots of meditations while making love, and one that always tickles me: "While sitting in an oxcart and swaying, go within the swaying." Meditation is a means to help us wake up, to be aware. Each of us may need different techniques, and different techniques at different times.

Nor is meditation a contest, an examination that one passes or fails. Nobody that I know can really "think about nothing." I certainly can't. That kind of freedom is a rare, momentary, and unwilled happening, a grace. All of us, including me, have minds that jump and veer and are constantly in motion.

That's why, I went on, I sometimes suggest that my patients begin by practicing expressive meditations — like chaotic breathing or very fast dancing, or simply shaking for ten or fifteen minutes at a time. The total immersion in physical activity fatigues the body, breaks up patterns of fixed and repetitive thinking. After a storm of activity there is the possibility of a calmer, clearer mind. Often, after months or years of this kind of practice, it becomes possible and desirable to use the quieter techniques that initially seemed impossible.

Leslie seemed intrigued, even excited. Maybe that was something she could do. "I really like the idea of dancing. I was always kind of embarrassed to do it around other people. I wasn't the prettiest girl, and the boys didn't ask me to, and I was kind of dumpy and awkward, and I didn't think I looked very cool, and also"—here she started to laugh—"I really wanted to dance with the girls, and that was definitely a no-no. But you know, sometimes when I'm by myself, and I'm so tense and frustrated and scared about what's happening to me, and I feel like I could scream, I put on really loud rock and roll and just move. So that's meditation?"

"Do it," I said, so happy to feel this secret energy in Leslie. "Do it every morning for twenty minutes. Close the door, put the music on, and dance like a madwoman."

Awareness and meditation are, for me, fundamental to the deep change that is necessary for healing. Chronic illness is a way of life as well as, or perhaps even more than a disease entity. Before we can be free of the symptoms of illness and the role of the sick person, we need to know what has precipitated those symptoms, and how we are responding to our sickness. We need to recognize in our own lives the psychological, biological, and sociological factors that may affect our health.

Awareness allows us to see where we are; to stand for a moment outside ourselves; to appreciate in a powerful, personal way how the world around us affects us; to observe the thoughts, feelings, and sensations that arise in us. Meditation is a state of moment-to-moment awareness that over time may help to dissolve physical symptoms and habitual ways of thinking and acting. Both awareness and meditation enable us to experience the way our mind may limit or free us. Together they prepare us to use our mind to make the deep changes in thought, feeling, and action that are necessary for our healing.

To her joy and amusement, Leslie did dance. Every morning at home and, after some bouts with embarrassment, even on the road, at friends' houses, and in hotel rooms. She was turning the power of her will from making it in the world to taking care of herself. With the dancing came a sense of pleasure in her body, a growing confidence in its reliability. She lost weight, stood straighter. The lines that had deeply creased her forehead became less pronounced. Her complexion was clearer.

And so was her mind. The dancing helped Leslie to release her nervous energy and to feel less anxious. With the decrease in anxiety, she was able to step back from the patterns of thought and action that had dominated and encased her life. She felt less driven to do what was expected and more capable, when she fell back into old habits, of seeing what was compelling her. Keeping a journal helped too. She wrote in it most mornings, after her yoga and dancing.

Though she was feeling better, Leslie was still preoccupied with the MS. Her journal entries reminded her of how pervasive her fear of it was: the slightest tingling in her toes was conjuring up visions of paralysis, emergency hospital treatment with intravenous steroids, and that terrible wheelchair. MS, like some great unpredictable beast, dominated Leslie's life. She not only lived in fear of its attacks but had learned to define herself by her condition. There were things she could and could not do, activities and emotions that seemed risky, rules that had to be observed or else violated at grave peril.

One day I said something that I thought would seem strange, even outrageous to her, because it flew in the face of what all the experts, all those neurologists, were saying. Leslie, I said, you've got to drop the MS before it drops you. The idea that any symptom-free period is only temporary, a "remission," that a relapse is always awaiting you, is so damaging. Forget about what the doctors have said, what the textbooks and pamphlets say. Their words are filled with fear. Their diagnosis is like a judicial sentence. Our minds, our expectations, can make a powerful difference, not only in how we feel but in whether we get well. Their dismal predictions and expectations are influencing your mind and may be damaging your body.

I'd gotten accustomed to backing up my statements with facts and stories, and so I began to tell Leslie about my meetings, thirty years before with Henry Beecher, who was then the professor of anesthesiology at Harvard. What I'd learned from him about placebos had made a major difference in the way I thought about all medical treatments, and I had a sense it might be helpful to her too.

Dr. Beecher had explained to us that the word *placebo* means "I shall please" or "I shall serve" in Latin. Early nineteenth-century physicians had defined placebos as inert substances, given "more to please than to benefit the patient," and had understood that this pleasing by itself sometimes produces improvements. Later, pharmacologists who understood the effect that placebos can have began to use them as "controls" in experiments on new drugs.

In such experiments some patients are given the drug to be tested, while others are given inactive pills or injections—placebos—made up to resemble the drug. Neither the physicians giving the drugs, nor the patients receiving them, nor the people evaluating their effects, know which is the drug and which the placebo. These studies are controlled and "double blind." The difference between the effectiveness of the drug and the placebo, as measured by impartial observers, is regarded as the true effect of the drug.

Beecher, who had an original way of looking at medical problems, had become fascinated not by the power of the drugs in which the pharmacologists were interested but by the ability of the placebos to simulate their effects. He had reviewed the available medical literature and discovered that placebos are, on the average, 35 percent as powerful as drugs that are known to be effective—*regardless of the drug being tested or the condition being treated*. I told Leslie that I had been particularly impressed that placebos, when tested against morphine, our most powerful analgesic, can in 30 to 40 percent of patients do as well as morphine in relieving excruciating pain.

More recently, other studies have shown that placebos—which are now sometimes defined as "the sum of all the non-specific interactions" between patient and physician—can be even more powerful. One review of several treatments that later proved to be *ineffective*—surgery for asthma, an invasive procedure for gastric ulcers, and three different treatments of herpes simplex virus—indicated that *70 percent* of the treated patients had "excellent or good outcomes." The power of their doctors' belief in these treatments, and their own belief in their doctors, not any effective ingredient in the therapies themselves, had relieved their symptoms.

There had also been, I added, a number of studies in which patients who believed they were receiving active treatments but were in fact receiving placebos experienced all the negative side effects—nausea, hair loss, and the like—that might be expected from the active treatment.

The point was, I explained to Leslie, that belief—in the efficacy of a treatment or indeed in the person giving the treatment—can have a powerful effect, and that that effect can be strongly negative as well as strongly positive. It seemed to me that if she chose to continue to believe that MS was going to be the chronic, debilitating condition that her doctors predicted, she was, in essence, administering a dangerous negative placebo, a nocebo, to herself.

"On the one hand," I went on, "you have to drop the idea that you have MS, with all that that has come to mean. You have to stop letting it, and your fears about it, deform your life. On the other hand, you have to become aware of when and why your symptoms come, and of what you can do to care for yourself better. In other words, you have to free yourself from MS as a dangerous thing, with a predetermined outcome. Instead, you can look at its symptoms as informative experiences, ones that help you to see when you are stressed and give you hints about what to do about it."

I'd thought Leslie might be shocked—most people are after years of being told how they should feel and what kinds of problems they might expect—and she was, but not for long. The idea of freeing herself from all the gloom and doom of her doctors, from those MS magazines with their wheelchair ads; from the dread of those stunning, damning pictures of the bright plaques in her brain, was definitely appealing. "You mean, live like I was free? Deal with what comes up, with how I feel, rather than what somebody else tells me? Understand that I've got the plaques but that I can also be well? Yeah, I like that."

I told Leslie that I thought a simple awareness meditation would help. I suggested that after her morning dancing, when she was feeling both calm and energized, she sit quietly. "Then," I said, "breathe slowly and evenly, in and out; notice the thoughts, feelings, and sensations that arise; and having noticed them, return to the breath." Sitting quietly, observing, she would become aware of what was actually going on in her mind and body. Little by little, I thought she would see how her fearful thoughts created uncomfortable sensations, which, in turn, produced troubled feelings. In time she would be able to detach herself from this vicious circle.

I suspected that this awareness and detachment would happen first during periods of meditation, but that then she would be able to bring them into her daily life. Slowly, she might find herself less anxious, less put upon at work as well as in her minutes of meditation. I hoped she would find freedom from both the damning diagnosis of MS and from the pressures and anxieties that contributed to her symptoms.

Leslie embraced this project. When I saw her every two or three weeks, she told me what she was discovering. She could see herself "tuning out," becoming "Leslie the machine."

She was also becoming more aware of how sensitive she was to every twitch and tingle, how the slightest altered sensation could precipitate a cascade of anxious thoughts and troubled feelings. She was noticing too the connections between the events in her life and her defensiveness with other people, and between emotional insecurity and physical reactivity. "Sometimes," she said, "it freaks me out. And sometimes I have to crack up laughing. It's so idiotic."

The more she saw, the more she began to feel there was something she could do about her situation. MS no longer seemed an implacable force and an impenetrable mystery. There were very real and predictable events, thoughts, and feelings that generally preceded and precipitated her symptoms.

Soon, Leslie even began to have some perspective on the panic she felt about the tingling and numbness. She could use it as a reminder, a signal to pay attention, to ask herself what was going on, to slow down if she was pushing too hard.

At first she continued to depend on her journal entries to reinforce her understanding. After a few months of awareness meditation, she was able to locate the sources of stress almost as soon as the symptoms arose. There was no question that they erupted around the times of those overburdened business trips. They also came when certain kinds of conflicts arose at work, most often when her boss acted like she wasn't living up to some idea he had about how and who she should be. The symptoms also emerged when she felt torn between her desire to spend more time with her lover, Kate, and her need to maintain the schedule and role of the corporate lawyer.

None of this was really new. She had had, at one point or another, inklings of almost everything that she was confiding to her journal and to me. But now it had a different kind of force. These were no longer fleeting impressions, easy to bury in the avalanche of doing corporate business and "maintaining a relationship." They were strong, clear feelings, churned to the surface of her mind by her morning movement; they were observed and felt in the minutes of her quiet meditation. There were undeniable associations between life events, feeling states, and physical symptoms.

After a year, Leslie was feeling, as well as looking, much better. The "MS-y sensations" were far less severe and lasted less long, and the threat of the illness had receded. But some symptoms were still there, and she had to ask herself why she was continuing to live in a way that wasn't good for her. Leslie hadn't had much use for psychotherapy—it had seemed like a rich person's indulgence—but she did feel she needed to "talk over" a few things, and she wanted to do it with me.

Kate, she told me, was a carpenter, hated the city, and lived almost two hours away in West Virginia. She and Leslie never had enough time together, and there was always the tension—two different households, two ways of living. Kate's indifference to money and her obvious but unspoken disdain for Leslie's job made Leslie feel ashamed and then angry. Leslie told me that Kate was willing to "borrow" money from her to repair her old truck. And if Leslie wanted to have a vacation or even a good meal out with Kate, she had to pay Kate's way. She resented Kate for putting her in this position and was angry at herself for being resentful. Sometimes they had terrible, tearful fights, and Leslie had the sense that things would never be right. Then, too, she would feel weaker, more symptomatic.

The more aware she became and the more pain Leslie felt about her life, the more certain she was that something had to change. "For so long I felt helpless," she told me, "bouncing between trying to keep up with everything and worrying about when the symptoms would hit. Now I know I've got to do something and that I can, but it terrifies me."

"What do you want to do?"

"Well, there's no question, the job's got to go." Leslie still enjoyed the challenge of solving legal problems, but she realized that neither the problems nor the solutions had any meaning for her. Actually, she wasn't even sure she should be working on them. She was "a working-class girl"; her father had always been "a union man." What was she doing slaving away to put more money in the hands of people who did their best to keep people like her in their place? Sure, it had been necessary to make money to pay off her debts, and the excitement of making so much money, so much more than her father or anyone else in her family had ever dreamed of making, had been intoxicating. But she was over that.

Sometime, without ever having realized it, Leslie had crossed the line from determined striver to debilitated drudge. She felt stiff and uncomfortable in the trendy restaurants she could afford, and she was always in a hurry when she drove her fancy car. Why, she had to wonder, did she have to drive two hours just to see the woman she loved? Why was she always feeling like she wasn't doing what she wanted? What kind of a life was that?

While her questions hung in the air, I said to Leslie that it was exactly the kind of life that might make her more vulnerable to MS. I told her about work that George Solomon, who had observed the role of the hypothalamus in regulating immunity, had done with women with rheumatoid arthritis. During the 1960s Solomon had observed that certain women who had the "rheumatoid factor" in their blood developed symptoms of rheumatoid arthritis while their sisters, who had the same genetic background, did not. The difference, he discovered, was psychological. The sick sisters "felt inhibited, trapped, and tense," while the healthy ones were able to express their anger and felt freer and more joyful.

Leslie was "blown away. I'm not going to be anybody's 'sick sister,'" she announced. She began in earnest to think about jobs she would really like and where she wanted to live.

Clearly, like Kate, she preferred the country. She wanted to use her legal skills to help ordinary people, maybe work for a union or do environmental law. She and Kate began to discuss moving in together, and where they would like to go, and what they would do when they got there. As they took trips to other states, scouting possible jobs and homesites, and discussed their future, the quarrels between them dissipated. It seemed that as Leslie's commitment appeared stronger, Kate's dependency diminished. They were no longer straining against each other, vigilant for signs of indifference and exploitation, but planning together. They traveled to rural areas all over the country, getting the feel of New England, the South, and the Southwest.

As Leslie began to look for another job, the tension she felt at work decreased. She knew now that it was only a matter of time before she would be free. Her symptoms dropped another notch in intensity and frequency.

Nine months after she began to look for another job, Leslie found one. She would be working for a legal services office in rural Colorado, helping poor people deal with banks, bad debts, and family crises. She would make less than half of the money that the hotel corporation had paid, but it felt like more than a fair exchange. The work seemed honest and useful, and the hours reasonable, and she could live somewhere beautiful. She wouldn't feel tense or trapped anymore. Kate was really excited too—she'd met a contractor who liked her carpentry—and she and Leslie were looking for a house they could fix up together.

Leslie called from Colorado after six months, just to check in. She'd had a few symptoms during the tumult of moving but had had none since they'd set up house. "None, zero, no tingling, no weakness. I still do the dancing a few times a week, and I do the awareness meditation every day," she reported, "and Kate and I walk in the mountains, and I really like the work. It's so beautiful."

A year later I got a Christmas card. It read: "Merry Christmas. I'm well. Love, Leslie, your former MS patient."

NINE

Self-Care as Primary Care:
The Power of the Mind (II) ∽

AWARENESS AND MEDITATION were, for Leslie Newman, catalysts sufficient to create psychological transformation and physical healing. In many instances, however, I use other techniques as well, other ways to mobilize the mind to affect itself and the body. These approaches include relaxation therapies, biofeedback, visualization, and hypnosis. Each has individual characteristics that make it useful in particular situations. All are integral to the mind-body approach that is central to the new medicine. And all, like awareness and meditation, have been helpful to me, personally as well as professionally, at different times in my life.

The first technique I learned, in the early 1970s, was Edmund Jacobson's *progressive muscular relaxation*. In 1908 Jacobson, a physician who taught at Harvard, observed that strong mental or emotional stimuli affect the contraction of the skeletal muscles as well as the smooth muscle in the body's internal organs. Angry words or loud noises may make us furrow our brows and/or contract the muscles in our intestines. Jacobson reasoned that if we could learn to relax the skeletal muscles consciously, the smooth muscles of the internal organs, which are under control of the autonomic nervous system, would relax along with them.

The technique that Jacobson devised to help his patients do this was simple and intelligent. He asked people to create more tension in their muscles, then to let go of the tension. By using activity to create relaxation, he bypassed the contradictory and hard-to-follow order to "try to relax." When I first heard about it, this process reminded me of the chaotic breathing I had begun to do—coming to stillness through effort. I tried it for myself and found I could do it, and that it was indeed relaxing. I began to teach it to my patients.

When I use this progressive relaxation procedure, I ask people to begin at their feet and move upward, contracting and relaxing specific muscle groups. I tell them to contract the muscles as they breathe in, and release the tension on the exhalation. I guide them, beginning with the feet and moving up to the calves and thighs, then to the muscles in the genitals and anus. Next come the abdominal and chest muscles, then the shoulders, upper arms, forearms, and hands, and finally the neck, face, scalp, and back. I ask people to breathe slowly and deeply, contracting and relaxing.

Progressive muscular relaxation allows us to experience and reclaim our body and to affect it in a positive and immediately perceptible way. It also feels safer the relative passivity of concentrative or awareness meditations sometimes makes people uncomfortable. Progressive relaxation gives us something to do while we're learning to relax. I use this technique often with individual patients and in workshops with hundreds of people.

I began to learn about biofeedback—literally, the feedback of biological information—soon after I started working with progressive muscular relaxation. It's never been as personally congenial to me as meditation, hypnosis, and other mind-body approaches, probably because it interposes technology between me and my bodily processes. Still, over the years I've come to understand biofeedback's enormous power to facilitate the mind's capacity to control a vast array of physiological functions. I've also learned to appreciate its role in making the mind-body approach more accessible to technology-trusting Western physicians and patients.

In 1961, when Neal Miller first suggested that the autonomic nervous system could be as susceptible to training as the voluntary nervous system, that we might learn to control our heart rate and our bowel contractions just as we learned to walk or type or play tennis, his audiences were aghast. He was a respected researcher, director of a laboratory at Yale, but this was a kind of scientific heresy. Everyone "knew" that the autonomic nervous system was precisely that—automatic, beyond our control. The fabled feats of Indian yogis—their claimed ability to slow the rate of their heart and their breathing and to profoundly alter their body temperature—were regarded as a masochist's perversion, a charlatan's tricks, or neurological accidents.

Miller persisted. He was convinced that the difference between the autonomic and voluntary nervous systems was not so much one of kind but of opportunity. The skeletal system is subject to visible and immediate correction from the environment: seeing the disastrous results of your looping forehand encourages and enables you to shorten your swing. The results of the autonomic nervous system's actions are not immediately apparent. We don't see or feel or hear anything when our blood pressure rises.

Miller believed, and soon proved, that if he simply offered a perceptible recording of autonomic behavior—sounding a high-pitched tone, for example, till elevated blood pressure decreased or cold hands warmed—people would be able to use this information to correct their internal functioning. This procedure, which Miller first demonstrated in dogs and then in rats—teaching them to salivate both more and less, to raise and lower their heart rates—is biofeedback.

Biofeedback worked. People learned to use it to lower blood pressure and to increase hand temperature. Soon enough, clinicians began to use it for common and debilitating problems. For example, since the arterial constriction that is prominent in the first phase of migraine headaches also causes cold hands, feedback of information about finger temperature can be used as a form of treatment for migraines: the patient who learns to raise the temperature in her hands by relaxing the muscular walls of the blood vessels there is automatically doing the same thing with the blood vessels in her head.

Over the last thirty years, physicians, psychologists, and "biofeedback technicians," in tandem with engineers, have developed sensors and procedures that have enabled hundreds of thousands of people to become aware of and to control even the most obscure aspects of their physiological functioning. For example, people can now use readouts of tension from their urethral and anal sphincters to control urinary and fecal incontinence, conditions that often resist all other medical and surgical interventions; and some epileptics can now use biofeedback from electroencephalograms to calm the irritable brain tissue that produces their seizures.

Biofeedback not only produces replicable and powerful changes in many people's physiology and improvement in their symptoms, it also gives them a sense of connection to and control over their internal processes. This sense of mastery often generalizes to other aspects of their lives: people who have practiced biofeedback for a specific condition find it far easier to induce a relaxed state when confronted with any kind of stress. In time, many people who use biofeedback monitors learn to effect the same kinds of changes without them, using the power of their minds alone.

Biofeedback is precise and potent. Hypnosis and imagery are poetic, equally powerful, and so far as I am concerned, even more versatile ways of mobilizing the mind to aid in healing.

As best we can tell, Siberian shamans and African witch doctors, medicine men and healers around the world, have successfully used hypnosis and imagery for thousands of years. They have induced trance with drumming, dancing, and psychedelic plants and, in this state, evoked and prescribed a variety of powerful visual, kinesthetic, and auditory experiences.

Hypnosis is a state of attentive and focused concentration in which "subjects," as those in hypnotic trance are called, are relatively unaware of but not completely blind to their surroundings. It is not, as its name suggests, physiologically or experientially similar to sleep. (*Hypnosis* comes from the Greek *hypnos* or "sleep.") If something demands attention, the hypnotized subject can readily arouse herself to react to the situation.

In hypnosis we're highly responsive to suggestions, though we cannot be, as popular folklore and fear would have it, forced to follow suggestions against our wishes. Generally speaking, hypnosis is characterized by absorption (in the words presented by the hypnotherapist); dissociation (from one's ordinary critical faculties); and responsiveness.

After an initial period of relaxation and quieting, hypnotherapists use an "induction" to create a deeper state of relaxation, or trance. There are probably almost as many inductions as there are hypnotherapists, but common ones include concentration on a spot and instructions to roll the eyes up or imagine one is descending stairs. When the subject is in a deeply relaxed or trance state, the hypnotherapist gives suggestions to mobilize the mind's capacity to explore and affect itself and the body.

Modern hypnosis began in the 1770s with the Swiss physician Franz Anton Mesmer. Mesmer believed that he could successfully treat patients with an "animal magnetism" that he transmitted from his own to their bodies. He inaugurated what was to become a notorious career in Vienna by helping an Austrian woman who appeared blind to regain her sight. Not long after, he moved to Paris, where he staged dramatic public healings. He submerged sufferers in tubs of iron filings and, to the accompaniment of dramatic music, waved his hands—made "magnetic passes"—near them. People cried, laughed, and convulsed. Some recovered from previously incurable illnesses.

When a skeptical French royal commission, which included Benjamin Franklin, the chemist Antoine Lavoisier, and Joseph

Guillotin, investigated Mesmer's miraculous results, it concluded that there was no evidence for the magnetism he claimed. His cures, they decided, were the result of "expectation" and "suggestion." Mesmer believed they would be healed, and was able to mobilize their belief and somehow to create the alterations in mental and physical processes that resulted in a real improvement. The royal commission saw themselves as debunking a clever charlatan. We can, two centuries later, applaud them for describing two of the prime ingredients of successful hypnosis and of medicine itself—expectation and suggestion.

Mesmer's successors earned the same mixture of adulation and opprobrium that he did. In the mid-nineteenth century, shortly before general anesthesia became available, John Elliotson in London and James Esdaile in India both performed numerous major surgeries using mesmeric passes. Their patients experienced far less pain, had fewer infections, recovered faster, and had a significantly lower mortality rate than patients of other surgeons. Though their successes were widely noted in the popular press, their medical and surgical colleagues were both skeptical and hostile. Even James Braid, who gave hypnotism its name and regarded it as a purely psychological phenomenon, was treated with, at best, indifference.

By the late nineteenth century, hypnosis began to be regarded as a subject worthy of scientific scrutiny. The celebrated Parisian neurologist Jean-Martin Charcot described hypnosis as a disease state akin to hysteria, while in Nancy, Auguste Liebault and Hippolyte Bernheim explored and emphasized the power of hypnotic suggestion.

Freud, who studied with both Charcot and "the Nancy school," initially embraced and then rejected hypnosis. He found some patients quite difficult to hypnotize and was distressed by the powerful, sometimes erotic feelings that trance evoked in others.

Though Freud later praised its utility, his abandonment of hypnotic suggestion for his own method of free association helped once again to cast a shadow on the therapeutic possibilities of hypnosis. Not only was hypnosis not taught during

tric residency, it was generally dismissed as a dan-
authoritarian procedure and/or a stage magician's

In spite of medicine's low regard for hypnosis, a few physicians continued to use it therapeutically, particularly for
pain relief. It wasn't, however, until World War II that the
first signs of the current revival of interest in hypnosis
appeared. These were the discovery of the utility of hypnotic
techniques in the treatment of what was then called battle
fatigue (what we now refer to as post-traumatic stress disorder), and the appearance on the American psychiatric scene
of a uniquely gifted and influential practitioner and researcher,
Milton Erickson.

Psychiatrists used hypnosis to help soldiers recover and
reintegrate the traumatizing battlefield experiences that they
had repressed, and return to action. Meanwhile, Erickson, who
also founded the *American Journal of Clinical Hypnosis*,
introduced a more congenial approach to the use of hypnosis: though he was every bit as much of a performer as any
stage hypnotist, he used a less authoritarian, more conver-
sational style of hypnotic induction. He helped make hypnosis
a creative part of, rather than a radical departure from the
ordinary process of psychotherapy, and he encouraged the
present generation of hypnotherapists (most of them non-
medical psychotherapists) to understand that all hypnosis is
actually self-hypnosis. The therapist is a guide and a catalyst, helping the subject make use of his or her own innate
capacities for exploration and change.

In the years since then, an enormous body of clinical and
research experience has demonstrated the power of hypnosis to affect virtually every aspect of physical and psychological
functioning. Hypnosis has been shown, in a number of studies, to reduce severe pain by an average of 50 percent. It has
been used, successfully, to decrease anxiety, remove phobias,
improve immune functioning, diminish the destructiveness
of severe burns, control reactions to poison ivy, decrease vomiting and nausea in chemotherapy patients, improve eczema
and psoriasis, cure warts, and even increase breast size.

Obstetrical studies have shown that hypnosis can produce significant decreases in length of labor and pain in childbirth. Modern heirs to Elliotson and Esdaile have successfully used hypnosis when general anesthesia has been considered dangerous or undesirable. Experimental work has demonstrated the power of suggestion to increase or decrease the rate and amount of bleeding, to produce or remove blisters, and to induce or relieve allergic reactions.

In my own practice I may use hypnosis in situations where other practitioners might work with biofeedback—to help people alter specific biological functions that are otherwise difficult to bring under control. In a single session in her hospital room, I was able to teach a young woman who was in excruciating pain from an ulcerated and inflamed large intestine to control both her pain and the fear she had of her upcoming surgery. I've used hypnosis to help patients reduce the severity of asthma attacks, to increase the numbers of dangerously depleted clot-forming blood platelets, and to speed up the healing of fractures and sprains.

I also look to hypnosis when self-awareness, meditation, and relaxation—coupled with all of the other therapies I use—don't resolve a specific psychological or physical problem. I help people go into trance and ask them to go back to the time when they first experienced the present difficulty. This "regression" is surprisingly easy for most people. It is as if something inside them were just waiting for help in exploring and resolving an issue that had long troubled or disabled them.

Then, in trance, they are able to recall memories—of events, thoughts, and feelings—that they associate with their present problem. Next, I may help them put the traumatic events of the past in a more instructive or hopeful context. This kind of "reframing" lends a psychological support that in turn makes a real difference in the patient's present life.

I use this process to help people explore the emotional factors that may be contributing to physical illness, as well as to address disturbing and difficult-to-resolve psychological issues. It is certainly not a panacea—some problems are terribly recalcitrant—but it often helps people understand and deal with dehabilitating symptoms that have resisted all other kinds of therapy. My work with Claire, a shy thirty-one-year-old married woman whom I was treating for depression, anorexia, bulimia, and a fear of crowds, is an example.

After some months of psychotherapy, journal keeping, and meditation, Claire had begun to feel more confident about herself. She was less depressed, had put on some weight, was vomiting less often, and was dealing with her daily life far better. She no longer panicked when guests were coming over, and she was able to speak more firmly and confidently to her husband. She was even able to go to the meetings that were necessary for her work and to the theater she loved. But she was still extremely anxious. When she was among a large group of people, she felt dizzy, her hands dripped with sweat, and her heart pounded in her chest.

Hypnotic regression revealed an incident at a circus when she was ten years old. Amidst the noise and the crowd but out of sight of her parents, a man dressed in a clown suit had forced her to perform oral sex on him. Though she had consciously "forgotten" the incident, the emotions that she associated with it had become attached to crowds in general. As she recovered the memory, she was able to share the fear, pain, confusion, and humiliation with me. "Imagine," I said while she was still in trance, "if you had felt comfortable enough to share this experience with your parents, if they had been the kind of people you could have run to and cried with." As Claire imagined this scene, rushing to her parents, embracing them, telling them of her fear, confusion, and hurt, tears of relief streamed down her cheeks. She was able, soon after, to venture out into crowds with little anxiety.

Hypnosis is, if anything, even more useful with kids than adults. Young children haven't yet accepted the rigid distinction between "make-believe" and "real life" that grown-ups have and so are able to make full use of their imaginations. A nine-year-old was able to use an image of warm friendly sunshine to quiet panic attacks that had made being alone unbearable. An eight-year-old, whose previous psychiatrist had wanted to prescribe Ritalin for the "attention deficit disorder" that was disrupting his schooling was able, after a single session, to summon an imaginary "power animal"—a large comforting dog—to help him focus his scattered mind.

As these examples reveal, the use of imagery is central to hypnotic suggestion. In fact, though imagery therapists and hypnotherapists work hard to distinguish their practices, it is all but impossible to differentiate the therapeutic use of imagery from hypnosis. The physiological characteristics seem to be identical; profound relaxation facilitates both processes. People who have the capacity to image well are good hypnotic subjects, and suggestions for imagery are indistinguishable from those used in hypnosis. Finally, the changes that they produce are all but identical.

Imagery makes use of our human capacity for internal control in a direct and unmediated way. Imagery includes words and thoughts that represent all the senses, including hearing, touch, and smell, and therefore differs from visualization, which refers only to seeing with the mind's eye. Imagery is also a powerful common ingredient in a variety of modern mind-body approaches, including meditation (focusing on a candle flickering or hearing a mantra), biofeedback, hypnosis, and autogenic training or AT.

Autogenic training, which was developed by a German neurologist, Johannes Schultz, in the 1930s, is one of the simplest, most widely used, and best-researched forms of imagery. Making use of a sequence of seven phrases that describe bodily feelings—"my arms are warm and heavy," "my legs are warm and heavy," and so on—it is sometimes used as a prelude to biofeedback. It is also, on its own, capable of inducing deep states of relaxation and relieving a variety of physical symptoms.

The capacity of imagery to exercise a potent effect on many aspects of our mental and physical functioning may well be related to the close proximity, in the brain, of the areas for imaging to the hypothalamus and the emotional centers.

You can experience the immediate effect of an image on your autonomic nervous system functioning simply by closing your eyes and imagining that you are sucking on a glistening yellow wedge of lemon. Within seconds most people will feel their salivary juices flowing. To test the emotional power of images, all you need to do is recall the face or voice or smell of someone you love, or the threats or gestures of someone you fear.

Imagery, which seems to bypass conscious censorship, can also give us easy access to our unconscious and our intuition. I find it extremely useful as a tool to help people understand why they are anxious or are experiencing a particular physical symptom. In some situations describing the work I do as imagery has certain advantages: it doesn't carry with it the fears of being controlled that the word *hypnosis* still sometimes evokes.

Sit comfortably, I will say. Close your eyes, take a few slow, deep breaths, and visualize the reason why you are uneasy or not feeling well. Many people will immediately come up with an image. Sometimes it's the precise cause—an anxious bureaucrat feels his boss standing over him. Sometimes it's fanciful or symbolic—a medical student with chest pain sees an unfaithful lover squeezing her heart in a vise.

I often use imagery to help people to explore options for future action—about life issues as well as medical problems—allowing a possible course of action to unfold in an imagined story. Not long ago, I did a workshop on "Reviving the Spirit of Medicine" for health professionals, many of whom were struggling to infuse their work with the spirit and approaches of the new medicine. After talking about the necessity for making this spirit an integral part of their practices, I invited them to see how this might happen. They were eager to do so.

I began, as I often do, with progressive muscular relaxation. After ten minutes, most everyone in the room was sitting quietly and breathing slowly. I told them then that we all have parts of our mind that are wiser than our conscious mind. "Many of Freud's followers," I went on, "have encouraged us to think that the unconscious is just a garbage heap of everything that we've repressed. But in fact, the unconscious is also a rich source of creativity and wisdom. It is a repository of all the intuitive ways of knowing that our culture, and particularly our medical training, have ignored or disparaged. All we have to do is get out of the way a little, and it will tell us what we need to know."

I asked them then to call on this unconscious mind, to allow it to help them image their work as it was now, to let the scene unfold as it needed to, then to write down what they saw or heard or felt. Next, I asked them to image what they wanted their work to be, then write that down as well. Finally, I asked them to image how they were going to get from where they were now to where they wanted to be, then write that down.

The results of this simple twenty-minute exercise were very interesting. One of several people who shared their experiences told the following story: "I see myself in the hospital where I'm a resident," she began, "and I'm in my green scrubs, moving from the ward to the OR with my head down, then back to the ward, from bed to bed and to the nurses' station, just like I do. Then it starts to speed up, and my arms and legs are pumping up and down, and I'm running at triple speed, yawning and lying down and bouncing back up, drinking coffee and eating doughnuts and talking fast to people, not really looking at them, and hurrying away, and zipping in and out of the OR, just like a cartoon character or Charlie Chaplin in *Modern Times*." She took a deep breath. "That's exactly how I am now.

"Next, I saw myself as I was going to be, or as I wanted my work to be, and it was totally different and amazing. I was standing with these three other women, in this big airy space, with light streaming down on us from a skylight. We were wearing loose, flowing dresses, talking to each other, giving advice and listening. They were my partners—and I knew one was an ob-gyn like me, and the other two were midwives—and it was like we were sisters. Then we turned, slowly, and all our movements were so graceful. I went into my office, and there were plants and flowers all over, and I sat down and began to talk with this young pregnant girl, and it all felt so natural.

"I was a little nervous when it was time to do the third image, because I couldn't imagine how I could get from where I am now to where I saw myself going. So I took a few more deep breaths, and as you said, I asked that part of me that knows more than I consciously do to help out. And after a minute or so, the image came to me. And it was so simple.

"I was sitting at this conference, just like I am now, and I was opening my eyes and looking around, then reaching out my hands, and there were other people—women and men too—who were taking my hands, and each other's, and we were all in a circle. And it felt really good, but I couldn't believe it could be so easy, so I said, 'That's it?' And this gentle reassuring voice inside me said, 'Yes, that's it. That's all you have to do. Just open yourself to other people right here at this conference. Just begin now, and take it one step at a time, and know it's possible.'"

The images this resident created were "guided," but the guidance was loose, general, and gentle. Imagery can also be carefully shaped by a physician or therapist to address particular problems: to help people prepare for childbirth, or for painful medical procedures like pelvic examinations, burn debridement, and cyst removal. To do this, I ask people to visualize what's going to happen while they're in a relaxed state. After a few "rehearsals" they begin to experience a sense of comfort and mastery. A number of studies have shown that when the event does take place, fear, pain, and discomfort are significantly and measurably decreased.

Imagery techniques can have powerful biological consequences. We haven't yet found direct evidence that imagery can alter the course of life-threatening illnesses, but we now know, for example, that a combination of relaxation and imagery can help people with cancer and AIDS increase the numbers and activity of their immune-enhancing white blood cells. Imagery, it seems, can also be stunningly specific: psychologist Jeanne Achterberg, who did some of the first studies on the use of imagery in cancer, discovered that people could use different images to exert measurable effects on different kinds of white blood cells. One set of images raised the count of neutrophils, while another activated the production of lymphocytes.

All of these approaches—relaxation, biofeedback, hypnosis, and imagery—enable us to use our mind's extraordinary capacity to affect our bodies. Each of them can be taught. And all of them are central to the care we can learn to provide— for ourselves and others.

TEN

Self-Care as Primary Care:
Touch, Movement, and Breathing   ⌇

"E NLIGHTENMENT," a Zen master once said, "is simply this. When I walk, I walk. When I eat, I eat. And when I sleep, I sleep." The master was referring to a quality of attention that must be paid to life's most ordinary activities. He was also reminding his questioner, and us, of the central importance of these activities to all our lives.

For the most part, modern Western medicine has ignored the quality and therapeutic power of these vital functions, and of touch and breathing as well. It has focused on their quantity and on the ways they are deformed by pathology. Physicians may measure the numbers of calories patients consume, their respiratory rate, and the "timed vital capacity" of their lungs. We listen to see if the sounds of the breath are diminished by fluid accumulation or inflammation. During neurological examinations we observe whether a patient can stand upright and walk heel to toe without falling to one side. We prick his skin with a needle and brush it with a feather to assess whether his sense of pain or his sensitivity to light touch are diminished by disease.

The new medicine, by contrast, assesses the quality as well as the quantity of these essential functions, the way we make use of them every day, as well as the obvious problems that may occasionally arise. It is interested in how we are moving and breathing, and what we eat and in what combinations. It understands also that touch and movement, breathing and eating, are tools for healing—tools that each of us can learn to use wisely and well—as well as essential elements in sustaining ourselves. This understanding represents a significant reversal of conventional medical wisdom—and a major step toward appreciating, enjoying, and healing our bodies and ourselves.

TOUCH

Touch, not sight or sound or even smell, is the oldest of the senses. It is present in the six-week-old, inch-long embryo. It may also be the source of the other senses that, during the course of evolution, may have differentiated from the skin and its receptors.

Though touch is fundamental to life, its use for comforting or healing is largely ignored by conventional medicine, and in many quarters it is even feared. Concern about "inappropriate touching"—unbalanced by examples of appropriate touch—makes many doctors painfully stiff and awkward. For psychiatrists, the situation is even stranger: there's a virtual taboo against any kind of touch at all. And yet touch is necessary to our survival and so vital to our healing.

In the 1930s René Spitz, a psychoanalyst, noted that many infants who were raised in spotless, up-to-date "foundling homes" had difficulty feeding and developed more slowly than they should. A number died, and most seemed in later life to be less socially adept than their noninstitutionalized age-mates.

One year, while on vacation, Spitz visited a dilapidated, dirty Mexican orphanage. To his amazement, the infants there seemed to do far better physically and emotionally than the ones he cared for in the north. Spitz searched for the reason and discovered that every day women from the nearby village came to feed, fondle, rock, and sing to these babies. It was loving touch, Spitz concluded, that was, quite literally, saving these children's lives.

In the 1950s, University of Wisconsin psychologist Harry Harlow added the weight of experimental evidence to these clinical findings. He discovered that monkeys that were separated from their mothers at birth never developed normally. All had marked inhibitions and peculiarities in their social conduct. When he constructed cloth mothers for infant monkeys which had been separated from their biological mothers, he was able to observe the attraction and effect of touch: these young monkeys rarely left their cloth mothers except for brief periods of feeding. In experiment after experiment, the desire for touch—not food—seemed to be the strongest motivator of their behavior.

Not long afterward, at Case Western Reserve Medical School, pediatricians Marshall Klaus and John Kennell took a close look at the then conventional medical practice of anesthetizing laboring women and separating them from their newborn infants. Klaus and Kennell studied the effect of skin-to-skin contact (holding and stroking) between mother and infant in the hours after birth and concluded that this kind of intimacy established "a mother-infant bond" that was predictive of closer and better long-term interaction. They soon discovered that contact during these hours improved the babies' growth and development and decreased the number and frequency of their childhood illnesses.

Subsequent studies on animals have confirmed and extended these findings. Newborn rat pups that were removed from their mothers and not handled by humans showed fewer receptors for adrenocortical hormones in their brains. Later in life they exhibited a markedly increased sensitivity to stress. In another study rat pups removed early from their mothers showed significant decreases in growth hormone and delays in development.

Some human young who have been deprived of maternal contact suffer even more dramatic kinds of defects. One notable example is *psychosocial dwarfism*. This is a condition of decreased levels of growth hormone and markedly retarded growth, apparently caused by severe emotional neglect.

Taken together, these studies raise important questions about the emphasis on technical efficiency in childbirth and the kind of institutional care we give our young. They have encouraged obstetricians to allow mothers and their infants to remain in contact after birth and have made more intimate contact a larger part of the care of institutionalized and hospitalized children. They also have helped to pave the way for a new appreciation for the therapeutic power of touch throughout the life cycle.

The *mind-body* approaches discussed in the last two chapters mobilize the mind—through awareness, biofeedback, relaxation, meditation, imagery, and hypnosis—to transform itself and the body. Touch affects the same integrated mind-body system but addresses it through the physical body. The various approaches that make use of touch are sometimes called *body-mind* or *body-oriented therapies.*

Massage, the best-known and most widely used of the touch therapies, was until quite recently regarded by Americans as suspect, a fringe practice. It was quirky, foreign, at best an indulgence of the rich, and almost certainly sexual—in some of our states massage of men by women or women by men is still a criminal activity, prosecuted under the same laws as prostitution.

The celebration of the physical and sensual that marked the cultural changes of the 1960s helped make massage more acceptable to Americans. People who felt more comfortable with their own sensuality and sexuality were less fearful of touch and, therefore, more able to distinguish its therapeutic from its erotic uses and to appreciate both. Once people experienced the pleasure, relaxation, and therapeutic value of massage, they began to explore a variety of other body-mind therapies—including Rolfing, the Alexander technique, the Feldenkrais method, and Reichian body work.

I began my experimentation with these approaches with my own body, in the bathtub. I took long hot baths with the pound of Epsom salts that Dr. Singha had recommended. I reached down to rub the soles and the tops of my feet, exploring the tender and tight places, stretched my arms, and arched my back. I reached around or over to hold tense tissue and to press my fingers into muscles I had seen in anatomy books and dissected in a cadaver but never really felt.

A whole new world began to open up under my fingers and in my hands. In spite of being both a doctor and an athlete, I hadn't paid much attention to the quality of my physical body, its shapes and textures. I noticed for the first time that the muscles in my shoulders were hard and sensitive. My hamstrings were tight. Some parts of my feet were easily hurt by vigorous massage, while others were soft and resilient. I realized, to my surprise, that rubbing one part of my body deeply could release tension in another; that moving an arm or a leg in this direction or that subtly affected every other aspect of my posture and every part of my body.

Soon afterward I went to a massage therapist. I began with Swedish massage, a basic system that is the most widely used approach in the West and the one I am still most likely to recommend to my patients. This set of techniques was developed, not surprisingly, in Sweden, in the early part of the nineteenth century by Per Ling, a fencing master and gymnast who borrowed liberally from approaches long used in China.

Swedish massage consists of five basic strokes, or hand movements, including the long gliding strokes of *effleurage*; the kneading movements of *petrissage*; the striking motions of *tapotement*; the compression and pressure of *friction*; and the shaking motion of *vibration*. These are variously used to soothe or stimulate tissue, to increase circulation in the muscles and around the joints, and to improve the flow of blood and lymph toward the heart.

At first, I felt uncomfortable on the massage table. It was difficult for someone used to doing, and doing for himself, to just lie back and let someone else work on him. I soon got used it. Massage dissolved tension in my tight calves, allowed my shoulders to relax and settle back, and created soft spaces where my vertebrae had seemed to crowd my head. My lower back felt both less stiff and less vulnerable when I received regular massage. Sometimes I drifted off to sleep. Always I felt looser and livelier when I got off the table.

In recent years researchers have begun to confirm massage clients' impressions about its beneficial effects. Massage does indeed relieve the "symptom distress," the discomfort, of people with cancer and back injuries. Regular massage has been shown to lower blood pressure and heart rate in the elderly. It can alleviate depression and anxiety in adults on coronary care units as well as in adolescents hospitalized on psychiatric wards. And it will decrease the stress response in most people.

Some of the most dramatic effects, however, have been demonstrated on premature infants. Tiffany Field and her colleagues at the University of Miami's Touch Research Institute showed that preemies who were massaged several times a day for ten minutes demonstrated a 47 percent greater weight gain and were able to leave the hospital six days earlier than age-mates who received only the customary hospital care. In a second study they demonstrated that massage had even more profound effects on the preterm babies of cocaine-using mothers: in addition to the expected weight gain, these high-risk infants developed more quickly and had far fewer post-natal complications than nonmassaged babies.

Massage also conveys a welcome emotional message. By its very nature, it communicates caring, overcomes the feelings of isolation that make illness unbearable, and provides a bridge of trust that allows people to communicate their fears. I know that during some confused and lonely times in my life, the deep, attentive, wordless touch of a massage therapist has provided comfort and helped reassure me about my own endangered connection to others. It is also a wonderfully satisfying way for people to help—and give to—one another. In another of Field's studies, in which elderly people massaged babies, the beneficial effects were striking for both groups.

As I learned about and experienced massage, I found myself increasingly surprised and troubled by my own and my profession's ignorance. Every other healing system in the world includes at least some forms of massage and musculoskeletal manipulation. Why were we so confident about penetrating the body and all of its orifices, yet so diffident about using touch to help it?

Soon I was exploring other body-oriented therapies. All, I discovered, had in common an appreciation of the inseparability of mind and body; an understanding that emotions and thoughts take on a physical reality in tight muscles, restricted movements, and physical dysfunction; and a conviction, based on experience, that working with and reeducating the physical structure can also profoundly alter the mental and emotional life. Each has its own special way of addressing the body, and one, I soon found out, may be helpful when another falls short.

The Alexander technique caught my attention first. It was created by F. Matthias Alexander, a touring Australian actor who lost his voice and, after fruitlessly seeking medical help, cured himself. Alexander discovered that the way he held his head—pulling it back and down—constricted the muscles in his throat. With the aid of mirrors, he taught himself to hold his head in a more relaxed way, to speak and stand and move with less effort.

Having successfully treated himself, he began to help others, then to teach some of them to become teachers of his method. His famous pupils, including George Bernard Shaw, the novelist Aldous Huxley, educator John Dewey, and Nobel laureate Nikolaas Tinbergen, spread the word: Alexander lessons help you to abandon habitual constricting postures and patterns of movement; they create a sense of expansiveness and lightness in the body and, in turn, the mind; the technique is gentle and aesthetic.

Some Alexander lessons take place on a massage table. The practitioner's hands subtly teach the shoulders how to relax, and coax the muscles of the chest and throat to soften and widen. Other lessons are given in the home or office. The teacher's hands on your body show you how you sit at your word processor, bend over to pick up your child, or use a dental drill. Then, moving you softly, subtly, they demonstrate how the same activity can be done with much less strain.

Moshe Feldenkrais, like Alexander (and many other pioneers of the new medicine), initially developed his method to deal with his own disability—a knee that he had torn up playing sports. Feldenkrais, who was both brilliantly analytic and wonderfully intuitive, discovered that he could create and teach movements that would reeducate the brain and in turn enable it to communicate in new ways with the rest of the body. He taught in one-to-one, hands-on sessions and in classes where students practiced the movements he demonstrated.

Feldenkrais's methods were original and dramatic, and the results were striking. Stroke victims and people with cerebral palsy often recovered functions they had been told were forever gone. Ordinary healthy people discovered they could expand their repertory of movements and, in the bargain, their own sense of psychological as well as physical possibility.

If Feldenkrais was a kind of wild somatic poet, Ida Rolf saw the body through the lens of a great architect or engineer. Rolf, who was in fact trained as a biochemist and was inspired by her studies of osteopathic manipulation and yoga, developed a way of manipulating the myofascia—the tough connective tissue that covers and separates the layers of muscles. By urging the fascial layers apart and freeing them up from the muscles they enclose, Rolf sought to return the body to its natural alignment with the forces of gravity.

During a course of "basic ten" Rolfing sessions, jammed joints, confined ribs, and tight pelvises are opened. Emotions that may be connected with particular body parts—for example, the terrifying memories that lodge in the rigid

137

pelvis and tense thighs of the adult who was sexually abused as a child—may be evoked and released. Before-and-after photographs demonstrate that people who have been Rolfed show remarkable changes in posture. They stand straighter and seem more balanced on their feet. Many say they feel looser, more flexible, and freer in their minds as well as in their bodies.

Rolfing, Feldenkrais work, and virtually all the other modern body-mind or body-oriented therapies owe a considerable debt to the discoveries and practices of Wilhelm Reich. Reich, a German psychoanalyst who was one of Freud's most gifted pupils, won his master's praise by writing some of the first and most important papers on "character," that complex of perception and feelings, opinion and behavior, that defines who we are. Reich's interest in the analysis of character—as opposed to specific neurotic or psychotic symptoms—in turn led him to examine the resistances with which we defend ourselves against change.

In time he observed that these resistances have physical as well as emotional and characterological manifestations. Reich believed he could see and feel these rigidities of thought and inhibitions of feeling in the constrictions of the body's structure and the contours of its muscles. He called them *armor* and addressed them with breathing exercises, specific postures, and deep probing touch, as well as the verbal interventions of psychotherapy. This kind of body work releases physical and emotional constrictions, dissolves the armor, and makes way for the free flow of what Reich named *orgone energy,* the same vital force that the Chinese long before had called *qi.*

I've found all of these approaches helpful—to myself, as well as to my patients. I've used them separately and in combination. Sometimes one seems most appropriate, sometimes another. I like to match them to the particular problem I or my patients are experiencing and also to our personalities: perhaps Alexander technique for a sensitive aesthetic type who is beset by the constrictions of habitual postures or who needs gentle guidance in realizing the connection between mind and body; Rolfing for the patient who needs to have someone else untie resistant physical and emotional knots; Feldenkrais work for a student hopeful of undoing the knots himself; Reichian therapy for those who are eager or desperate to move beyond the limits of words and verbal therapies; and massage—both Swedish and the "deep tissue" kinds that borrow from Rolfing and Reichian approaches—for anyone who would like to let go of the tension in tight muscles.

But these are generalities. Having experienced each of these modalities, I've developed a sense of when one is most useful and when another, a sense that in time many of my patients come to share. All of these approaches, at different times and in different ways, help us to undo what has been done to us or what we have done to ourselves. All help us to discover new ways of knowing ourselves as beings whose bodies are intimately connected with our minds and alive with emotion and intelligence.

MOVEMENT

The fetus in the womb moves in response to sensation. In our cerebral cortex, the area that controls motor functioning lies adjacent to the one where sensory impressions are received. Movement and touch are also deeply connected metaphorically and linguistically. We call our feelings "emotions." If our emotions are aroused, we are "moved" or "touched."

As children, we move with extraordinary freedom. Our movement grows from the basic activities, the reflexes and random motions that are built into our biological structure. Out of them, we fashion an extraordinary array of feeding and finding behaviors and facial expressions. We push and probe with our mouths, tongue, fingers, hands, and feet. We kick and scream; scan with our eyes; crawl toward or recoil; and explore everywhere. After a while, as our nervous systems develop further, we learn to play. We run and fall down, pick ourselves up, and move on again.

Very soon, movement is shaped by the demands and exhortations of our families, schools, and societies. Just as we are not supposed to touch some parts of our body, so our movements are constrained. Boys are meant to walk and sit one way; girls another. Certain kinds of emotions and interests, usually ones that indicate our acceptance of and pleasure in the world of the adults around us, may be expressed physically, others may not be. For too many hours each day, we are confined to desks in schools and forbidden to fidget. We are questioned, corrected, or even hit, when we so much as let our eyes wander.

For some children, sports is a release, a time when limbs are freed for running, throwing, tumbling. Too often, and often too soon, children internalize the expectations and judgments of adults. It is not enough to play. We have to play well. Children who are not "good" in sports, not as interested and coordinated as their age-mates, are sometimes cruelly mocked. I remember in fifth and sixth grade the boys who dropped easy passes or flailed at the soccer ball were called "fags." Those of us who were "good" bore another kind of burden. Our pleasure in movement was quickly shaped to particular purposes. We were urged to strive not only to be good but to be best. It was competition, far more than excellence, that ruled our playing fields.

Physicians are notorious for their fascination with sports—particularly golf, a source of many stories about not being able to find a doctor on Wednesday or Thursday afternoons. But though they may enjoy sports, doctors generally have little understanding of how movement—the walking of the Zen master or, for that matter, tennis or golf, yoga or t'ai chi—may be used to relieve illness or enhance health and well-being.

Recently, as the literature on the beneficial effects of exercise on cardiovascular functioning has expanded, there's been some shift. Twenty-five years ago, patients who'd had a heart attack were ordered to "remain at bedrest": one false or hurried stop, it seemed, might doom them. Now they are told to begin to exercise soon, often within hours of their attack. Every physician now knows that aerobic exercise—exercise that consumes large quantities of oxygen and lasts long enough to allow the oxygen to reach muscles and increase the heart rate—can help prevent and treat coronary heart disease.

Aerobic exercise decreases the high blood pressure that strains the heart and pounds the blood against the vulnerable inner lining of the arteries. It lowers heart rate, raises the concentration of artery-protecting high-density lipoproteins (HDL), and encourages smokers to cut down or stop. Interestingly, the major decline in cardiovascular disease in the United States in the last twenty years is well correlated with the increased interest in jogging and fitness.

Other facts about exercise are also becoming more widely known and shared, particularly by physicians who specialize in the new field of sports medicine. In menopausal women, weight-bearing exercise (walking, jogging, and the like) seems not only to protect against cardiovascular disease but to significantly decrease the risk of osteoporosis.

Recent studies showing the beneficial effects of aerobic exercise on immune status are far less well known but may be equally important. Those who do regular but not excessive aerobic exercise show increased levels and activity of a variety of immune cells and substances, including cancer-fighting natural killer cells and interferon. This translates into real improvements in health. For example, people report they have far fewer colds when they run regularly than when they are inactive. And HIV-positive individuals who exercise regularly not only exhibit higher levels of vital T-4 lymphocytes but also seem to be disproportionately represented among long-term survivors of the viral infection.

In addition to these direct effects on physical functioning, exercise exerts powerful indirect effects through its capacity to reduce stress and improve mood. Aerobic exercise increases blood flow to the brain. It releases endorphins, the brain's own natural morphine, and increases the level of norepinephrine, a neurotransmitter that is often depleted in depression. In experimental studies, people who exercise regularly are less likely to exhibit the stress response of increased cortisol and norepinephrine when confronted with frustrating tasks or harsh criticism.

These physiological changes have real-life consequences: some clinical studies have shown that regular jogging effectively reduces anxiety, while others suggest it may be as good a treatment for mild to moderate depression as either psychotherapy or antidepressants.

All these positive effects on stress and mood are good in themselves. They also help protect against such physical illnesses as hypertension, heart disease, and diabetes, which are exacerbated by anxiety and depression. Exercise also enhances our self-esteem, our pleasure in our bodies, and our sense of control—all of which also contribute to improved mood and diminished stress.

It turns out it's also possible to obtain many of these same physiological and clinical benefits from exercises not generally regarded as aerobic. For example, the postures of hatha yoga have been shown to improve cardiovascular functioning and decrease blood pressure in hypertensives. They also improve breathing capacity in asthmatics; decrease blood sugar levels in people with diabetes; and diminish anxiety and improve mood. Similarly, the gentle movements of t'ai chi, a meditation and martial art that tens of millions of Chinese practice daily, improve respiratory function, decrease stress, and elevate mood.

Each of these approaches also has particular virtues that are different from those of conventional aerobic exercise. Yoga, for example, is wonderfully useful for people with the stiff joints and inflexible muscles of arthritis; t'ai chi has a powerful effect on improving balance and muscular control in the elderly.

All exercise can be useful, but it's also important for it to be appropriate and fun. Individual differences are paramount.

Jogging is great therapy for depression—but not if you dread stepping into your running shoes. Age has to be taken into account as well as physical condition and psychological make-up. Yoga was perfect for David Donne. It worked powerfully well for his arthritic joints and suited his precise and patient temperament. Dancing was great to help Leslie Newman loosen up emotionally as well as physically.

I often ask people with asthma to begin to do yoga. Then, as they feel more at home in their body, and less frightened of losing their breath, I may suggest jogging or dancing. T'ai chi is wonderful for most older people and patient younger ones, but it's often too slow and frustrating for young type As and troubled teenagers. And because our need for and pleasure in particular forms of exercise change from time to time, I check in periodically to make sure that something that once was useful continues to be.

When I ran the Adolescent Service at St. Elizabeths, I encouraged all kinds of physical activity. We started with basketball and morning stretching and yoga for all the patients. We had softball and touch football for everyone, and weightlifting and dancing pretty much whenever anyone felt like it. Then, at the suggestion of an overweight attendant, we started a jogging group for girls and female staff.

After a few months I got the idea to bring in a kung fu master to work with the young people. I told the staff that I thought kung fu might give the teenagers a controlled outlet for their rage and frustration. It promised the kind of strength that would serve them well on their very rough streets, yet it exacted a high price of discipline for obtaining that strength.

The dominant staff response was terror and outrage: I was putting lethal weapons into the hands of crazy young criminals. "You're teaching them to kick and kill" was a common cry. I believed—and on a few rough days prayed—that long before any of the kids could do any damage with kung fu, they would be so steeped in its philosophy of purely defensive action, so accustomed to its discipline, they would be highly unlikely to harm anyone.

To my great relief, this proved to be the case: incidents of violence, levels of medication, and enforced confinements in the "seclusion room" all decreased after we began our lessons. Most everyone seemed to look forward to the twice weekly workouts. They were incredibly demanding physically but strangely nonstressful. The routines were so hard, the speed and balance so difficult to maintain, that nobody had much time to be self-conscious or check out anyone else. Staff participation created a shared learning, a rough equality that was rare in the experience of these young people. We were beginners too, like the kids, and we huffed and puffed and toppled over right along with them. The fact that Dennis, the kung fu master, was young, black, at once encouraging and demanding, and handsome didn't hurt either. The boys wanted to be like him, and many of the girls, between rapid-fire push-ups and backward kicks, developed a serious crush.

At St. Elizabeths, in the medical student teaching I do, and in my work with individual patients and groups, exercise and movement are neither peripheral nor optional but an absolutely essential part of treatment. They improve physical functioning, favorably alter brain chemistry, and help create a sense of mastery and pleasure in and satisfaction with our bodies. They allow and encourage a freedom and joy that many of us have forgotten. They create experiences—the excitement of learning together in a group, the quiet satisfaction of solitary practice—that may deeply change the way we feel about our bodies, ourselves, and others.

BREATHING

Using exercise and movement therapeutically requires a certain level of choice and commitment. Breathing, by contrast, is inevitable, automatic. The infant coming into the extrauterine world is announced by her first crying breath. Once the process has begun, it continues, as indefatigably, and usually as exempt from conscious control, as the beating of the heart. Like heart rate, it is regulated by centers at the very base of the brain, in the medulla oblongata, an area of our most primitive functions. Yet breathing, observed, made conscious, and controlled, can also be a powerful tool for healing.

We breathe in two phases, inspiration and expiration. In inspiration, the dome-shaped sheet of muscle called the diaphragm constricts and descends, leaving a vacuum into which the lung tissue, filled with air, expands. On expiration, the diaphragm rises and the area of the lungs contracts. The air, which is about 20 percent useful oxygen and 80 percent inert nitrogen, is inhaled through the nose, where it is cleansed of some of its impurities. It enters the trachea and from there descends into the two major bronchi, which in turn divide further into even smaller tubes. These bronchioles end finally in tiny saclike alveoli. Oxygen diffuses across the walls of the alveoli into the capillaries, where it attaches to the iron-based hemoglobin molecules in the blood's red cells.

The blood flows from the lungs to the left side of the heart, which propels it through the arteries and the smaller arterioles and capillaries. The oxygen diffuses across the walls of the capillaries into the tissue, where it fuels the metabolism of every one of our body's cells. At the same time, carbon dioxide, the waste product of that metabolism, diffuses into the bloodstream. The carbon dioxide attaches to the hemoglobin molecules for the return trip, via the veins, to the right side of the heart and then to the lungs, where the blood is once again oxygenated.

Gravity dictates that the blood flow in the lower part of our lungs is far greater than in the middle and upper portions. This means that this lower portion is the most efficient place for exchanging oxygen and carbon dioxide. As babies, we make excellent use of this capacity. Our breathing then is diaphragmatic: the diaphragm descends maximally, and oxygen is able to diffuse easily into the blood-rich capillaries of the lower part of the lungs.

As we grow older, we shift to thoracic breathing, preferentially filling the less efficient middle and upper portions of the lungs. We make this shift for a variety of reasons that are in part related to both stress and cultural conditioning. As we repeatedly experience the fight-or-flight response, we learn to tighten our muscles and breathe more shallowly. On top of that, we are taught by our society to suck in our guts and puff out our chests—a posture totally at variance with our need for oxygenation. Finally, many of us, because of embarrassment during our adolescence or too much time spent hunched over desks, develop a stooped posture that further diminishes our lung capacity.

The end result is that we constrict our musculature and breathe more shallowly, into the less efficient middle and upper parts of our lungs. This taxes the lungs, which must move faster to ensure adequate oxygen flow. Shallow breathing also strains the heart, which increases its rate to provide enough blood for oxygen transport and raises its pressure to pump the blood through the arteries.

I use breathing exercises often to help people break up these habitual, inefficient, and constricting patterns of inspiration and expiration; and to enable them to relearn the deeper, more efficient, and relaxing breath of infancy and early childhood. I often teach the yogic "complete breath." This simple exercise can be done sitting or lying down. I ask my patients to inhale deeply and slowly, allowing their diaphragm to descend and the belly to expand. Then I suggest that they allow a wave of air to ascend from the belly, slowly filling the middle and upper parts of the chest. In expiration, I explain, they can allow the wave to recede from top to bottom.

Practicing this complete breath for ten or fifteen minutes twice a day, or for several minutes many times a day, can begin to reverse years of bad breathing habits. It increases lung capacity, slows heart rate, decreases blood pressure, and reduces anxiety. This kind of breathing also reinforces our sense of control over our body and our emotions. I accomplished the same thing with David Donne by asking him to make his belly soft as he breathed deeply. With David, I used a mantra—the words *soft belly*—along with a visual image of his belly, to reinforce his practice.

The chaotic breathing that Dr. Singha prescribed for me—that I sometimes use with anxious, rigid, or depressed people—accomplishes something similar in a different way. Here fast, irregular breathing disrupts habitual muscular and postural patterns and urges the lungs to exchange larger volumes of air. After weeks or months of practice, the patterns break and deep diaphragmatic breathing begins automatically to reassert its rightful claim.

Breathing slowly and deeply changes everything. The body is pulled toward the earth as the belly expands. Each exhalation drains away tension as it releases carbon dioxide. Focusing on the slow rhythmic inhalations and exhalations, the mind begins to match its rhythms to the breath. Thoughts, normally so immediate and insistent, seem less pressing. The pain and tension in muscles, the constriction in the gut, the compulsive need to eat, the asthmatic's desperate hunger for air, and the anxious person's worries: all seem less overwhelming. We begin to experience a sense of detachment, to observe rather than feel victimized by our concerns. Sometimes a smile rises irresistibly to our lips. It's so simple.

I add other techniques as well, ones I've borrowed from pranayama, the yogic breathing exercises; Chinese qi gong; and Tibetan and Middle Eastern religious practices. Alternate nostril breathing, a yogic practice, is one that I frequently use. It helps to break cycles of anxiety and gives asthmatics a greater sense of control and security. In this technique you breathe in one nostril, covering the other; next, you hold the breath; then you exhale through the other nostril, holding the first one closed. Then you reverse the process, inhaling through that second nostril, holding the breath, and exhaling through the first. You can begin by counting slowly to four to time each part of the breath, and increase the count as you feel more confident. This technique works, in part, by synchronizing electrical activity in the two halves of the brain.

I also use breathing in combination with imagery or, as in Reichian body work, as part of psychotherapy. Many people find that "breathing into" a part of the body that is tense—imagining that the breath is actually going directly there—will help to dissolve that tension. Sometimes emotions and memories that are connected with that part of the body begin to surface. Someone with asthma may feel the fear that seems to live in the muscles of her chest, see the images that once provoked that fear. These images may then be experienced, explored, discussed, and understood.

We need, paradoxically, to remind ourselves often about breathing, our most automatic and vital process. This is especially true in times of stress, when our tendency is to revert to a shallow, inefficient thoracic breathing that serves only to compound our anxiety. Then it's important to become aware of what we are doing, to remind ourselves to return to the deep, slow, physiologically sound diaphragmatic breathing of childhood. Sometimes I suggest my patients make signs to post in their office, at their computers, or in their bedrooms—signs that simply say, "Breathe!"

ELEVEN

Self-Care as Primary Care: "When I Eat, I Eat" ∽

I REMEMBER in grade school we used to say a blessing before lunch. Often, ravenous after a long morning of heavy listening, I was impatient. Occasionally, repeating the familiar words of thanks, smelling the platters of food waiting in the kitchen, I had such a feeling of joy.

I loved those meals beyond any culinary reason and have loved other meals before and since, meals that are earned by hunger and graced by good feelings and my own or other's good company. Eating is a communion with Nature—or God—from whom both we and our food come, with ourselves, and with those with whom we share food. Eating and drinking are the way that Christians know their God most intimately. Eating and drinking are central to the celebrations of Judaism and to Thanksgiving, our most joyous secular holiday.

Often, however, our relations with food are distorted. As children, many of us drank anxiety and sorrow with our mother's milk, or more likely with someone else's "formula." Later, we sat stiffly, terrorized by the inquisitors who preside over too many families' dinner tables. We learned to hurry through food as if it were a chore blocking our way to the real business of the day; to stuff ourselves against the threat of anxiety; and to starve or vomit ourselves into anorectic acceptability. When we are young and vulnerable, we are teased and tricked into eating foods whose greatest virtue is the money they make for their manufacturers.

Most of us eat too fast as well as too much—almost seventy million Americans are more than 20 percent above their ideal weight—and there is increasing evidence that obesity predisposes us to a variety of illnesses and that weighing less contributes to longevity. As adults, we unconsciously perpetuate the habits of childhood or, making food a battleground, struggle against them. Just as we have forgotten how to touch and move and breathe, so too we have lost the capacity simply to eat or, for that matter, to select and prepare foods.

When I work with diet, I am using foods and herbs and spices in ways that are most appropriate for each person. I may eliminate foods that for one reason or another seem to be deleterious; and I suggest vitamins, minerals, and other food supplements that make up for deficiencies or enhance functioning. There is convincing scientific evidence for most of these therapies, and hundreds or thousands of years of experience back up others. But beyond any of these specific prescriptions, I am aiming at something else: I want people to discover the great joy of eating and to reclaim the intuitive knowledge of what and when and how much is good for them to eat.

When someone calls for an appointment, I inevitably tell him that he is going to have to take a look at his diet, that I may suggest a time of fasting and perhaps major long-term changes. If he asks why, I explain that our modern diet is a deep violation of our evolutionary programming, that most of us are eating in ways that are at dramatic variance with our biological needs, and that these derelictions have caused us great harm.

True humans, *homo sapiens,* developed approximately 40,000 years ago. They, like our more remote Paleolithic ancestors, ranged far and wide in search of food. Archaeological evidence suggests they ate a diet that was based largely on strikingly fat-free wild game, a wide variety of plants with an extremely high content of fiber and vitamin C, and few grains. Ten thousand years ago, with the rise of agriculture and a less nomadic way of life, much of humanity shifted to a grain-based high-fiber diet, with less meat and fewer kinds of plants.

The planet's remaining hunter-gatherer societies—in Africa, Australia, South America, and the Arctic—consume diets that resemble our collective ancestors'. Similarly, some tribal groups continue to eat as the early agriculturists did.

When Denis Burkitt, an English surgeon, went as a missionary to rural Africa some years ago, he was puzzled. Where, he wondered, were all the patients he was accustomed to operating on or visiting in the medical and surgical wards of British hospitals? The African people were plagued by a variety of bacterial and parasitic infections, but they were, to a remarkable degree, free from the diseases—hypertension and cardiovascular disease, cancer, diabetes, inflammatory bowel disease, asthma, and arthritis —that beset our modern industrialized world. These illnesses, Burkitt, came to believe, are "diseases of civilization." He concluded that they owed their prevalence, if not their origin, to our modern, highly processed, low-fiber, fat-heavy diet.

It is difficult to cleanly separate dietary change from the stress, alienation, inactivity, and pollution that accompany modern industrial society. Still, epidemiological evidence strongly suggests that traditional hunter-gatherer and agricultural societies developed diets that are well suited to human biological programming. Diabetes, cancer, and heart disease, for example, are as rare among some American Indians who preserve their traditional diet as they are among rural Africans. These conditions, are, however, quite common among Indians—in some instances far more common than among Caucasians—who have shifted to more typical modern American fare.

Though the hunter-gatherer or "Paleolithic" diet is virtually impossible for modern *homo sapiens* to achieve—very few of us have access to the large amounts of game and wild plants on which it is based—the early agricultural way of eating provides a reasonable example for us to emulate. In recent years a number of studies have confirmed the health-promoting utility of regimens based on large amounts of grains, fruits, and vegetables and very small quantities of fat and/or animal products.

Some of the early studies on Seventh-Day Adventists, a religious group that is vegetarian but consumes milk products and eggs (they are called lacto-ovo-vegetarians), demonstrated significantly lower blood pressure and cholesterol, as well as lower rates of breast, bowel, and prostate cancer than both a comparable group of non-Adventist meat-eaters, and Adventists who ate some meat. More recent studies on people who follow the Japanese macrobiotic diet—based largely on grains and vegetables—that George Ohsawa created, have produced still more impressive cardiovascular statistics.

Even less stringent regimens, which include meat but are based on large quantities of vegetables, legumes (beans, peas, and lentils), and complex carbohydrates like pasta, and small amounts of animal fat and refined sugars, seem to have significant health-enhancing effects. Epidemiological and clinical studies on one of these regional ways of eating, the so-called "Mediterranean diet," have demonstrated a lower incidence of both intestinal cancer and diverticulitis, an inflammatory bowel disease, in those who follow it. The Mediterranean diet also has been shown to help prevent a second heart attack in people who have recently suffered an initial one.

All of this evidence shapes and lends weight to the recommendations that I make. So, too, do studies on some of the specific elements in diets that are health enhancing or health threatening. In recent years I've been particularly impressed by the data on the beneficial effects of fiber, soy products, fatty fish, onions, garlic, ginger, and olive oil; and by the hazards of overconsumption of refined sugar, caffeine, milk and milk products, and food additives.

High-fiber diets improve bowel functioning generally and may diminish the risk of gallstones and kidney stones. Regular intake of oat bran fiber decreases the level of "bad" or low-density lipoprotein (LDL) cholesterol, and may raise the level of "good" high-density lipoprotein (HDL) cholesterol as well. Wheat bran significantly reduces the occurence of colon cancer in people who already have rectal polyps.

Soy, a staple of traditional Asian diets, not only decreases total and LDL cholesterol, as other beans do, but appears to be a valuable anticancer food. Studies showing the significantly decreased incidence of breast cancer in Japanese women who consume high quantities of soy are particularly impressive. This protective effect is presumably due to soy's high content of *phytoestrogens,* plant estrogens that, like the drug tamoxifen, inhibit the stimulating effect of human estrogen on the development and progression of breast cancer. Soy is also extremely high in protein and serves as an excellent and often tasty substitute for meat and milk products.

All fish contain significant amounts of omega-3 fatty acids, which dilate blood vessels, decrease the clumping of clot-forming platelets, damp down the inflammatory response, and generally protect us against the development of hard, plaque-filled atheroslcerotic arteries. The fish highest in omega-3s are fatty and come from cold deep waters: mackerel, tuna, herring, sardines, salmon, and anchovies among them.

Onions, which have for millennia been used therapeutically by people all over the world—and which figured prominently in my first experiments with food—are now coming into their own scientifically. They have been demonstrated to have anticancer properties, to increase HDL cholesterol, and to decrease the risk of blood clots. It turns out, too, that they really can help prevent allergies and asthma attacks.

Garlic, which has also been long seen as a great healer as well as a culinary treat, has in recent years had its effectiveness confirmed for an astonishing variety of conditions. It helps control infections, reduces cholesterol levels, decreases elevated blood pressure, enhances immune functioning, and may even improve mood. And ginger, which has traditionally been used to improve digestion, turns out to be as good as powerful drugs in controlling nausea and vomiting.

Olive oil is, as anyone who has ever visited that part of the world knows, a major ingredient of the Mediterranean diet. It is a monounsaturated fatty acid, which means it has only one chemical bond in its structure that is not "saturated" with hydrogen atoms. Animal fats by contrast, are saturated and are hard at room temperature, while polyunsaturated fats like corn and safflower oil remain liquid. Whereas saturated fats raise LDL cholesterol and polyunsaturated fats decrease HDL cholesterol, olive oil seems to have only beneficial effects: it lowers LDL and tends to raise HDL. It also seems to have a specific protective effect against the damage that LDL causes to arteries.

It's comfortable for me to promote foods that have health-giving properties, but it always makes me a bit uneasy to warn people *against* consuming anything. I don't want to add to the chorus of prohibitions that scream at us from the pages of diet books and the popular press. These nagging voices prey on our seemingly endless capacity to worry about and condemn almost every aspect of our lives. They also contribute to a judgmental attitude that, I'm sure, is at least as destructive as the most careless diet. It's far better to eat an occasional steak or hot fudge sundae or to drink a potent cup of espresso than it is to pine away for these foods or sneer at those who are happily consuming them.

Still, because it's so easy for us to become habitual and unthinking users of foods that in large quantities may be detrimental, I want to mention some of them.

Until recently, most scientific studies disputed parents' oft-made observations that sugar—in sodas, candy, and cakes—made their kids "hyper." More recently, some impressive work has demonstrated that in some children sugar, which is not as well metabolized by the young as by adults, does indeed produce hyperactivity. In large quantities refined sugar, which provides plenty of calories but is otherwise "empty" of nutritional value, strains the insulin-producing capacity of the pancreas. I've also observed that sugar can be responsible for exacerbating some people's inflammatory conditions—arthritis and irritable bowel among them.

Caffeine, which has come to be many Americans' "drug of choice," is highly addictive. A number of people suffer severe withdrawal symptoms—headache, fatigue, depression, muscle pains—when they abruptly stop their coffee or indeed their caffeinated tea intake. Caffeine also gives some people headaches and makes others quite anxious. Coffee in particular irritates the stomach and may stimulate the development of cysts in women's breasts.

Milk and milk products, which are promoted and advertised with almost as much zeal as tobacco products, also may contribute to a number of problems. Many people cannot easily digest milk sugar, lactose, and develop symptoms of diarrhea when they take milk products. Others, including most particularly infants, have problems with the protein in cows' milk. Milk may also produce allergic reactions, including arthritic flares, and may be in part responsible for the congestion in those who suffer from sinus problems. Nor is milk necessary for adults or even children. There are a number of other good sources of calcium, including fish, beans, and leafy vegetables.

Food additives, preservatives, and colorings, most of them synthetic, are used by manufacturers to enhance the taste, prolong the shelf life, and alter the appearance of food, not to improve its nutritional value. Not surprisingly, a number of them can cause adverse effects. The most dramatic examples are the headaches and flushing that monosodium glutamate (MSG) produces in susceptible people; the asthma and allergic reactions caused by sulfites, which are added to some dried fruits and wine; and the headaches that may result from aspartame, the artificial sweetener that is present in many diet drinks and foods.

As a general rule, I suggest that people who want to eat a healthier diet include large quantities of fiber-rich raw fruits and vegetables, as well as a morning helping of wheat and oat bran. I recommend that they use fish, particularly fatty fish, and soy products as primary sources of protein and decrease their intake of beef, pork, and lamb, which are high in saturated fats, as well as of milk and milk products. Onions, garlic, and ginger by themselves and as ingredients in cooking other dishes are high on my list of recommended foods. Though other oils and butter are delicious and certainly fine for occasional use, I suggest olive oil for regular cooking and salad dressing. I often advise people to eliminate or cut way down on refined sugar—a little honey or maple syrup, both of which at least retain their native vitamins and minerals, is better—caffeine, and food additives, colorings, and preservatives.

These general guidelines, are, however, only that. In nutrition as in every other aspect of our lives, each person has unique needs and requirements. Often, for longer or shorter periods of time, I suggest particular diets for people with specific chronic conditions and constitutions.

An initial period of fasting—usually one or two weeks on a single food—is useful for many people with chronic illness, and shorter fasts are sometimes helpful. Though we haven't adequately studied what happens, it seems that fasting gives the body a time to heal itself—the demands of digestion and metabolism are markedly decreased—as well as an opportunity to remove toxic substances, like pesticides, herbicides, and drugs, that have long been stored in the liver and fatty tissue. Sometimes people who are fasting will smell the odor of ether, which years before was given to them as an anesthetic and was subsequently stored in their fat cells.

This process of cleansing and detoxification seems to be innate among animals who are sick and a routine practice for people who fall ill in some tribal societies. It has been used for therapeutic as well as religious reasons in many cultures for millennia. Still, there is woefully little scientific literature available on the process or its effects. One of the few studies published, which was done in Japan some years ago, did show that several weeks of fasting—on water or fruit and vegetable juices—was generally helpful for chronic illness. This was true whether the condition was asthma or chronic pain, cardiovascular disease or a bad back. Interestingly, many of the beneficial effects lasted long after the period of fasting ended.

Fasts on single foods, or "mono fasts," are helpful for specific conditions. So far as I know, none has received the kind of investigation it deserves. Nevertheless, they've been used by healers and herbalists for centuries. Among them are watermelon for poor kidney function and kidney stones; boiled onions for chronic bronchitis; and hot water, lemon juice, cayenne pepper, and maple syrup as a "liver cleanser."

I've used these three and many more, including the memorable but uncomfortable pineapple fast, with patients like David Donne, for more than fifteen years. In every case I've tried them on myself before ever suggesting them to anyone else, and in no instance have I suggested that anyone do a one- or two-week fast without my close supervision: during this process of physiological rest and detoxification, a "healing crisis"—a chronic illness becoming acute prior to an improvement, like the one I experienced on pineapple—is common. There are other things to pay attention to as well. A medication level that has been adequate may, during a fast, become excessive and dangerous. In addition, some people, particularly during the first three days of a fast, may feel tired and depressed, irritable or weepy. It looks and feels as if both mind and body are cleaning themselves out.

In addition to the specific effects, fasting has other long-term benefits. It seems to clear the palate as well as clean out the body and purge the mind. Old eating habits are broken, at least for a while, and an intuitive sense of what is right to eat emerges. We may find ourselves thinking, "I really need hot food or something sweet or salty." We taste and appreciate it more, eat it more slowly, and need less of it. And we don't seem to get stuck again quite so easily. Instead of thinking, "I'm in this restaurant, and I've always liked the steak and baked potato," it's more like, "Let's see what I really want to eat today, right now."

Twenty years ago, when I first began to prescribe specific foods, herbs, and spices, people looked at me in the strangest way: it was as if I had emerged, with leaves and roots in my hair and the mystery of the dark woods in my voice, to announce that ginger works for stomach problems; that garlic and onions forestall the flu; that romaine lettuce broth can be used for sleep; or that yogurt may be placed intravaginally to dispel a yeast infection. Though they are not yet a part of conventional medical practice, these and many other home remedies are fast becoming staples of the popular pharmacopoeia.

In the years since then, both Western and Chinese herbs have also become a significant part of my practice. In many instances they accomplish what drugs cannot—gradually enhancing physiological functioning or building up the body's defenses—or they achieve the same results with fewer side effects and at less expense. For the most part, I use them in time-honored combinations, ten or a dozen together. Here I'm just going to mention the therapeutic properties of a few particularly useful plants that have, in recent years, been scientifically documented.

The liquid extract of the leaves of ginkgo biloba has been shown in many carefully controlled studies to improve circulation and mental functioning in the aged. Rehmannia, a widely used Chinese herb, is effective in regulating blood sugar in people with diabetes and hypoglycemia and in reducing the inflammation and pain of rheumatoid arthritis. Saint-John's-wort really does have the antidepressant qualities that herbalists have long attributed to it. Ginseng root is a good stimulant, an antidote to the effects of stress, and an immune enhancer. Echinacea, a common Western herb that many people are now using to prevent and treat the flu, has been demonstrated to have both immune-stimulating and antiviral properties. Saw palmetto berries seem to be just as effective as prescription drugs in reducing enlarged prostate glands, but cost far less.

The failure to thoroughly investigate and make full use of the therapeutic properties of foods, herbs, and spices is sometimes attributed to the uncertainty and possible danger of using substances that cannot be precisely measured. This is a problem, but I also think the reluctance reflects an uneasiness on the part of the medical establishment.

It is as if these hard-to-calibrate substances were an affront to the ordered authority of the physician and the power of the pharmaceutical industry. And indeed, the use of homely, widely available plants *is* a kind of challenge to those who adhere to and profit from a rigid and inflexible model of doctor-controlled medicine. They are democratic tools for health. They do not require a prescription, cannot be patented, can often be widely and inexpensively grown, and can be easily used by anyone. Their use raises questions about the superiority of extracted and synthesized drugs. It is an emblem of popular medicine, and a sign that people are reclaiming power over their own bodies.

The use of vitamins, minerals, enzymes, amino acids, and other nonprescription supplements may be even more of a problem for biomedicine and its practitioners. This is not surprising. Each year the evidence for their effectiveness is accumulating, and popular acceptance and use is skyrocketing. These substances, packaged as pills and capsules and advertised as therapies for specific conditions, look like and are used in ways that are similar to the medicines they claim to supplement or replace. They are, in short, therapeutic and economic rivals. Their use has also been complicated by extravagant claims and by incidents of dangerous abuse and careless or ignorant overuse.

Because of their potency and the potential side effects of overuse, I tend to use these supplements more sparingly than

I do foods or even herbs. Still, scientific evidence, human need, and personal experience have led me to prescribe some of them regularly and others occasionally, and to encourage my patients, students, and colleagues to learn more about them.

Though scientific data and popular interest have significantly increased, the amount of information that medical students receive about supplements—or indeed, the entire field of nutrition—is hardly greater now that it was thirty years ago when I was in school. The problems of obesity and eating disorders are acknowledged, and an occasional but casual nod may be made to the benefits of a high-fiber diet, but usually that is all.

Students, now as then, are told that virtually everyone in this country receives an adequate supply of vitamins, minerals, and other nutrients. Vitamin deficiencies—the scurvy that lack of vitamin C produced in eighteenth-century sailors, the bone-deforming rickets of children deficient in vitamin D—are said to be historical curiosities or remote Third World problems. There are no discussions of the therapeutic use of supplementation, except in the case of the skid-row alcoholic, or the genetically or surgically altered patient or pregnant mother. Questions about "megavitamin therapy," Linus Pauling's studies on vitamin C, or reports in the popular press are treated casually by lecturers or even with contempt.

In fact, we have little reason to be so sure of our nutritional ground. To begin with, Roger Williams's work on biochemical individuality suggests that we really don't know if the Recommended Daily Allowance (RDA) is adequate to meet the needs of particular patients or, indeed, anyone. Secondly, the more-than-adequate levels of vitamins and minerals that many of us believe we obtain may be inadequate during times of physical or emotional stress. And finally and most surprisingly, large numbers of us are not, even at the best of times, taking in the RDAs for some essential vitamins and minerals. Some recent studies have indicated significant deficiencies in major portions of the population. Up to 71

selenium with breakfast. Most people probably ought to add a B-complex vitamin (larger than "recommended" amounts of folic acid, B6, and B12 seem to help prevent heart disease) and a multimineral—with iron for women who are still menstruating, without it for postmenopausal women, and men—once a day with food.

If supplements have sometimes evoked strident debates, discussions of food allergy have on occasion provoked frenzies. Traditional physicians are likely to see food allergy as a relatively uncommon and limited phenomenon, whereas clinical ecologists (who are concerned with the wide variety of possible environmental insults) are inclined to suspect that food allergy may contribute to almost every chronic illness. In fact, people with several widespread conditions exhibit a high degree of sensitivity to some common foods.

A recent British study showed that 56 percent of patients experienced exacerbations of their rheumatoid arthritis when they ate wheat products, and 54 percent when they took corn in any form. Similar kinds and even higher levels of food sensitivity have been repeatedly documented in hyperactive children. In one clinical trial, some 64 percent reacted negatively to milk and milk products, and 59 percent to chocolate. A landmark study by Dr. Joseph Egger, at the Hospital for Sick Children in London, demonstrated that an astonishing 93 percent of children with severe migraines could become symptom free by avoiding the foods that triggered their headaches.

Over the years, I've been impressed by how prevalent such sensitivities are, in adults as well as children, and by how seldom they are detected and treated. Sometimes the skin scratches that allergists use don't reveal the sensitivity. Then it's possible to employ tests based on saliva or blood. But most often, at least initially, I simply ask people to eliminate the most likely culprits—wheat, milk, sugar, food additives, and sometimes corn, citrus, and eggs—for a period of time. If they notice a decrease in their symptoms, I may ask them sometime later to reintroduce these foods one at a time. Then we can tell—by the provocation once again of symptoms—which of them may be at fault. In time, as these people improve their overall diet and health and enhance their immune functioning, many are able to tolerate, at least occasionally, foods to which they were previously quite sensitive.

It's not pleasant for most of us to stop eating foods we love— an interesting and often noticed phenomenon is that we tend to be addicted to precisely those foods and drinks that are most harmful to us—but it's usually even less desirable to suffer from chronic digestive problems, asthma, or pain. And once we've experienced how much better we feel when we're not eating certain foods, we're in a position to make truly informed decisions about our diet. Now the choice and the treatment are ours.

I'm grateful daily for supplements but recognize that they are an emblem of the difficult world we live in, and of our vulnerability. They are forced on us by our need to maintain ourselves in the face of chemical, biological, and social stresses, or by specific conditions that require them. Using food, herbs, and spices, on the other hand, is different, and far more satisfying.

Sometimes the early stages are difficult. After all these years and many useful and even interesting fasts, I cannot say that I really enjoy the process. Nor do I like to eliminate foods from my diet or ask others to do so. Still, I have learned to find a satisfaction in the discipline this requires, as well as in the significantly better health these diets bring.

In the long run, though, there are other, equally great rewards in making, as Hippocrates advised, "food our medicine, and medicine our food." Over the years I have found that my pleasure in the smells and textures and tastes of food, herbs, and spices has steadily grown, and that this pleasure has helped to reconnect me to the natural world from which our food comes and to my own physical being. Combining, preparing, and eating foods has become an aesthetic pleasure and a meditative experience as well as a therapeutic boon.

TWELVE

Other Medicines ⌒〜

ALL OF THE WORLD'S traditional healing systems are based on an understanding that modern biomedicine has largely forgotten, an understanding to which the new medicine has only recently and tentatively begun to recall us. Classical Chinese medicine, Indian Ayurveda, Persian Unani, American Indian, Siberian, Central and South American, Australian, and African healing: all tell us that we are part of a larger world and, indeed, a small version, a microcosm, of it.

We are made of the same stuff as the earth, water, and air around us. We are as connected to the cycles of our planet's seasons, the quadrants of the compass, and the hours of each day as we are to the ebb and flow of the blood and chemicals in our bodies.

These ancient systems tell us that we are spiritual beings, emanations of something beyond us, as well as bodies and minds. We are connected to one another, to the earth, and to that beyond in ways that are more powerful and deeper than any of us may know. Disease, they explain, represents an imbalance within ourselves and between ourselves and the natural, social, and spiritual world. Our health and our healing depend not only on careful diagnosis and expert intervention but on a restoration of that balance.

Each system has its own richness and resonance, a language, practice, and theory that reflect the particular time, place, and people where it began and grew; each system also has its archaeological aspects. It includes, as it develops, the most useful or sometimes just the most persistent or impressive elements of earlier times and other cultures. In many traditions, older beliefs in divine healing, soul loss, and demonic possession—legacies of the first tribal societies, and of the shamanic healers who served and helped create those cultures—persist alongside later formulations of natural causes and rational cures.

The influences of other cultures are also apparent. Techniques that prove potent in one civilization diffuse with trade and study to another. Some historians believe that "traditional" Chinese breathing practices and exercises, called qi gong, owe their origins to Indian pranayama and yoga; that some of the surgical procedures that were the glory of Greek medicine were first learned from Egyptian physicians.

Until the last ten or fifteen years, however, most of the beliefs and practices of the world's traditions were strangers to one another. All were mere curiosities to the biomedicine that has come in the last half century to so thoroughly dominate medical practice, discourse, and policy in the United States. Thirty years ago, when I first became interested in the Chinese worldview and the Asian medicine that embodies it, I was unable to find more than a few obscure references in English. Five years later, I could unearth only two books on acupuncture, both of them dense and difficult.

Today quite literally hundreds of books are available on every aspect of Chinese medicine. The focus is on acupuncture in all its many forms, but there are dozens of handbooks on the use of finger acupressure, moxibustion (the use of heated herbs on acupuncture points), and tongue diagnosis. There are rival translations of basic texts, like the two-thousand-year-old

Yellow Emperor's Classic of Internal Medicine, comprehensible versions of ancient herbals, and lavishly illustrated modern compendiums. New Age bookstores, and even chain stores in malls, stock a wide variety of manuals on the breathing practices of qi gong and on t'ai chi; some on tui na, the Chinese form of massage; a few volumes on the way the Chinese use foods therapeutically; and an almost infinite variety on how following "the Way"—the Tao—can help to bring health, happiness, contentment, long life, and ever-increasing sexual pleasure to modern Westerners.

The other healing traditions are also becoming more widely known and accessible. When I was preparing to go to India in 1979, I had to search through histories of medicine to find information about Ayurveda. Such academic surveys treated this immensely powerful healing system as a quaint artifact, an archaeological remnant. When I arrived in India, I discovered that Ayurveda was offering primary health care to the majority of people on the subcontinent. And today, thanks in large measure to the efforts of Maharishi Mahesh Yogi, the creator of transcendental meditation, and to Deepak Chopra, a Western-trained physician and best-selling author who was his student, Ayurveda is also thriving in the West.

Chinese medicine and Indian Ayurveda, the drumming and dancing of shamanism, the sweat lodges and purgations of American Indian healing, the foods and baths of European naturopathy, the orishas or spirits of West African healing, the little pills of European homeopathy: all are offering modern North Americans something that we are missing in our health care and in our lives. Often it is answers to the unanswerable questions that specific illnesses raise: How do I treat my cancer when Western medicine says nothing more can be done? What about wasting conditions like chronic fatigue syndrome for which there are no conventional answers? Whom or what do I turn to when I feel a confusion so pervasive, a despair so deep, that neither psychotherapy nor psychopharmacology can effectively reach me?

Some of the approaches—Chinese medicine and Ayurveda are the best examples—are richly elaborated healing systems that are in many ways more comprehensive, if on occasion less appropriate and potent, than our own biomedicine. They are, as our research is beginning to show, more useful for many chronic illnesses than anything Western medicine has to offer. Other approaches—homeopathy, the manipulative therapies of chiropractic and osteopathy, the *curanderismo* of Latin America, the indigenous healing practices of various American Indian tribes—offer particular approaches and techniques that afford improvements and sometimes cures that are unimagined by conventional physicians. All of these yield perspectives that can enlarge our understanding. All may be seen as parts of the greater synthesis that is the new medicine.

In this chapter I want to focus on two of the modern alternative healing approaches, the manipulative therapies and homeopathy, and on one of the great healing systems, classical Chinese medicine. Taken together these three systems give a fair sample of the range and benefits of the other medicines—of the new ways of thinking and being they demand, and of the therapeutic possibilities they make available to us. I choose these three because they are becoming increasingly well known and widely practiced in North America and because I use them myself and with my patients.

THE MANIPULATIVE THERAPIES

My bad back opened the door on a new therapeutic world. Dr. Blood's osteopathic manipulations had clearly been helpful. What, I wondered, were they all about? Where had osteopathy come from, and why had I and the medical profession as a whole been so ignorant about it, and so ignorantly prejudiced against it? And what about chiropractors, those men and women about whom M.D.'s spoke with undisguised and unembarrassed scorn? Did these people also know and do something that I should experience? How were they different from osteopaths, and why?

My initial investigations were very practical. At various times on trips across the United States and on other continents, my back would trouble me. Plane rides and long drives were often the culprits, but too many busy days and nights sometimes brought on pain, stiffness, and suffering. It was never nearly as bad as the first time, but I definitely wanted relief. I would ask my hosts for a referral or I would stop in at the local health food store, or sometimes I just looked in the Yellow Pages for somebody.

At first I sought out osteopaths, but often, especially in rural areas, chiropractors were easier to find. Like physicians of any variety, some members of both professions turned out to be helpful and knowledgeable; others were not. Occasionally I came across someone whose hands seemed touched by grace. When, in the late 1970s, I was asked to direct the Special Study on Alternative Services for President Carter's Commission on Mental Health, I also started reading about the origins of and differences between the two professions.

I discovered that movement of the vertebrae and other bones, as well as joints, muscles, and other "soft tissue," was integral to most cultures' therapeutic systems. It had long been a part of Chinese medicine and Ayurveda—some of the most surprising and effective "manipulations" I would ever experience were at the hands, and feet, of my yoga teacher in Delhi—and it was a feature of Hippocratic practice as well. It was, however, reintroduced into Western medicine only a little over a hundred years ago.

In 1874 Andrew Taylor Still, a dissatisfied physician, became the first *osteopath* (from the Greek *osteo,* or "bone," and *pathos,* "suffering" or "disease"). Still, who had lost several members of his family to meningitis and pneumonia, was deeply disturbed by the inadequacies of contemporary medical and surgical practice. At first he turned to magnetic healing, based on Mesmer's work. He learned from Mesmer's American heirs that imbalances or inadequacies in a person's "magnetic fluid" were responsible for disease, and that they could be rectified by passing one's hands over the body of the afflicted person. Still seemed to have become particularly interested in a magnetic healing technique in which the practitioner rubbed his hands along the patient's spine.

In time, Still altered and expanded on Mesmerist doctrines. He came to believe that Mesmer's fluid was blood, not magnetic charge, and that the treatment of all diseases depended on reestablishing unimpeded blood flow. After observing some itinerant nonmedical "bone-setters," he became interested in how rapidly flexing and extending the spine could reestablish blood flow. This emphasis on altering the body's skeletal structure to affect its functioning became the hallmark of the treatment that Still would espouse and teach. In 1892 he created the American School of Osteopathy at Kirksville, Missouri.

Not long afterward, Daniel David Palmer, a grocer who was also a magnetic healer, used manual thrusting movements to move the thoracic vertebrae of Harvey Lillard, a janitor. Palmer's maneuver restored the hearing that Lillard had lost seventeen years before, and provided the basis for a new profession, which he named *chiropractic* (from the Greek *cheir*, "hand," and *praxis*, "practice" or "action"). Lillard's and future patients' problems were said to be the result of "subluxations," partial displacements of vertebrae from their normal positions. Palmer believed he could manipulate these displacements and thereby remove pressure from the nerves on which they impinged. Within two years, Palmer had founded a school, Palmer College, to teach his methods.

Over the years osteopathy and chiropractic have developed a variety of manipulative techniques. Though each profession works hard to distinguish its philosophy and approaches from the other's, there are many important similarities. Both believe that structural abnormalities in the spine and joints can produce functional problems and eventually disease by affecting the nerves and circulation that supply the internal organs as well as the musculoskeletal system. Both believe that reversing these structural abnormalities allows the body's natural healing forces to reassert themselves. Both have greatly augmented their founders' original approaches: High velocity, low amplitude thrusts now coexist with a variety of low force approaches and stretching and holding techniques which are designed to aid the body in gently restoring its own structural integrity. And both professions are still unsure about the origin of the disconcerting cracking or popping sounds that characterize many manipulative maneuvers: Are they produced by bones moving suddenly on bones, or by air being expressed from the mobilized joints?

Still, in spite of their obvious common ground, there are clear differences and enduring disagreements between chiropractors (D.C.'s) and osteopaths (D.O.'s). Even though many of the techniques seem quite similar and are in fact freely used by members of both professions as well as by M.D.'s like me, there are ongoing quarrels about which ones are more effective and which profession should be credited with their creation. Osteopaths tend to feel that chiropractors are undereducated, while chiropractors often feel that osteopaths are insufficiently trained in manipulation. Both groups are impatient with the manners of the other.

Osteopathy has maintained Dr. Still's uneasy and ambivalent connection to orthodox medicine. Though it long resisted biomedicine's drug therapies, it has come in the last forty years to make full use of them. Though it regards itself as an evolutionary advance on medicine—a more integrated and inclusive kind of practice, one that emphasizes primary care rather than specialization—it still sometimes sees itself as orthodox medicine's poor, less well-funded, less prestigious relative.

In fact, in the last thirty years osteopathy has done its best to emulate medicine and to obtain the status and prestige of its sister profession. Osteopathic schools have significantly raised their admission standards, and their curriculum is in most respects identical with conventional medical training. Manipulation, once the cornerstone of osteopathic practice, is now merely an adjunct to it, valued by some students but largely, sadly, ignored by the majority. Osteopaths have the same kinds of postgraduate residency training as M.D.'s—a year of internship in an osteopathic hospital is required, after which the osteopath can seek specialty training in either an osteopathic or a medical program. Graduates, like M.D.'s, are licensed to prescribe medication and do surgery. In some states—California is one—the osteopath is allowed to exchange his D.O. degree for an M.D. degree.

Chiropractic, like Palmer himself, developed entirely outside orthodox medicine, and its philosophy and practice are at variance with and in opposition to it. For many years M.D.'s viewed chiropractors as actual outlaws and often instigated criminal prosecutions—for "practicing medicine without a license"—against them. Palmer was the first to be jailed, but many others, perhaps thousands, followed. As late as 1971 the American Medical Association's "Committee on Quackery" declared that its "primary mission" was "first, the containment of chiropractic, and, ultimately, the elimination of chiropractic." And until a 1991 court decision (*Wilk et al. v. the American Medical Association*) compelled an end to the practice, physicians who referred patients to chiropractors did so on pain of censure—or worse—by their own medical societies.

Working outside and in defiance of the medical establishment, chiropractors learned to mobilize political constituencies as well as displaced vertebrae. They developed a much stronger and more insistent focus on the power of spinal manipulation to treat illness and improve health than did osteopaths. Early in chiropractic's history, however, conflicts arose between those who used only manipulation, the "straights," and those who combined it with a variety of other dietary and physical therapies, "the mixers."

For a number of years, the chiropractic course of study was less rigorously scientific than both medical and osteopathic education. In recent years that gap has closed. The chiropractic basic science curriculum (anatomy, physiology, and so on) is currently similar to that of medicine and osteopathy. Their clinical training is still, however, quite different.

Chiropractors now rarely train in hospitals (large numbers of them once did), and they are not licensed to prescribe drugs or perform surgery. For contemporary chiropractors, manipulation continues to be not one technique among many but the cornerstone of their therapeutic approach. Their education, which gives them far more instruction in manipulation than even osteopathic students ordinarily receive, reflects this emphasis. Though some struggles between straights and mixers persist, most recent graduates combine manipulation with a variety of other nonpharmacological remedies—including nutritional supplements, herbs, acupuncture, and massage.

Though osteopathic manipulation and chiropractic have always been appreciated by significant sectors of the population, manipulation has been consistently ignored or scorned by all but a few orthodox M.D.'s. The reasons for this schism between medicine and manipulation are not altogether clear. It undoubtedly had something to do with the rebellious origins and independent development of osteopathy and chiropractic, as well as with medicine's economic self-interest and its insistence on being the final arbiter of what is correct and proper in the healing arts. It was in part a result of the paucity of credible research in osteopathy and chiropractic, a lack that was perpetuated by medicine's control of research funding. It was also, however, a product of class distinctions and snobbery, and of a dogmatism that gives me pause every time I hear medical orthodoxy make unequivocal statements about any unconventional therapy.

Chiropractors, at least until very recently, usually occupied a lower social status than M.D.'s. They were often, like Palmer himself, from the Midwest and its small towns. They usually had less formal education than their medical counterparts and were of a practical rather than an abstract or intellectual cast of mind. Osteopaths also tended to be from middle America and sometimes had entered their training after having been denied admission to medical school. Chiropractic was hence labeled by medicine, and by the segments of public opinion that medicine shaped, as a fringe practice, maybe even a kind of unsubstantiated folk belief. Osteopathy, preoccupied with assimilation and unsure of its status, was stigmatized as a "second-best" medicine, its distinct manipulative practices ignored or dismissed.

Perhaps these prejudices, together with the unwillingness of medicine to cede a portion of the economic or theoretical pie to any rival profession or technique, help explain why manipulation, its theoretical implications, and its remarkable therapeutic results were so long ignored by the majority of the American people.

Orthodox physicians were, and often still are, taught that the vertebrae and the bones that make up the skull do not move, except under extreme and pathological conditions. We learned, too, that only those findings that were visible on the kinds of X rays we were taught to order were real.

So, like some tribe that is conditioned to see only a certain range of the visible spectrum, we were simply unable to see or feel what is obvious to any unprejudiced observer, or to listen to the testimonies of chiropractic and osteopathic patients. Vertebrae that appear normal on our X rays may indeed be out of place. Manual adjustments may restore them to a more appropriate location and make those who experienced these "lesions" feel better. The bones of the skull do appear to exhibit subtle movement.

In recent years the testimonies of satisfied patients—as many as fifteen million people may visit the nation's 45,000 chiropractors each year—have been amplified by a number of laboratory and clinical research studies. Osteopathic researchers have demonstrated subtle rhythmic movements in the cranial bones of cats, while chiropractors have shown decreases in nerve conduction in patients who have been diagnosed as having subluxations.

Reports from both the chiropractic and osteopathic literature suggest that manipulation may relieve headaches, diminish chronic pain, and at least transiently decrease high blood pressure. Most importantly, there have been a number of impressive studies—in Canada, the United States, England, and

Holland—that demonstrate the effectiveness of manipulation in the treatment of low back pain. In many of these studies, chiropractic care has been shown to be far more effective and satisfying to patients than hospital outpatient care.

In the last several years the body of research on manipulation for low back pain has been gathered together and evaluated twice. Separate panels of M.D.'s, D.O.'s, and D.C.'s have reviewed the scientific literature—twenty controlled studies plus fifty more were surveyed for the RAND Corporation and an even larger number for the U.S. government's Agency for Health Care Policy and Research. These panels have come firmly and inescapably to the conclusion that, at least for low back pain, manipulation is a safe and effective treatment. My own experience doing manipulation over the last fifteen years confirms this conclusion. It also suggests that were the same kind of careful research done on such other conditions as neck and head pain, we might discover that manipulation has a much wider range of effectiveness.

I'm certainly not the best or the most experienced manipulator I've known—my training has come, sporadically, from Dr. Singha, Dr. Blood, and assorted osteopaths and chiropractors whom I've consulted and studied with over the years. Yet I've had results that are enormously gratifying to my patients and me. My success with low back pain is the most consistent, but I've also helped many people recover from long-standing, serious upper back pain, from whiplash injuries, frozen shoulders, and carpal tunnel syndrome.

I've seen remarkable changes in people who were suffering from horrible, debilitating migraine headaches for years— headaches that sent them whimpering to bed three, four, even seven times a week. These people have been diagnosed in leading medical centers and treated, unsuccessfully, with the latest drugs. After two or three manipulative treatments, some, though certainly not all, are virtually symptom-free. They stay that way, needing only occasional visits to readjust necks that tend under physical or emotional stress to turn and twist out of place.

Manipulation also produces the occasional miracle. One was set in motion the day when, five years ago, I received a call from Mrs. Nkomo, the wife of an African diplomat. For a month her eight-year-old son, Jacob, had been having terrible headaches. They began when he awoke and ended late in the evening, when he would suddenly and inexplicably fall down unconscious.

Jacob had been hospitalized twice. The first time was for a week. He had multiple X rays, CT scans, and electroencephalograms (EEGs) of every description. There were no fractures in his head or neck. The CT scans were normal. There were slight abnormalities in his brain waves, but they were not particularly distinctive.

Antiseizure medicines were prescribed, one after the other, then one with the other. They made Jacob drowsy and nervous but did nothing to decrease his pain or relieve the seizures. After two weeks back home, he was rehospitalized, retested. His mother was now told that he had narcolepsy, an illness in which people are suddenly overtaken by sleep. He was taken off the first set of medications and put on another.

Jacob's headaches and periods of unconsciousness continued. He became more and more baffled and fearful. His mother never left his side and often woke at night to make sure he was still breathing. At the suggestion of one of his neurologists, they moved into a hotel for a while to escape the paint fumes in the ambassadorial residence. The headaches and seizures continued. Jacob's hospital, doctor, and hotel bills mounted to $40,000.

One day while watching Jacob playing listlessly with another child, Mrs. Nkomo burst into tears. She told the woman on the bench next to her about Jacob's fits. The woman was a patient of mine and suggested she call me.

Jacob was holding his mother's hand and trembling when he entered my office. A thin, handsome boy, he carried his head at a slight angle. Dark skinned, he showed still darker circles under his eyes.

"What happened a month ago?" I asked.

"Nothing," he said with a slight British accent. "Everything was quite normal."

"What about a month or two before that?"

"Nothing really."

"A blow to the head? A fall?"

"No," he said. "Only one thing. I was hit with a ball, a softball, in the head. I wasn't looking."

"And what happened?"

"I had a headache afterward for a while, and it came and went."

"And then?"

"And then I started going unconscious. I haven't slept well for a month," he added. "I'm very frightened."

"Did you tell the doctors about being hit with the ball?"

"Oh, yes, surely, but they said it couldn't be connected."

I asked Jacob to take his shirt off and lie down on my table. His heartbeat was visible, shaking the ribs of his thin chest. He was trembling more now, smiling bravely at his mother, who was as scared as he.

"You've both been through a lot."

They nodded almost in unison. I asked Jacob to turn over and felt the vertebrae in his back—several on his thoracic spine protruded a little too far—and then to lie on his back once again. I moved my hands up to his neck. I felt as if I'd touched fire. The second cervical vertebra had shifted to the right - so far it made a visible bulge in the skin. The third vertebra was turned almost as far to the left. He winced, pulled away, and apologized. "Sorry. That hurt so much."

I touched him there again, unbelieving. "Didn't anyone ever feel his neck?" I said to myself, knowing even as I asked that no one had, or that if they had, their beliefs and their X rays had convinced them that they could not be feeling what they were. I thought about the medieval physicians who had believed Galen's description of the liver rather than their own eyes.

I put my hands on his thin neck and on his head and turned his head quickly, to bring the second vertebra back into position. A noise exploded from Jacob's neck, and his mother jumped, as if a shot had lifted her off her feet. I said something I hoped would be reassuring and repositioned my hands. Jacob smiled bravely. I turned his neck the other way to reposition the third vertebra. Again a loud crack.

Then Jacob was crying out: "My head doesn't hurt," he said in a sweet high voice. "My head doesn't hurt." He was smiling and looking up, as if to see where the pain had gone or maybe where help had come from. His mother was laughing and crying, and I was grinning with tears standing in my eyes—feeling so pleased for Jacob and his mother, so sad and angry at such unnecessary suffering.

Jacob's headaches and the seizures might have continued for years. More tests would have been done, and more medication prescribed. The whole structure of his life might have been warped by a condition that could easily have been treated by a pair of moderately well-educated hands. The problem was so simple, so straightforward when one was looking for it, but was completely invisible to those who weren't.

I told Jacob to take hot and cold showers—to relax the muscles and improve the circulation to his neck—asked his mother to call me the following day, and made an appointment for the end of the week.

When she called the next day, Jacob was fine. "He's reading his books again," she said, as if he had walked on water. When he picked up the phone, he told me proudly that he had "only a very mild headache and no spells." I asked Jacob's mother to discontinue his medicine.

When I saw Jacob three days later, he was feeling well, but his vertebrae were a little out of place. I adjusted them and we made an appointment for the following week.

I've continued to see Jacob in the five years since then, once a month for a year and then every two months or so. He had one very brief episode of headache and dizziness about eight months after our first visit. It seems to have been precipitated by a rough soccer game. I adjusted his neck that day, and he's never had another "spell" since.

HOMEOPATHY

Manipulation makes sense. Its absence in conventional Western medicine is anomalous, even aberrant, a by-product perhaps of our attachment to and dependence on technology, and our nervous avoidance of using our hands to help others' bodies. In spite of organized medical efforts to suppress its use and stigmatize its practitioners, it has flourished.

Homeopathy is, as they say, something else again. Where manipulation had always been an integral part of healing systems, homeopathy arose full-blown in the early nineteenth century from the mind and practice of a single German physician, Samuel Hahnemann. Though it draws on the ancient doctrine of similars—the belief that "like cures like"— and resembles vaccination in some respects, its use of minute doses of those similars was, and is, utterly strange to the conventional medical and scientific mind.

Even if we don't know exactly what is popping and cracking when an osteopath or chiropractor works on us, we can make a pretty satisfying guess, and we can, in any event, see and feel the changes. It is above all concrete. Homeopathy, by contrast, is abstract, improbable, even mysterious. How can a substance that may no longer contain any molecules of its active ingredient—as is the case with many repeatedly diluted homeopathic remedies—possibly do what homeopathic remedies are supposed to do? And yet they can and do produce demonstrable physiological and clinical changes.

Hahnemann, like Still, was deeply dissatisfied with the orthodox medicine of his time. Though important advances were being made in pathologic anatomy and physiology and in the classification of disease states, treatment was still a crude and largely ineffective affair. Bloodletting and purging were widely used, as were toxic heavy metals such as mercury, often with disastrous consequences. Hahnemann was troubled enough by medicine's shortcomings to leave a successful practice and earn his living translating classical medical works into German.

While working on a book by the British physician William Cullen, he read that cinchona bark achieves its success against malaria because of its bitter and astringent properties. This made no sense to Hahnemann. He knew that cinchona was far less bitter than other substances that were quite ineffective against malaria. Why and how, he wondered, posing one of those open-ended questions that seem so often to pave the way for profound change, did cinchona work?

Hahnemann approached the matter as directly as he could. He ate the bark for several days and, much to his fascination, developed exactly the same pattern of periodic fever and chills, apathy and irritability, that characterize malaria itself. Hahnemann concluded that cinchona acted so successfully on malaria because of its "similarity" to the illness—because it could, in a normal person, produce the same set of physical and mental symptoms as the illness for which it was a treatment.

This "law of similars" is the first principle of homeopathic practice and the rationale for Hahnemann's famous "provings." Over the course of his lifetime he, his family, and his disciples ingested, or "proved," dozens of other substances, many quite toxic, and carefully recorded the symptoms they produced. These comprehensive and detailed "symptom pictures"—and the many more from later homeopathic provings—form the basis for the homeopathic *materia medica*. The homeopath's job, according to Hahnemann and his successors, is to take a detailed history—of mental predispositions and emotional reactions as well as physical manifestations—and to match the patient's unique symptom picture to the remedy whose proving most closely resembles it.

This process of matching constitutes the second of the three principles of homeopathy, the concept of the "single remedy." Hahnemann and the "classical homeopaths" who have most strictly followed his teachings believe that there is one remedy that particularly characterizes each person. This is their "constitutional remedy." It is often used at the beginning of treatment and may be repeated at later times.

As other illnesses occur, and other symptom pictures emerge, other remedies appropriate to these unique symptom pictures are also prescribed, one at a time.

The use of small or "micro" doses is the third of homeopathy's principles and the hardest for the Western scientific mind to grasp. Hahnemann was troubled by the toxic over-medication so common to his time and by the "aggravations" of symptoms that often followed even small doses of the medications he prescribed. Accordingly, he was concerned to prescribe no more than the necessary amount of his remedies. As he experimented, he discovered that smaller and smaller doses were effective.

Soon some of Hahnemann's followers were observing that the potency of homeopathic medications actually increased as they became more dilute. In fact, the most potent medications were those that were so dilute that it was highly unlikely that even a single molecule of the original remedy remained in the pill or liquid.

Hahnemann tried his remedies on people with a variety of illnesses, apparently with great success. Soon homeopathy's clinical achievements, its benign remedies, and its elegant conceptual system were arousing interest in Europe and America. Some physicians were attracted to the approach, and many prominent lay people—among them Nathaniel Hawthorne, Harriet Beecher Stowe, Henry Wadsworth Long-fellow, and William James sought out homeopathic treatment. The medical establishments in Europe and the United States were not pleased. They viewed homeopathy as both an ideological and an economic threat, and they lost no time in denouncing it as "unscientific," "cultish," and even "devilish."

In spite of this organized opposition, however, the practice of homeopathy spread. Like Hahnemann, his followers saw it as a less toxic alternative to the dangerous "heroic medicine" of the time. Besides, homeopathy appeared to work: during the Austrian cholera epidemic of 1831 and again in the American epidemic of 1849, those who were treated with homeopathic remedies seemed, according to surveys done at the time, far more likely to survive than those treated by conventional methods.

By the end of the nineteenth century, homeopathic medicine was a prominent feature in the medical landscape in Europe and the United States. In 1900, according to *Divided Legacy,* Harris Coulter's encyclopedic history of homeopathy, 10 percent of all American physicians called themselves homeopaths. They were trained in twenty-two homeopathic medical schools, practiced in more than a hundred homeopathic hospitals, published their studies in twenty-nine journals, and prescribed remedies that were dispensed by more than a thousand homeopathic pharmacies.

Homeopathy's ascendancy was soon halted by a combination of forces. The length of time required for homeopathic history-taking and prescribing discouraged some practitioners. Improvements in conventional medicine, particularly the abandonment of its most toxic remedies, made its practice more appealing. And powerful drug companies, which vigorously opposed their homeopathic competitors, weighed in against the upstart profession. The single most significant factor was the publication, in 1910, of the Flexner report.

This document, prepared by educator Abraham Flexner for the Carnegie Foundation, is regarded as a landmark in medical education and, indeed, in the maturation of the profession. Flexner assessed the laboratory and clinical facilities and faculties of all the American medical schools and made definitive judgments about which were and were not acceptable. He used as his measure the example of Johns Hopkins, with its rigorous academic standards, its impressive full-time faculty, and its devotion to research in the basic sciences.

From the point of view of most medical historians, the Flexner report established standards that promoted the rise of modern biomedicine and insured the demise of "inferior" institutions. Contemporary homeopaths, and later historians of homeopathy, saw it as the scourge of their independent profession and an elitist power grab.

The Flexner report generally gave low marks to homeopathic medical colleges. Most had only part-time faculties, and many were deemed to devote insufficient attention to the laboratory sciences. Their concern with homeopathic prescribing was not regarded as a substitute for more conventional pharmacological approaches. Because only graduates of institutions with high marks were permitted to sit for licensing exams, some homeopathic schools shifted their post-Flexner emphasis toward the basic sciences; homeopathic perspectives and prescribing suffered as assimilation proceeded. Other schools simply went under.

By 1923, the number of homeopathic medical schools had declined from twenty-two to two, and the U.S. branch of the profession was in eclipse. By 1950, all of the homeopathic medical colleges had closed. When I first began to investigate homeopathy twenty years later, there were probably fewer than a hundred practicing homeopathic physicians in the United States.

In the mid-1970s, as part of my search for more effective and less harmful therapeutic ways, I—and many of my equally curious colleagues—rediscovered homeopathy. It was certainly strange to our Western scientific eyes, but it was also, at least potentially, a nontoxic, inexpensive alternative to conventional medical therapies. It seemed holistic in its emphasis on understanding the mental, physical, and spiritual aspects of each person's condition and in its appreciation of individual differences and uniqueness.

Homeopathy was also curiously literary. Each symptom picture has a particular personality. The Sulphur type, that is, the person for whom sulphur is the appropriate constitutional remedy, is lean, hungry, disorderly, stooped, prone to skin problems and infections, and preoccupied by abstract concepts and occult concerns. Homeopaths nickname him or her "the ragged philosopher." The Rhus Toxicodendron (poison ivy) picture is of a depressed, restless, fearful person, a man or woman with stiff joints, headaches, and chronic skin problems, slow to start in the morning and better with movement and as the day passes. For me, it was fun to think about and imagine or remember these people—a couple of men I used to run into late at night in Cambridge bookstores were certainly Sulphur types. And it was fun and, so far as I could tell, quite safe to experiment with low-potency homeopathic remedies.

Once I understood the basic principles, I had only two questions about homeopathy, but they were big ones: Does it work? and how could it possibly work?

The answer to the first, at least at this time, is "apparently" and "probably." Every experienced homeopath has stories of someone who was utterly changed, physically and mentally, by a minute dose of the single appropriate remedy. And on occasion I have felt a subtle but real, though not long-lived, shift in the way I feel after a single dose of a carefully chosen substance. But there are not, so far as I know, any really good scientific studies on the efficacy of constitutional prescribing. On the other hand, there is a substantial body of rather well-done research on the use of homeopathic remedies to address specific symptoms, biological reactions, and disease states.

This kind of isolation of a specific symptom from the total picture—prescribing Rhus toxicodendron for the pain and swelling of fibrositis—would undoubtedly be distressing to Hahnemann were he here to observe it. Nor would he like the use of a combination of eight remedies to treat varicose veins. But these two examples of recently published studies are helping to provide the data that demonstrates the effectiveness of the medicine he created. The study on Rhus tox, which was published in the *British Medical Journal,* showed a significant decrease in painful and inflamed areas quickly following the medication. The German work on varicose veins demonstrated that patients who received the homeopathic remedies improved by 44 percent while those who were given placebos actually got worse by 18 percent

Similarly well-done studies on other remedies have demonstrated the effectiveness of Oscillococcinum (a dilution of duck's heart and liver) in treating flu; Arnica (a common root known as leopardsbane) and Hypericum (the very same Saint-John's-wort that is useful as an herbal treatment for depression) in decreasing postextraction dental pain; microdoses of a combination of pollens in relieving hay fever; Arnica, Rhus tox and Bryonia (or common hops) in diminishing the symptoms of rheumatoid arthritis; and most recently, a selection of remedies in decreasing the severity of children's diarrhea.

Research has also shown similar results on animals—Caulophyllum (blue cohosh), for example, has significantly lowered the rate of stillbirths in a strain of pigs prone to them. In addition, carefully controlled laboratory investigations have revealed that homeopathic remedies can inhibit viral growth and stimulate enzymatic and immune activity.

Taken together, this work has gone a long way to legitimizing homeopathic prescribing and has encouraged health food stores and pharmacies to fill their shelves with easy-to-use, low-potency combination remedies keyed to particular symptoms or diagnostic categories.

My own experience with homeopathic remedies is mixed. Sometimes the combination remedies work rather well with adults; sometimes they work for a while, then seem to lose their effectiveness; and sometimes they don't even touch the symptoms. On the other hand, I have been enormously impressed by the power of homeopathic remedies in treating children.

My most dramatic successes have been with children with chronic middle ear infections (otitis media). These kids—I've had four in my practice—each had had four to six bouts of otitis media a year for several years, and their pediatricians had put them on every antibiotic known to be remotely effective. Their mothers were desperate, and all the kids seemed to be getting progressively worse.

In each instance I selected the remedy according to rather simple homeopathic criteria—Pulsatilla (windflower) for the whiny, clingy child; Chamomila for the angry demanding one; and Belladonna (a poison in large doses) for the kid with a high fever and a red face. In three out of four of these cases, the child, parents, and I were rewarded with a remarkable cure: no more ear infections. Now, it's true that I restricted the children's milk and milk products and occasionally some other foods, but none of these dietary changes had ever before produced such remarkable results.

These and similar results—I have seen flus stopped in their tracks, vicious migraines abate, prolonged menstrual periods abruptly end, and hay fever symptoms all but disappear— have been absolutely necessary to convince me to continue to learn about and use homeopathy. This is because even after many years of experience and careful reading of the best scientific studies, it is still so hard for me to actually believe that it works; and because we are still groping so tentatively to figure out why it works.

Still, though I'm skeptical, I'm excited about the possibilities of homeopathy. At low potencies the remedies are utterly nontoxic. They're easy to learn to use, for ordinary people as well as physicians. They're quite cheap—only a small fraction of the cost of conventional drugs for the same conditions— and finally, and most important, they often do work.

I've also been stimulated by speculation about their mode of action. Maybe the remedies resonate with the body's electromagnetic field and somehow "dissolve" the patterns of illness that manifest in that field. Maybe they leave a kind of electromagnetic memory trace in the water in which they've been diluted; perhaps their extreme dilution enables them to cross the usually impenetrable blood-brain barrier and enter the smallest structures within each cell.

These theories, and preliminary experiments performed to validate them, offer not only possible explanations for the improbable success of homeopathic substances but new ways of understanding how mind and body are integrated and how other therapeutic approaches may "work." Mind and body may well be two aspects of a common electromagnetic field. Acupuncture, like homeopathy, may exert its effects by altering that field, and so too may laying-on-of-hands, the practice in which one person with a healing intention gently touches another. Indeed, this concept of a field that is susceptible to subtle influences hints at an explanation for the ways all our interactions—our words, our attitudes, and even our thoughts—may influence each other's physical and emotional states.

CHINESE MEDICINE

To appreciate musculoskeletal manipulation, we must expand our notions of what can be done to and with the physical body. To use homeopathy, we must open ourselves, at least provisionally, to the realm of the improbable. To begin to understand the power and utility of Chinese medicine, a system that is twenty-five hundred, perhaps five thousand years old, we must enter a whole new world. The laws and measurements are different, the language is strange. Substances that are so far invisible and unmeasurable are said to interact with and govern the visible, palpable world. The organs we know so well from our anatomy and physiology books are not, we are told, what we have come to believe them to be.

In Western medicine there is one pulse; we time its rate and check if it is strong and regular. In Chinese medicine that same pulse, palpated on the radial arteries at the wrists, resolves itself into a dozen parts—or according to some variations, far more—each revealing facts about physical and mental functioning that are unavailable to even the most sophisticated Western diagnostic methods.

Moving back and forth from Western medicine to Chinese medicine is a bit like journeying from a modern industrialized city to an ancient and elegant rural world, or like staring at one of those drawings in a Gestalt psychology text. Look at it one way, and it is clearly a gray vase against a white background; allow your eyes to move out of focus, and it is, just as clearly, two white faces gazing at each other across a patch of gray. A single discrete diagnostic entity in Western medicine—a migraine headache or a stomach ulcer—may, when observed through the eyes of Chinese medicine, reflect half a dozen distinct processes. Conversely, one Chinese category—say, "qi deficiency"—may be implicated in conditions as varied as diarrhea, depression, and vaginal prolapse.

I fell in love with Chinese medicine twenty-five years ago, drawn for reasons I am still not sure I totally understand. My mid-1960s contact with macrobiotics and its founder had piqued my interest. I had felt light and alert after eating those straightforward, delicious meals, and as a critical and curious medical student, I had been attracted by the possibility of another conceptual system, so different from our own, that could help and make healing happen.

A few years later, I found myself fascinated by the medical and political possibilities of the Communist revolution in China. Here was a people—this was long before the terrifying truth of the Cultural Revolution emerged in the West—who were committed to making health care available to all and to enabling ordinary people to learn to care for themselves and educate others.

The Chinese understood, as I was beginning to, how powerfully social structures and attitudes could affect our outlook and our health. They were creating changes, in the hospital, the clinic, and the countryside that made it possible for doctors and patients to relate as equals. They were insisting on attitudes that would give more dignity to patients and imbue doctors with more respect for those they cared for and for those whose labor made their work possible.

I enjoyed reading about the peasants who learned to be "barefoot doctors," bringing combinations of Western and traditional Chinese care to their remote communities; about hospital administrators and chiefs of medicine who were, in an effort to make the medical profession more egalitarian, compelled to spend a day a week sweeping floors and cleaning toilets; about patients going on ward rounds with doctors and nurses, confidently questioning insensitive treatment and arrogant words.

I was also, by 1971, beginning to get interested in acupuncture. I didn't like our conventional ways of dealing with the biological aspect of psychiatric problems—the antidepressants and tranquilizers always seemed to have more harmful "side effects" than anyone, except the patients who took them, wanted to acknowledge. I had begun to hope that maybe acupuncture would offer another, "nonharmful," way to improve biological functioning.

Certainly the reports coming out of China were exciting. First there was that famous front-page article by columnist James Reston in *The New York Times,* in which he described how acupuncture had relieved his pain after an emergency appendectomy. Then there were the pictures of Chinese surgical patients, slim needles in their limbs, sipping tea while surgeons probed their open chests. Soon I was looking at reports in the English-language *Peking Review* on the successful acupuncture treatment of "deaf-mutes" and people with arthritis and asthma.

I felt the ground shifting slightly under my feet as I raced through digests of these studies. What I was reading seemed so improbable from the point of view of Western medicine: children deaf from birth or early childhood who were hearing again, people crippled with arthritis who could walk, and asthmatics who were abandoning medication on which they had long depended. The methodological flaws gave me pause—these studies were not based on comparisons with "control" groups of patients who didn't receive acupuncture. The possibility that all this was the result of a placebo response was never far from my skeptical mind.

On the other hand, I could understand that the Chinese, with a billion souls to succor, didn't have the luxury to use more careful methodologies. Unless I labeled the whole enterprise as fraudulent, I had to be impressed with the numbers—often thousands of patients in a single study—and the results. The placebo problem concerned me longer—until I read a study on the successful treatment of laminitis (inflammation of the hooves) in oxen. Oxen, I knew from personal acquaintance, were unlikely to be much influenced by the acupuncturist's belief in the power of his needles. Even allowing for poor study design and some exaggeration, something positive and promising and quite mysterious to me was clearly going on.

By the time I met Dr. Singha in 1973, I was ready to find out more. Other Americans who were becoming interested in acupuncture journeyed to China, Japan, or Macao or studied in Europe, where interest in acupuncture had persisted since the Jesuits returned with knowledge of it from seventeenth-century Asia. I meanwhile followed Dr. Singha—who had spent several years in the schools and monasteries of China and Japan—as he led me into the mysteries of the Chinese way.

In the more than twenty years since then, I've had ample opportunity to organize my thoughts, to compare his often cryptic comments with the classic texts and the dozens of commentaries that are now available. Principles I couldn't take on faith have become part of my worldview, and many statements I initially mistrusted have been borne out by my own clinical practice and the dozens of careful scientific studies that have appeared since then.

The world of Chinese medicine is indissolubly connected to the larger world we live in. The principles according to which our bodies and minds move and maintain their balance are the same as those that govern the form and function of the natural world. Our changes reflect and depend on the changes in that world. We live, when we are healthy, in and according to the Tao, "the way." It is like a river, flowing, ever changing, ever new. And it is, as Lao-tzu, its great sage and poet, wrote, also impossible to define: "The way that can be described is not the way." Definition, or even its attempt, removes us from the flow. Experience, made possible by our hands and eyes and heart, opens us to it.

The Tao expresses itself in the world in polarities that are complementary. The Chinese call them yin and yang. *Yin* means "the shady side of the hill." It is feminine, damp, dark, slow, deep, and down. *Yang,* "the sunny side of the hill," is masculine, dry, bright, quick, superficial, and up. Everything on our planet, our entire universe, including the organs in our body, the pathogens that afflict us, and the moods we experience, may be described as either yin or yang. Yang diseases are usually acute and are characterized by fever, sweating, constipation, a dry mouth, dark urine, heavy breathing, a rapid pulse, and irritability. People suffering from yin conditions feel chilly and have loose bowels, shallow breathing, a slow pulse, and a feeling of lethargy. These conditions are usually chronic.

Yin and yang are not, however, static. Yin becomes yang, as the night gives way to the day, and yang in turn becomes yin, as the light yields to the dark. Each contains the other within it, just as each half of the famous black and white yin-yang symbol contains a small circle of the other's color: the first glimmerings of dawn are there in the darkest night, the shades of evening immanent in the midafternoon sunlight; the soft marrow is at the center of the hard bone; the strong closed form of the fist opens to reveal the soft emptiness of the palm; and the acute injury gives way to the chronic nagging pain. Each of the polarities is defined in relation to the other: five o'clock in the afternoon is yang in relation to seven at night, but yin when compared with high noon; the chest is yang in relation to the abdomen, yin to the head's yang.

Human beings are a field in which the eternal play of yin and yang takes place. We are also, simultaneously, and in the kind of paradox that is so prevalent in the Chinese worldview, mediators between the heavenly destiny that is yang and the earthly nature that is yin. Other perspectives, including our own Judeo-Christian tradition and the Western science that arose in it, tend to split the heavenly from the earthly and the realm of mind and spirit from matter. We approach the former through faith, the latter by scientific analysis. The Chinese and the medicine they fashioned see man as the cauldron in which spirit and matter, aspiration and limitation, are mixed.

The Chinese way of knowing is not primarily analytic. The verb *to know* is constructed of characters that represent both "the Tao" and "to know." To know is to know the Tao, and knowing comes through living in and through the Tao.

The first Chinese physicians were monks. They lived in a pastoral world, alert to the ebb and flow of nature. They practiced meditation, going within to experience the energy, the qi, that animated all the processes in their minds and bodies. They came, so far as I am able to tell, to know the bodies they lived in not primarily by dissection of the dead or experimentation on the living but through introspection and observation. They felt, in the stillness of long hours of undisturbed sitting and quiet walking, of simple work and attentive eating, the functioning of their organs and the ways they affected one another. And they came to sense the subtle connections between the organs in their bodies and the times of day, the seasons of the year, the colors of the spectrum, and the plants and animals among which they lived.

The Chinese medicine I am learning and practicing comes from the experience, several thousand years ago, of these adepts and from the refinements made by all the generations of their students since then. It is based on a system of substances, influences, and categories that is not easily accessible to contemporary Westerners but that would have been quite comprehensible to Hippocratic or Galenic physicians who used the language of "humors" and "airs" and character types, of "pneuma" or spirit, and "psyche" or soul.

There are, the Chinese tell us, "three treasures"—shen (mind or spirit), qi (energy), and jing (essence). Though these three are the "fundamental" substances of life, qi is regarded as the most basic, the one of which the others arᵉ manifestations. The written character for qi suggests its dynamic capacity for change; it includes the characters for "uncooked rice" and for "steam"—for a solid substance, the vapor that its cooking produces, and the process of transformation that produces the vapor.

Qi is "the root of a human being." It is the refined energy that nourishes the body and mind, as well as the dynamic functioning of all the organs. It circulates constantly, through the lines on the body, the "meridians" on which the acupuncture points lie, energizing the organs in turn. It is also the nutrition that is extracted from food, the process of nourishing the internal organs, and the force that propels the blood and animates the lungs. And qi is the shield that protects the person against adverse climates, microorganisms, and stress.

Jing is the essence. In its "pre-heaven" manifestation it is the precious substance that nourishes the embryo during pregnancy and helps sustain the organism throughout life. In its "post-heaven" form it is extracted from food and stored largely in the kidneys, where it is said to sustain growth, development, and reproduction. It nourishes the mind and protects the body. Jing and qi are the material foundation of the more subtle and refined shen, or spirit. The spirit depends on them and will flourish if they are healthy and abundant; it will decline if they are not.

In addition to these three, the Chinese describe two other vital substances, blood and moisture, or bodily fluids. Blood, regarded as a dense form of qi, flows with it throughout the body, nourishing organs. Both blood and bodily fluids are extracted from food. The fluids are repeatedly purified and transformed into urine, sweat, saliva, and all of the body's other lubricants and secretions, and these in turn lend the tissues their suppleness.

The body's organs—the heart, lungs, liver, kidney, and so on—are both the source of the vital substances and the sites at which they act. The Chinese regard these organs as like and yet different from the organs we see when we open our anatomy books. They partake of something larger, a fundamental category of experience variously called a "phase" or "element," in which they are linked to specific emotions, times of day, seasons, colors, tastes, sounds, and the like. There are five of these elements—wood, fire, earth, metal, and water. Each element nourishes the one that succeeds it, as wood feeds fire, or as the mother feeds the child, and each governs or controls another element. Fire, for example, controls metal.

Each element has its own particular picture. Metal, for example, is the element of fall. Its emotions are apprehension and sorrow; its qi is highest between the hours of three and seven in the morning, when the associated organs, the lungs and colon, are said to be functioning at their maximum strength. Metal "types" tend to restrict their emotions and suffer when events elude their control. Metal is the mother of water (water condenses on metal), and it controls (cuts) wood. Asthma is often (though not always) a "metal" condition, as are irritable bowel syndrome, colitis, and anxiety. The skin is connected to the metal element, and its ailments reflect imbalances in the metal organs: constipation or poor breathing patterns may contribute to acne or eczema.

The Chinese physician assesses the state of the fundamental substances and the vitality of the organs by carefully listening to, observing, and touching his patient. The voice tells one story—the metal type, or the person with a metal ailment, speaks with a crying sound. The shape and color of the various parts of the face and the smell of the body give other information.

According to the Chinese, each part of the body is a microcosm of the whole, a map on which the signs of imbalance and illness may be read. The tongue, barely noticed now in the West, offers a window on the body's recent functioning and long-standing problems. Its size, shape, fissures, furrows, coats, textures, and colors and its degree of moistness and dryness yield data about which substance and organ may be malfunctioning. The lungs, which sit in the chest, are read toward the front of the tongue, while the functioning of the colon and kidneys, which are lower in the body, can be determined by the appearance of the root of the tongue.

Areas of tenderness and tightness in the belly, sounds, discolorations, and hollows there, will yield other clues about blockages in the flow of qi, blood, and moisture. The pulses, the most subtle and complex of the diagnostic guides, will fill in the gaps, telling the skilled practitioner—by their size and contours, their solidity, tension, or hollowness—not only which organ and substance is disordered but what illnesses have and may in the future afflict the patient.

Years ago, when Dr. Singha suggested that the lung is the "mother" of the kidney and that somehow the kidney is connected to the back, I was incredulous. But today words and concepts like these have become as much a part of my vocabulary as the stages of embryonic and fetal growth or the physiology of the fight-or-flight response. I look at the coating of the tongue—if the illness is hot and acute, it is likely to be yellow; if cold and chronic, then white—and check for the tight lumpiness of qi and blood stagnation in my patient's belly as attentively as I might listen for a murmur in her heart or feel for enlargement of her liver. I ask questions that arise in both the Western and the Eastern halves of my mind. I see and hear with Chinese as well as American eyes and ears, and I record what I have learned in such a way that, most often, each set of information enlarges and enriches the other.

It is satisfying to know from the trembling tongue that qi is depleted; or to see, in the dark circles under a man's eyes, a weakness in his kidney long before it shows up in the lab values; or to feel in the pattern of the pulses the "empty heart fire" of the depressed and anxious ex-addict. It is useful as well. Once I know this information, I can find the combination of acupuncture points that are most likely to make a difference. When all is going well, I feel like I am composing a melody or improvising a solo. The needles, like the jazz musician's notes and chords, seem to find their own way.

As the years have gone by, I've begun to make use of other aspects of Chinese medicine as well. I work now with some of the thousands of herbs, minerals, and animal substances of the Chinese pharmacopeia and am deeply impressed by the sophistication of the system that determines their use. Some herbs produce heat, others cool; some tonify qi, others disperse it, and each has a particular affinity for specific organs. With David Donne, for example, I prescribed a combination of herbs designed to dispel dampness and wind, to warm blood, and to tonify the qi, particularly in the kidney and spleen. Acupuncture redistributes the flow of qi and alters the functioning of all the vital substances and organs. Herbs, the deep treatments of Chinese internal medicine, nourish, balance, and sustain them.

The breathing exercises, movements, and visualizations of qi gong and its sister art t'ai chi work directly on qi, and have added another dimension for me and my patients. They energize asthma-weakened lungs, bring suppleness back to stiff limbs—my own injury-damaged knees bear mute but enthusiastic testimony—decrease stress, and improve our sense of balance and confidence within and in the world. After half an hour of qi gong or t'ai chi, most anyone will breathe more slowly and deeply, and feel lighter on her feet and clearer in her mind.

Chinese massage, tui na, along with other forms of hands-on therapy based on the system of acupuncture points and meridians perform similar functions. And the Chinese world-view—with its abiding appreciation for working with, not against, Nature's changes, for using all her bounty to help us regain harmony with our own nature—provides a wonderful and reassuring complement and counterpoint to the powerful interventions of Western medicine.

I would not rely on the Chinese approach if my blood pressure were so high that I might soon have a stroke, or if my system were overwhelmed by a bacterial infection, or if I were bleeding from an ulcer-ravaged large intestine. This is where Western medicine shines. But the Chinese approach can serve, over time, to establish a sound physiologica' basis for forestalling future episodes, and to help wean people like David Donne and Ty Collins from the drugs on which they have come to depend.

Chinese medicine can also work powerfully well in cases where our medicines are ineffective or are only of symptomatic use. David Donne's and Leslie Newman's cases are good examples, but there are dozens of others. In the course of a few weeks or months and without harmful side effects, I've used the Chinese approach to dry up the secretions of years-long asthma. I've seen it improve immune functioning in patients with AIDS and eliminate the hot flashes of a traumatic menopause. It can increase the energy and improve the overall well-being of cancer patients undergoing radiation and chemotherapy, settle the contractions of an irritable bowel, and restore long-flagging sexual interest and potency.

So far, medical research has not addressed itself to this kind of comprehensive therapeutic approach. This is unfortunate, because Chinese medicine is not just acupuncture or herbal therapy or dietary changes or qi gong but an integrated synthesis of all of them, in which each aspect works to augment the others. To be sure, we have not found conclusive support for some of the more dramatic claims—the regular restoration of hearing in deaf-mutes, for example—that emerged from China in the early 1970s. Still, we have begun, in our own careful way, in our laboratories and our clinics, to establish some of the means of action of acupuncture and to document the effectiveness of specific needling and herbal treatments.

The most consistent findings may provide a part of the scientific explanation for those remarkable pictures of tea-sipping surgical patients. Acupuncture points are areas of increased electrical conductance. They have higher concentrations of several different kinds of nerve fibers and a more abundant blood flow than the immediately surrounding tissue. Stimulation of these points alters the conduction of nerve fibers and produces a release of pain-reducing and mood-elevating peptides—endorphins, enkephalins, and serotonin—in various areas of the brain and throughout the body.

These changes in nerve conduction and brain chemistry are in turn presumed to be at least partly responsible for the surgical anesthesia and the powerful relief—of migraines, menstrual problems, and severe back and neck pain—that have been observed in clinical studies in United States as well as in Chinese hospitals and clinics. They are also likely the means by which acupuncture has enabled tens of thousands of addicts to detoxify from a variety of drugs, including heroin and cocaine, and have helped keep recovering alcoholics from resuming drinking.

This research doesn't, however, explain why and how acupuncture can alter the patterns of the EEG, or improve ease of breathing in some asthmatics, or stimulate the kidneys to work more efficiently, or augment immune functioning, or indeed, relieve inflammations in the hooves of oxen. We still don't know why and how specific points exercise particular and powerful effects on distant organs, or how each part of the body could be represented and read out on the surface of the tongue or at the radial artery.

Similarly, the research on herbs tells us that each has specific chemicals with specific effects. (For example, a number of mushrooms, including the shiitake and maitake varieties, that are traditionally used in the treatment of cancer and now have been introduced into AIDS therapies, have immune-enhancing properties.) It doesn't, however, begin to address the question of the correspondences between the Chinese theory of their action and the Western chemical analysis, or the reasons why apparently improbable combinations of herbs, minerals, and animal products may have the powerful, mutually enhancing, "synergistic" effects they do.

We are, in fact, just now beginning to grapple with questions like these. We are trying to find a way to comprehend a system that says that qi is the enlivening and modifiable force behind all of our body's and mind's activities; that the activity of each organ is somehow connected to the larger rhythms of the days and seasons; and that one organ may indeed be the mother of another.

While we are slowly groping toward some kind of common language and perspective, and planning and performing the next wave of scientific studies, ten thousand of us are practicing acupuncture in the United States. We are living out the next step in the evolution of Chinese medicine, working to find new and useful ways to marry ancient therapeutic wisdom and modern scientific medicine.

THIRTEEN

Helping One Another ∽

I'M PACING AROUND at the front of the big room, a
microphone in my hand, looking out at a hundred and
twenty people. Almost all their faces are black and tan.
Many are in their twenties and thirties, their bodies hard and
strong, their faces bright and clear; others are much older;
some are just teenagers. They all seem a little large for the
metal chairs they sit in.

Some of the people are dressed for office jobs. There are
a couple of Muslims in bow ties, but most everybody else is
in casual clothes. There are a few men and women, young
and old, who weigh too much. And there are two or three
very thin people, their faces blotched, their cheeks sucked
in behind mouths that seem irrevocably pursed. Eighty percent of the people or more in the room—no one requires
disclosure—are HIV positive, and a number have full-blown
AIDS. Almost everyone here has been an IV drug user, and
many have done time in prison.

Georgette, bobbing and weaving, her mini-dreds dancing
with her, has just introduced me: "And this is Dr. Gawden,"
she says, pronouncing it always in New Yorkese. "He comes

up here to give us our talk on holistic medicine and how we can take care of ourselves. He's a national expert on alternative medicine," she continues, with a proprietary pride that makes me feel proud too, "and he's the chairman of our board. So give him a hand. And"—a little menace here—"listen up."

I watch Theresa, a tall young brown-skinned woman who is watching me through the eye of her videocamera, and the words begin to form themselves. At some point I will talk about the power of exercise and meditation to improve the count of T cells, so important as an indicator of immune functioning in people who are "positive," and to increase the activity of phagocytes, those white blood cells that gobble up hostile invaders. I'll also go over some basic information about nutrition, and the new studies showing that acupuncture and Chinese herbs can also strengthen the immune system.

Tonight, however, it seems most important to remind the audience in front of me of how valuable and helpful they are and can be to themselves and to one another. I want to tell them that what they are doing for and with each other in this program for addicts and ex-prisoners is absolutely integral to the physical, emotional, and spiritual healing process for all of us, black or white, rich or poor, "positive" or "negative."

"Why are you here?" I ask. "I mean, what made you sign up for this ARRIVE program?" Close to 90 percent of these people, many of whom didn't make it through high school before they went to prison or out on the street, will "graduate" with fewer than three absences, a better number than most colleges can claim. "What made you commit to coming down here, to the bottom of Manhattan, for three long evenings a week for eight weeks?"

The hands begin to go up, at first just a few, and then as each one is called on and shouts or mumbles an answer, more, till after five or ten minutes, it seems as if everyone wants to tell his reason. "To learn more about the virus." "To stay straight." "I heard you could get job training." "I heard you was good people." "Got to have good information." "My PO [parole officer] said I better"—laughter here. "I heard this was a spiritual program." "Talk to other people 'bout living with the virus." "Find a way to express yourself." "Be part of a support group."

"Yes," I say, "all those are good reasons, reasons to come and reasons to stay. That's what we're trying to do here—provide information, and help you stay straight and healthy, and give you the tools you need to find and keep a job and be a supportive community. That's why Howie"—my friend Howard Josepher, the ex-addict, "ex-offender," social worker who directs ARRIVE—"started the program." Years ago another kind of support group, a live-in therapeutic community for addicts, helped him turn his own life around. Now he's giving back what he got.

I'm feeling my energy buoyed by their attention, and it's helping me to find my theme—the need that all of us have, particularly when we are ill, for group support and its vast, still largely unexplored therapeutic potential. "In tribal societies," I begin, "healing was always a group thing as well as an individual one. Sure, for minor problems, a cold, a cut foot, a painful period, you'd just go to your granny or someone else's, and she'd know what to do." A lot of people nodding here, remembering, I know from past talks, their own grannies in the rural South or Puerto Rico or the Dominican Republic or the West Indies.

"But if something big happened—a life-threatening illness, or something chronic that wouldn't go away, or a long bad time of depression—then the official healer, the witch doctor or shaman or medicine man, would be called on. And he—or she, because of course women did this work too—would bring the whole family and often the whole tribe or village together.

"You see, their understanding—the understanding of all of our ancestors—was that illness, serious illness, didn't just happen in one body, the way our medicine says it does. They believed it was the result of something being out of balance between that person and the rest of the tribe, and that person and Nature, and that person and the gods. And the only way to bring the balance back to where it belonged was to get everybody together and to make right the things that were wrong.

"And the way this was done, and the way I've seen it still done in villages in the rain forest and among some of our North American Indians, is for people to get together and get honest with each other, in a safe place and in a special way.

"The proper prayers are said first, and the forces of Nature and the gods are asked to help. Then everybody knows that no matter what, they're a part of the group, and that the hard or embarrassing things, the confessions—about how they haven't done the work they should have, or whose wife they've been with—that these things will not only be accepted by the gods and by the people, but that saying them is part of the healing process. Somehow, repairing the connection to their society, the body politic, helps repair the damage to the body of any individual who's a part of that larger body.

"And the amazing thing is, it often works. People get better—and the tribe or village is a happier place afterward. And of course, we've forgotten this.

"What happens," I ask, bringing it back home now, "when you get sick, really sick, here in New York City?"

A black man in the front row, ponderous as an oak, elevates an arm as big around as my thigh. "You must be joking, man," he begins, his voice as deep as his body. "I walk into the hospital the other week, looking the way I do—however else could I look?" he adds, nodding at the appreciative laughter. "And I tell them I'm positive, that I've got the virus, and I've got a bad cough and fever, and that I'm concerned it might be pneumocystis pneumonia or TB, trying to explain and be helpful and let them know that even though I'm big and black, I ain't stupid. And I'm feelin' kind of dizzy anyway, so maybe I'm swayin' a little, but I swear they start backin' away, as if they sure I'm going to do something, maybe fall on them and crush them and bite them to death all at the same time. And finally they say okay, we admit you.

"Ain't no one around because it's Sunday. So I'm by myself till the next morning, and then there's this whole group of doctors and nurses and whatnot right beside my bed, and they talkin' 'bout me like I'm not even lyin' there, big as I am. After a while I ask a question, and it's like the bed spoke to them, they so surprised. Then it's 'Oh yes, Mr. Brown, your doctor will explain everything to you.' And I say, 'Pardon me, but who is my doctor, and why can't you tell me as long as you're here?' So they say they busy. Of course, it's the next day before anyone comes, and then he only says"—clearing his throat, and sounding like his voice has gone up into his nose— "'Oh yes, Mr. Brown, we surely will tell you what we know, just as soon as those tests come back.' And then scuttling away just as fast as his little legs can take him. Shee-it. Imagine what happen if I was really sick."

The place cracks up, so many people seeing themselves in Mr. Brown. Laughing together, they overcome for the moment the terrible isolation they have felt and no doubt, as HIV-positive poor people who shuttle in and out of the city's hospitals, expect to feel again and again.

Then the other stories come, about loneliness and anger on hospital wards, and in doctors' offices too, a sense of being wrenched out of one's world and isolated—"like a bug on a pin, man," as one young Puerto Rican guy puts it. Sure, they say, sometimes the doctors will talk to them straight and even, occasionally, to a relative or a lover, but it seems, even if occasionally kind, perfunctory. "It's like," one tired-looking young woman begins, "*you've* got the problem, or actually you *are* the problem, and we gon' put on our gloves and clean you on up and get you on out, like you was dirty or something." "Yes," a dozen voices chime in, heads nodding as if we were in church together. "That's the way it is."

I do not tell them then, though I could, that I hear the same kind of story several times a week in my private practice in Washington. Money helps, but it doesn't insulate anyone against the casual callousness, the condescension of a system that devotes far more attention to insurance forms and academic discussion than to patient care. And isn't *patient care* an interesting, doubly meaningful phrase?

For a moment I am thinking about my mother, a well-to-do New York lady, and the doctors' dismissal of her symptoms that they couldn't understand, and the barely concealed irritation of the staff at one of the city's premier hospitals, concerned only with her surgical wound and not with the frightened and wounded woman who'd just had the surgery.

My eye catches Theresa's behind the videocamera, and all the anger and sadness I felt listening to Mr. Brown and in the hospital with my mother really hits me. I'm remembering what Theresa told me not long before. "I was in Rikers," she began, naming one of New York City's grim prisons, trying to explain why it was so important for her to go back there now, to give information and support to the inmates, to bring the ARRIVE program to them.

"I was doing a state bit for drugging. I got to tell you it was hard, because a couple of years before that I was a corrections officer, right there at Rikers. So they kept me in isolation, because they said they were afraid some of the inmates might go after me. One day they called me down to the doctor's office, and he said 'You have AIDS, and here's your prescription for AZT, and here's your card.' Just like that. And then they took me back to my cell. And that's all I have to think about: I'm HIV positive, and I'm going to get AIDS, and I'm here in a jail cell by myself, and I'm going to die."

There are times in all our lives when we feel overwhelmed, confused, and isolated—by a disabling and frightening illness, or by a loss, or by a new experience, or by the recognition that it's time to make some kind of fundamental and as yet unknown change. It is then that support and community—being with people who are going through the same experience or have gone through it, people who can understand and accept you—can give courage and be especially healing.

This seems so obvious. For too many years, however, our medical system has ignored both the small world in which treatment is provided and the larger world in which we live—the forces in our lives that may promote health or contribute to illness. Because it has paid so little attention to everything outside the perimeter of diagnostic procedures and therapeutic regimens, it has also neglected the ways we can organize ourselves to help one another.

For the last thirty years, however, researchers have been accumulating facts and figures, scientific studies on "psychosocial factors in health and illness," that inform us of what we feel to be true—that we need each other. We are social creatures, sustained by support from our fellows, and devastated, biologically as well as psychologically, when that support is suddenly withdrawn or is chronically absent.

First of all, there's the anthropological and ecological data. Nothing in Nature lives in isolation. Every animal is connected by ties of need to others of its species and to the many other plants and animals among which it lives. We humans, perhaps more than all the other animals, need others to be with us and care for us. This is especially true during our infancy and early childhood, which are the longest and most helpless stages of any species on the planet. Yet we have ignored this fact of our collective evolutionary history as we've rushed to industrialize and urbanize our world.

Our not-so-distant forebears (and members of most present-day tribal societies) lived in multigenerational extended families, where aunts, uncles, and grandparents were no more than a shout away from children whom they helped to raise and guide, educate and protect. Here and now, in the United States, almost all of us live in small, historically unprecedented, two-generational groups that we call nuclear families, or alone with our children. Those of us who live totally by ourselves, in buildings where we hardly speak to other people—and in some cases do our best to avoid them—are in an even stranger situation. Nobody, except a few monks with a particular aptitude for solitude, has ever before lived this way.

Many of us, looking around for family and close friends, feel the strangeness of having to drive an hour to see someone we would love to pass the time with every day, of having to plan for months—playing phone tag, poring irritably over impossibly crowded appointment books—to see someone with whom we once shared meals and a room. My brother Andy, who's an anthropologist, tells me that if we were in Africa, where he loves to spend his time, we would live in the same compound of houses, cooking and sharing friends and children and animals, hanging out at lunch and at the end of the day. But he has tenure at a university in South Carolina, and my work is in Washington, and my mother, now widowed, and my other brother still live in New York.

Increasingly, we have come to understand that the social isolation that is an accepted part of modern urban life can be a cause of illness or at least a major contributing factor to it. The most dramatic studies are on people who have lost a husband or wife. Many of these couples have for years lived in nests empty of children, depending almost exclusively on each other for companionship and comfort. It should not be surprising, then, though it is certainly distressing, that the surviving partner is two to twelve times more likely to die in the year afterward than other people of the same age and social class.

It's not just the isolation of sudden loss that kills. It's also being alone and lonely. Surveys done in Alameda County, near San Francisco, in the 1970s showed that people who had friends and relatives around them died at half the rate—from all causes—of those who didn't. Women who were socially isolated were much more likely to die of cancer than those who had friends. And men who developed cancer died from it far sooner if they didn't live among a network of friends and family.

These findings have been repeatedly corroborated—in sociological studies of the health benefits of living in close-knit traditional communities, like the Italian-Americans in Roseto, Pennsylvania, whom I mentioned earlier; and in long-term surveys of patients of all ages. The conclusions are clear. Good social support supports us biologically. Its absence is dangerous to our health and contributes to our early death.

*   *   *

Most Americans have never heard of these studies, but they have certainly begun to feel the pain and discover the truth of these observations. In recent years people deprived of close-knit communities and extended families have created an incredible array of organizations to meet their needs for intimacy and support. Many of these groups have been formed to deal with common problems and shared diseases.

Alcoholics Anonymous, AA, and other twelve-step programs—so named for the twelve steps that alcoholics and others who are addicted to drugs, food, or dependent relationships take on the path to recovery—are probably the most popular and best-known support groups. There are more than 60,000 "meetings" or chapters worldwide, with as many as several million regular attendees. Each AA meeting is autonomous, and all are egalitarian—members take turns leading the meetings.

AA's success has encouraged the development of many other groups with a wide variety of approaches and structures. The support groups of the 70,000-member National Alliance for the Mentally Ill (NAMI), established in 1979, are organized and attended predominantly by parents of schizophrenics, but there is also a strong national organization that works closely with mental health clinicians and researchers. Professionals with an interest in particular illnesses have established and now lead groups for people with bowel disease, cancer, multiple sclerosis, and other conditions. Some psychotherapists have begun to specialize in group work with victims of child abuse and people who are bereaved. Some groups charge fees, and some, like AA and ARRIVE, are free.

The power of these groups to command allegiance and to offer emotional support is no longer in doubt—one study of a thousand battered women rated "women's groups" as far more helpful than doctors, nurses, and clergy. In recent years it has also become clear that these groups may contribute not only to emotional well-being but to physical change as well.

One of the largest of these programs is Stanford's Arthritis Self-Help Course; more than 120,000 people have completed its twelve-hour program (now offered across the country) of relaxation, nutrition, problem solving, and physician-patient communication. At the University of Massachusetts Medical Center, Jon Kabat-Zinn has created groups for people with chronic illness that offer a synthesis of discussion, mindfulness meditation practice, and instruction in hatha yoga. And at Harvard's Deaconess Hospital, Herbert Benson has developed classes in which education about particular conditions—chronic pain, hypertension, and infertility among them—is combined with relaxation therapies, physical exercise, and nutritional counseling.

Each of these programs has demonstrated significant physical as well as psychological benefits. Those who complete the Arthritis Self-Help Course have decreased pain and greater mobility. Chronic pain patients in Kabat-Zinn's program are less uncomfortable and use fewer medications, and those with chronic obstructive pulmonary disease experience fewer episodes of shortness of breath. People in Benson's groups have regularly lowered their pain levels, decreased their blood pressure, and—interestingly—significantly increased their fertility rate.

In the last few years two programs have presented particularly impressive documentation for the efficacy of group support even for people with potentially fatal illnesses: the ones organized by psychiatrist David Spiegel for women with metastatic (disseminated) breast cancer, and internist Dean Ornish's program for men and women with coronary heart disease.

In 1976 Spiegel, who is a professor of psychiatry at Stanford Medical School, created what he called "supportive/expressive" groups for these women. There were eighty-six in the study, all of whom received the best conventional medical treatment. Fifty of these women were also randomly assigned to one of the professionally led groups.

The support groups met for an hour and a half once a week for a year. The women in them had the chance to talk about their feelings about their cancer, to share their experiences in dealing with it and its treatment, and their fears of death.

They did some relaxation exercises and occasionally used self-hypnosis to control their pain and discomfort. Over time they came to care deeply about one another. They helped each other formulate questions for their doctors and sometimes even accompanied one another to appointments. When a group member died, they mourned together.

Spiegel expected that the experience of caring and sharing would help the women feel better, that the "quality" of their lives would improve. Indeed, his early studies showed that after the year of meetings, the women in the groups were "less anxious and depressed and were coping more effectively with their breast cancer."

A careful man and a skeptical scientist, Spiegel never imagined that these groups would have any effect on the cancer itself. However, ten years after the groups ended, when he followed up on his study, he found something quite remarkable: the women who had been in the support groups had lived *twice as long* as those who were not in the groups— an average of eighteen months longer. Spiegel was astonished. He analyzed and reanalyzed his data, but the results held and were published in the prestigious British medical journal *Lancet* in 1989.

Since then, another study has also suggested that support groups may significantly prolong the lives of cancer patients. Fawzy Fawzy, a researcher at UCLA, developed groups for people with malignant melanoma, a dangerous and often fatal cancer of the skin's pigment cells. The patients with melanomas met in small groups once a week for an hour and a half for only six weeks. They received some education about their disease, learned a few relaxation techniques, did some work on problem solving, and had a chance to share their concerns with one another.

Six months later, those who were in the groups had significantly better natural killer cell activity than those who received only conventional medical treatment. And six years later, group members had a far lower rate of tumor recurrence and a dramatically lower death rate.

Dean Ornish's work at San Francisco's Preventive Medicine Research Institute is, if anything, even more striking. Over the past ten years Ornish has demonstrated that a comprehensive group approach—which includes an extremely low-fat diet, aerobic exercise, smoking cessation, yoga, and meditation, as well as group support—can unclog plaque-narrowed coronary arteries.

Some of the people who originally came to Ornish's groups couldn't walk more than a couple of blocks—or in some instances, a couple of feet—without shortness of breath and chest pain. A number had their coronary arteries so narrowed that they were prime candidates for bypass surgery. Within weeks most were comfortably walking a mile or more.

The support groups met three times a week for a year. Many of the people in them had indulged in years of poor eating and sedentary stressed-out living. They went on very low-fat diets. They learned yoga and meditated. They prepared food and ate together. And once a week they met to share their concerns about their health and their lives.

The results, after a year, were remarkable. These people looked years younger and felt much better. Ornish's elegant scans show more blood flow coming to their hearts, while coronary arteries that were almost one hundred percent closed were now open enough to permit near normal functioning. By changing the way they ate and exercised and thought about their lives, by participating in a group that supported and sustained these changes, these men and women had actually reversed life-threatening heart disease.

I tell the people in the class at ARRIVE about these studies and suggest, just before class breaks, that the group support they are experiencing at ARRIVE may well be contributing as much to their health. Already there is some evidence, from Miami psychologist Michael Antoni, that a ten-week-long stress-management group can significantly increase the levels of helper T cells and natural killer cells in HIV-positive men.

Finally, I tell them about the common characteristics that George Solomon has identified in a group of people who have been HIV positive since at least 1979. These men all have a sense of responsibility for their own health, a feeling of meaningfulness and purpose in their lives, a good diet and exercise program, and an ability to communicate openly about their concerns. And, perhaps, most importantly, they all have strong, mutually supportive connections to other people who are HIV positive. The men and women in front of me nod in hopeful recognition. All these characteristics are highly valued and encouraged at ARRIVE.

After the break, even before the class has settled back into its chairs, a dozen hands are in the air. For forty minutes the questions come, measured, informed, very polite, but insistent. Many people want to know which herbs are most stimulating to the immune system. I focus on astragalus, ginseng, and aloe vera. Are antioxidants useful for those who are HIV positive? There is evidence that they are. Where can they find the best nutritionist or t'ai chi teacher?

Soon people get even more personal. Concerns about children fill the room: what do you do about asthma and hyperactivity and kids who wake up in the night crying because their father is dead and their mother is not feeling so good?

The atmosphere feels different now. It reminds me of the first meeting, several months before, of another support group. This one, at the Center for Mind-Body Medicine, was for health professionals who want to learn how to lead "mind-body skills groups"—for people with cancer, AIDS, and other life-threatening and chronic illnesses.

I had asked the nine women in the group to draw three pictures: of themselves; their "major problem"; and how they would be if the problem were solved. As each woman showed her drawing, commenting on it, the words became simpler and more direct.

The air then was quiet and receptive as Delia, a psychiatrist, held up what she had done: "This is me," she said. "I am all head and very strong, and here I am bombarded at work by paper I regard as garbage; and here I am, as I would like to be, head and body in proportion, dancing, flying, free." Then Leah, a social worker: "I thought I would draw my endometriosis, that's what I always say is the problem. And that's what's acceptable for a strong woman like me. Everybody knows how painful it can be. But what came out is my fear of being abandoned by my lover. Here he is leaving, and here I am crying and staring off after him. There, in the last picture, is how I want to be. I'm alone, standing firm on my own two big feet." So it goes around the circle, each person invited to explore and explain, revealing in pictures what she might well have censored in speech.

A similar process is taking place here at ARRIVE, with a hundred and twenty people. It is as if a layer of self-protectiveness—and self-protectiveness, evasion, and defensiveness are endemic on the street and in prison just as they are in the offices and homes of professionals in Washington, D.C.—has been removed and an unspoken invitation accepted.

"Is it true that positive thoughts really can affect the immune system?" asks a depressed-looking, middle-aged Hispanic woman. "Why is it doctors know so little about all these things we're interested in?" says a young black woman, as puzzled as she is put out. "Come to think of it, how come the things that we think are doing us good aren't covered by Medicaid and the things we're kind of suspicious of are?" And—this is a muscular young black man with jailhouse tattoos up to his elbows—"How come I haven't been able to cry since my mother died?" Finally, I am drawn back to where I began, to what I particularly want to talk about. "It feels good to be here, man," says the Puerto Rican who had felt like a "bug on a pin" in his doctor's office. "You know, asking questions like this and the sharing we do in our team meetings, and the way we tell each other about therapies that are doing us good. It's strange, man, but all these weird people"—his arm sweeps around to take them in—"they really do feel like family."

I take a deep breath. "I think that what happens is that at a certain time, usually only after we've been hit upside the head many times, when we see that whatever we've been doing isn't working, then by some miracle of exhaustion with all our struggles or God's grace or something, we're ready. Then at that point, if we really look around, openly and honestly, often enough there's something out there in the world: another person, or a book, or a program like this one, that's ready to help us make the change that everything in us has up to that very minute been resisting.

"I think that's what AA is saying when they talk about 'hitting bottom,' and that's what I see in the patients who come to see me and the ones who join our groups in Washington. They've tried every known conventional medical treatment and every kind of therapy, and they've experienced its limitations, and they want something more.

"At that point, if there's a group available, then it becomes possible to enter another world, to let go of the old ways and begin to feel your way into being the person you can be in that new group; to recover those parts you'd long ago stunted or stomped on or forgotten about.

"You come into a support group, and you see people who're just like you. In Washington in this group I'm leading now, it's professional women—nurses, social workers, psychologists, and doctors—who don't want to admit that they can't handle the illnesses in them and around them. These women have to be strong for everybody else and haven't been able to reach their hands out for help, even when they feel their bodies crumbling from the inside. They are so terribly jammed up emotionally and are hoping so hard to have the chance to let go.

"And here you are. You come to the first class, and you see people who were drugging and dealing and doing everything just as bad as you were, people who've got the virus just like you do, and the same fear that there won't be anything that will help, and the same desperate hope that just maybe this could make a difference.

"In Washington it's a circle of women letting go and sharing their pain and struggles, seeing that all of them have the same or similar issues, and admiring each other for dealing with them, and learning, to their surprise, that the others also admire them. Here at ARRIVE, it's realizing that the people in front of the room are just like you. And as you listen, you find yourself admiring them too. You feel more hopeful, because it's clear that what they've learned has made them stronger and more at ease and that this program, which you're now a part of, has something to do with it.

"In D.C., in that first meeting, we draw pictures of ourselves and our major problem and how it would be if that problem were solved. Everyone is hesitant and embarassed at first because they can't draw, and they live in a world that is intolerant of imperfection; and because they're used to being therapists and not patients. But then one person takes a chance, and the others take courage from her example.

"Here you get your start on intimacy in the first week when you play the 'name game.' Everybody introduces himself by giving a funny nickname. Like 'I'm Hot Howie'"—everybody is laughing now, remembering my friend, ARRIVE's fifty-five-year-old executive director, saying it. "And you see how funny it looks and sounds, kind of awkward and childlike. And you wonder, What is this shit? and what am I doing here? Then you do it, and it's like you've jumped over something and you're in a different place, and you look around, and there's everybody else, right along with you, just as silly and uncomfortable as you are. Here you are, a bunch of people who never belonged anywhere, and you start thinking, 'Maybe *this* is where I belong.'

"Then, in team meetings, you learn that you can ask for help and that other people are willing and able to give it. They may tell you which clinics have the best doctors and what therapies have worked for them and where you can go for good job counseling. You find too that it's okay to open up emotionally, and let out the angry, sad, frightened, or loving sides of yourself.

"I remember once in the group in Washington, Grace—a highly competent, always cheerful psychologist with terrible arthritis and migraines—telling us about her early years with her first husband. For twenty years she accommodated her every word and action to his needs. When the marriage fell apart, she closed her heart. She told us that everything we saw was a show and a protection, that inside she felt so alone, so incapable of asking for or receiving help or love. In that moment, in that vulnerability, all our love seemed to flow across the room to her.

"Little by little in these groups, we're able to strip away the defenses we no longer need. Then it's possible to let all the other parts of us get to know each other, to let them take their rightful place in us. It's possible in this soil to grow again, with support, like a vine held up by sticks.

"Not just any group will do, because some of them feel like places where you're held down, or you never get beyond listening to each other's misery. Other groups seem to exist only to keep you patched up. They just tell you to keep on doing what the doctor ordered. No, the kind of group I'm talking about is one that sees, and lets you see, what is deepest and truest and strongest, as well as ugliest and most scared in you, and says it's okay, then gives you concrete help and a chance to see who you can become and lets you have some practice being that person.

"I think it's so important too that this place is about learning—Howie calls it a 'learning community'—because that definition helps you to change how you see yourself; you're not an inmate or a patient or a client, not bad or sick or even a paying customer, but a student, someone who's learning. It's an empowering role, and a dignified one.

"That's the way our groups are in Washington, D.C. We call them educational too. Those of us who are leaders have learned the lessons that we're teaching, not just from books but in our own lives, and on our own bodies. We're still learning them. We're not different from you, the way it seems or is made out to be in most schools, but simply people who've been tackling the same questions, struggling a little longer to come up with answers.

"The people in the groups are students—not students of something abstract but students of exactly those things that are most important to them. The curriculum consists of information that will help them stay healthy and understand themselves better. These students—and we do these groups with high school kids and teachers, old folks and medical students, as well as people with chronic illness—learn about their minds and their feelings and their bodies. They learn how every aspect of life affects every other. Each gain that one person in the group makes is an inspiration to all of us. After Ann, a very tense social worker, was able to use biofeedback to control her migraines, then Grace, who thought she never could deal with hers, took heart and was able to do it too.

"Along the way another kind of learning takes place, because this isn't only about learning material that's valuable and healthy, or even learning that it's possible to learn and change, though that's vital too. This learning comes as we see that everyone in the group is both different from and like us and that both the similarities and the differences can teach us.

"Each of us is a mirror for the others. All those differences that we notice so easily and criticize so readily in others are actually reminders of parts of ourselves that we might not want to admit to. So when I find myself criticizing someone else's envy or getting angry at her self-pity, it's most likely because envy or self-pity is still an issue for me. When I begin to work these issues through somewhat, it turns out that I'm no longer so troubled by *her* envy or self-pity.

"It is as if the group has an incredible self-regulating, evolving intelligence, which uses each of its parts, each of us, to confront all of its other parts, all of us, with what we most need to learn."

Georgette is back in the room now, motioning to her wrist. There are fifteen minutes left, and it's time for a closing meditation.

I pause for a moment. "I think it's time," I begin, my head cocked, hamming it up, changing the pace a bit, as if the thought had come to me from the ether and not from the very visible Georgette, "for a closing meditation."

I ask everybody to stand and shake from the feet on up through the knees, into the pelvis and shoulders and head. "Shake that thing," I say, while they groan and laugh at my silliness and their own, encouraging them to get out the stiffness or the nervous energy that comes from being still for so long. Then everyone sits again, and I lead them in a quiet meditation, breathing slowly and deeply in and out, just as I do at the Center in Washington.

I go inside myself, breathing slowly, feeling my body rise and fall with the breath. In the stillness I feel connected to those others in front of me who are also going inside, as if the inside were a great welcoming room that all of us have entered together.

While I'm standing there breathing, I find myself in a reverie. What are the real possibilities, I wonder, of groups like this one, and like the ones we have at the Center? Every good group seems to be capable of enhancing its members' immune functioning and improving their mood and attitude. People in Dean Ornish's groups have reversed heart disease.

What if we intensified and extended the psychotherapeutic work we do and made much greater use of the mind's capacity to affect the body—not just through brief training in self-hypnosis or relaxation techniques but through intensive experience with biofeedback and hypnosis, and carefully individualized work with imagery? What about combining all of these with other aspects of the new medicine: breathing techniques, aerobic exercise, massage, disciplines like yoga and t'ai chi that mobilize the body to affect the mind, and nutrition and herbal therapies? Would the results be even better if we included family members in this work?

What if we really made full use of the kinds of group rituals, prayer, and atonement that are so integral a part of tribal healing and of programs like AA? What if we encouraged all those we helped to help others? What could we do if we really learned how to use and share the connection that we're all feeling now in this room, as a hundred and twenty of us breathe together, growing calmer and stronger?

FOURTEEN

The Healing Path ⤴

I N THE LAST THIRTY YEARS we have begun once again
to experience and explore the spiritual dimension of
health and healing. Long denied or suppressed in practice as well as in theory, it now insists on its rightful place
in medicine, as if it had, as indeed it seems to, a vital force
of its own.

In most tribal societies illness was (and still is) understood
as a spiritual as well as physical disorder, a sign of imbalance between the individual and the natural and spiritual
world, as well as within the individual. It was also regarded
as a signal, a "wake-up call," as well as a misfortune.

The healer would heed this call, interpret it for his patients,
and help them address and redress these imbalances. This
kind of understanding helped make illness comprehensible
to the patient and enabled him to give a larger meaning to
his suffering. It shaped the form and content of treatment.
It provided the basis of, and rationale for, future changes in
thinking, attitude, behavior, and functioning—a healing path.

The traditional medicines of the ancient Hebrews, of Classical Greece, China, and India, were similarly infused with

the spiritual. Health and illness were believed to be ultimately dependent on our harmony with forces greater than ourselves. These spiritual forces manifested in each of us as the "vital" element of our human functioning. To the Hebrews, spirit was *ruach*; in Hippocratic Greece, it was called *pneuma,* in China *qi* and *jing* and *shen,* and in India, *prana* and *shakti.*

Each culture also understood that this energy or life force was intimately connected with the breath, whose coming marked the beginning, whose end, the passing of life. *Ruach* is the Hebrew word for "breath" as well as "spirit"; *pneuma* is also the Greek word for "lungs." The same connection is preserved in English. When invigorated, we are animated; when we die, we "expire." The Chinese and Indian systems, in particular, developed elaborate breathing exercises to enliven the body and mind and to maintain the link between both of these and the spiritual dimension.

Christianity preserved and in some ways intensified this connection between the power of the spirit and the work of medicine. Jesus urged his disciples to demonstrate God's power and grace, as well as their own commitment to His service, through their healing work. He and they were said to have cured the lame, the blind, and the leprous simply by touching them.

In the centuries after Jesus's death, the organized Church institutionalized this mission. Health was most important because it enabled people to serve God more completely and effectively. Physical illness was understood as an emblem of sin. Priests and monks were trained as physicians. Their work was the restoration of the sinner to biological, mental, and spiritual health, to both wholeness and holiness. In time the Church established the first hospitals in the West.

In the late Middle Ages the Church renounced concern with the body and its illnesses and forbade its cloistered monks to study and practice medicine. Soon Cartesian science would provide the intellectual justification for severing the connection between the biological and the spiritual. From the seventeenth century on, illness was regarded as a purely physical phenomenon, subject to clear, if sometimes still undiscovered, laws of material cause and effect.

The scientific discoveries of the last three hundred years have continually amplified and reinforced this perspective. By the mid-twentieth century, the dominant biomedical perspective viewed illness as existing solely in the body of the sufferer. On occasion psychological factors were invoked as contributory. More often they were regarded as the consequence of the pain and suffering caused by the disease, or as themselves the product of a similar biological process. The spiritual dimension was considered irrelevant—"immaterial"—to the development and treatment of disease. Priests, ministers, and rabbis were welcome as visitors to the sickbed, but were actively summoned only when biomedicine had done its utmost and death, the realm to which the spiritual was largely relegated, seemed imminent.

All this has begun to change.

In the 1970s epidemiological researchers began to awaken from a long secular sleep. They noted the absence of concern with religion and spirituality in clinical studies, and began to examine and record correlations between "religiosity" and good health.

Some of the more impressive research has focused on the most obvious sign of religious commitment—regular attendance at religious functions. A number of studies have shown that simply going to a church or synagogue is correlated with a significantly decreased risk of developing cancer, hypertension, strokes, and colitis, as well as with a lower overall rate of mortality. Church attendance also seems to be a major factor in the prevention of drug and alcohol abuse and of adolescent suicide.

Clinical researchers have focused less on behavior and more on attitude, particularly on the power of belief to affect our biology and on the potency of prayer and spiritual healing in treating illness. Studies on the placebo effect (which I discussed in Chapter 8) have shown that our belief that a treatment, a pill, or a surgical technique may be useful, can indeed help us materially. They have reminded us that this capacity for belief—for faith and hope—that we usually regard as part of our religous life, is also a force for healing.

Recently studies on the effects of "distant healing" and "intercessory prayer" have brought other, far more provocative and controversial elements of the world's spiritual traditions back into the discussion of effective therapies and, at least potentially, within the compass of modern medicine. They suggest that the healing in which Jesus instructed his disciples might still be, two thousand years later, a vital component of health care.

There is a vast literature—some of it of as high a quality as any medical papers—that shows that we can, simply by intending to do so, make significant positive changes in the well-being of others and in nonhuman biological systems. It would appear that both men and women who are known for their "healing powers" as well as perfectly ordinary people are capable of accomplishing this.

Some of the early, carefully controlled research was done on "laying on of hands" by Bernard Grad, a biochemist, in the 1960s. Grad worked with a well-known healer named Estebany. In some of Grad's experiments, Estebany held mice that had been experimentally "wounded." The wounds of this group healed significantly faster than those of mice that were held by medical students or left alone. Next, Grad did a series of experiments in which Estebany "laid hands on" salt water, which was then given to sprouting barley seeds. The seeds that were given Estebany-treated water grew far faster and had higher yields than those fed untreated water. Later researchers devised similar experiments with Estebany and other healers that yielded similar results.

In the early 1970s Dolores Krieger, a professor of nursing at New York University, extended this line of research into the clinical setting. Initially she too worked with a gifted healer, but soon she became interested in whether ordinary nurses, like herself and her students, could achieve the same results. Over the years Krieger, her student Janet Quinn, and a number of other nurse-researchers have demonstrated that with a minimal amount of training in what Krieger calls *therapeutic touch,* nurses and others can be taught to have a positive healing effect on their patients. Study after study has shown that simply by relaxing and "intending" to help, then bringing their hands close to their patients' bodies, nurses can improve the mood and increase the level of the red blood cells' hemoglobin (taken to be a measure of general well-being) of hospitalized patients.

While these studies were going on, others sought to demonstrate that physical proximity isn't a necessary ingredient in healing. In dozens of experiments researchers like William Braud and Marilyn Schlitz demonstrated that people, both experienced and novice healers, could produce significant changes at a distance *simply by intending them.* They could alter another person's blood pressure and muscular activity, and affect such diverse biological proceses as the spatial orientation of fish, the locomotion of small mammals, and the rate of hemolysis (dissolution) of human red blood cells.

Others performed comparable clinical experiments on the power of "intercessory prayer." In the best known and so far most meticulously conducted, Randolph Byrd, a cardiologist at the University of California Medical Center, divided 393 patients (over a period of ten months) in a coronary care unit into two groups. One group was prayed for daily, the other received the same care but was not prayed for. Neither the patients, the intensive care unit doctors, nor the nurses knew who was being prayed for. The people doing the praying, the "intercessors," didn't know the patients but were given a slip of paper on which their first name and their condition were written. They were asked to pray for a rapid recovery and the prevention of complications and death.

The results, which were published in the *Southern Medical Journal,* were impressive. The patients who were prayed for had significantly fewer cardiac arrests and fewer episodes of congestive heart failure and pneumonia than those who weren't prayed for. They required antibiotics and fluid-draining diuretics much less often, and spent less time in the coronary care unit.

All of these studies, which are largely unknown to or ignored by mainstream medicine, have quite extraordinary implications for health and healing, as well as for our understanding of what it means to be human. They strongly suggest that there are forces above and beyond our physical condition, genetic makeup, and medical treatment that may have powerful positive effects on our well-being. Our capacity for faith and hope, our willingness to ask for help from another, nonmaterial, dimension, indeed our subtle connection to others who may be asking this spiritual world to aid us, can all help protect us from illness and produce very real improvements when we are sick.

This research, and the experience of clinicians who have been impressed by correlations betwen good mental attitude and clinical outcome, have formed the basis for a popular psycho-spiritual medical literature that has struck a deeply resonant chord. Books like Yale surgeon Bernie Siegel's *Love, Medicine and Miracles,* endocrinologist Deepak Chopra's *Quantum Healing* and *Ageless Body, Timeless Mind,* and internist Larry Dossey's *Healing Words* have become major best sellers. They add a spiritual leaven to a medical practice that is ponderously material; inspiration and buoyant hope where the medical establishment purveys only a cautious realism.

Siegel urges his readers to use their capacity for self-healing to become "exceptional" patients, determined and hopeful exceptions to the grim statistical picture, particularly for cancer, presented by most doctors. Chopra, drawing on a mix of modern physics, recent studies on healing, and the wisdom of Indian sages, writes that the mind can control the matter of the body. Dossey cites hundreds of studies on the power of prayer—of every kind and from every religious tradition—to create profound physical and psychological change.

These men, and others who have proclaimed similar possibilities, have been accused of glib and inappropriate use of statistics and physics; of arousing "false hopes"; and of placing blame for their illness on patients—"you're responsible for it and have failed if you don't recover," they are supposed to be saying.

In fact, they have brought to popular attention research that demonstrates the ways our attitudes and emotions can affect us. They have reminded us of the potential healing power of love and of strongly held belief, and the possibility of miracles—so far unexplained but not necessarily inexplicable cures. They have clearly provided, as physicians concerned with the spirit as well as the body and mind, a healing and inspirational presence. Many people tell me that these doctors and their books offer a complement to or a substitute for what they find lacking in their own physicians and their health care.

They help us understand that we are far more capable of change and physical reconstitution, even in the face of so-called "terminal" illness, than most of us realize. Each of them encourages us with some of the many thousands of carefully recorded cases of "spontaneous remission," instances where people with such terminal diagnoses as metastatic cancer have for reasons that no scientist has yet explained suddenly recovered. Each of them reminds us that we make a terrible mistake when we foreclose or diminish this possibility of remission by our attitudes about outcome or by too heavy a reliance on the statistics we are so fond of quoting.

For a person sick with cancer or AIDS or any other life-threatening illness, the most important question is not what percentage of people live and die in five years—the standard by which cancer and its therapies are usually evaluated. Their first question is or ought to be, How can I be one of those who survives? What can I do?

In too many medical offices realism has come to mean a grim sentence from a distant doctor, pronounced with an unearned and unjustified air of certainty. Some behave this way to forestall possible malpractice suits for "incomplete disclosure"; or in the name of the "reliable" statistics they have read. Some believe they are only reflecting years of clinical experience, while others are paralyzed by the prospect of possible or probable death. It's important for physicians to understand their motivations, and to transcend them; to recognize that their words and attitudes can be powerfully harmful or helpful. We owe it to our patients to acknowledge the gravity of their situation, yet still to come down firmly on the side of what may be possible; to address, revitalize, and mobilize their spirit, not ignore, trample on, and paralyze it.

All of us need to remember, also, that even when physical recovery is or seems impossible, the most profound kind of emotional, mental, and spiritual healing *is* possible. In fact, for all too many of us, it is only when we are up against the wall of our mortality, that we really address the changes we need to make. I've often heard it in my office—from people confronted by a diagnosis of cancer or Parkinson's disease or the devastation of a stroke—as well as from the HIV-positive people in the classes at ARRIVE: "Only now have I realized how precious life is, how much I want to clean up my act, take care of unfinished business, live, and be the way I really want to be."

In addition we need to remember to always be open to the possibility that out of the healing of our emotions and our relationships, of the lives it looks like we are soon losing, sometimes, for reasons no one can yet predict or explain, a genuine physical cure does happen.

Jane Archer is someone who has used illness to transform her life and has lived longer and better than any of her doctors expected. I first met her two years ago. David Donne had called to ask if I would see her. She was an old friend of his, a "really nice woman" who had breast cancer that had metastasized. He asked if I could please see her "soon." He was, he had to admit, concerned.

I've learned over the years to pay attention when someone whom I know and respect wants me to treat a friend or family member, when it comes from some deep sense that I'm the right person. Responding to these requests has become an article of faith for me. And so no matter how jammed my schedule or how long my waiting list or how unlikely the possibility that I may be able to help, I somehow manage to find the time. I don't think it's ever been a mistake.

The day Jane calls, I am able to find an opening in my schedule. If she will agree to meet with me during the time I'm teaching the fourth-year students at Georgetown, I tell her, I can see her next week. She very much wants to do that.

The tumor that was discovered in 1987 and treated with surgery, radiation, and chemotherapy has now metastasized to her lungs. Conventional medicine offers no hope for a cure and little in the way of slowing the cancer's progress. Her oncologist has prescribed tamoxifen, an estrogen antagonist, but this is at best only palliative, a stop gap. He knows nothing about the alternative therapies she asks about, except that he doesn't like them and doesn't want to hear about them. But now that conventional medicine has so little to offer, she needs to know if there is anything else she can do. She needs someone to help her sort out all the possibilities—the herbs and drugs and diets—she has read and heard about.

Students are no problem for Jane. The ones who examined her during her hospitalizations reminded her of her own children. She welcomes the opportunity to help young people who are going to be doctors to learn what it is like to be living with cancer and dealing with its treatment. She says this in a kind and matter-of-fact way, reminding me without saying it directly, that medical education often overwhelms students with techniques and details at the expense of ordinary human understanding.

A week later, Jane comes to the psychiatry department's conference room. She sits squarely in her chair, her handsome blond head inclined slightly, in the dark, quietly tailored suit and white blouse of the Washington matron. Her voice is even, all but accentless. There is about her a stillness that I mistake for stiffness until, after a while of asking and listening, I feel its quiet strength. Though the story she tells begins conventionally enough, it too seems to grow and change until the room is filled with the earned gravity of her words and her sure presence.

"I began dating Jeffrey at fifteen. It was a 50s fantasy, a straight path through college and to marriage. There were no choices, but I didn't imagine there could be any. He went to business school, and I got my master's degree. I was glad to be out of my parents' house. All my friends were getting married, and everyone expected Jeffrey and me to do it as well. Jeffrey and Jane.

"Marriage was about getting ahead financially. We moved to the suburbs, and I began to have children and to raise them. I participated in all the community activities, was a room mother at school and active in the PTA.

"I was a good daughter to my own mother and a dutiful daughter-in-law, having all the holiday meals at our house, never complaining when his mother or mine forgot to recip-rocate or even call to say thank you. My husband's business flourished, and I entertained all of the important clients. We ate a little too much and drank a little too much and social-ized with people I wouldn't have chosen to see if I'd had the opportunity to make that choice. Jeffrey and I were both on the same track, except he was in front and I was following. Jeffrey and Jane."

Things changed for Jane as the children grew older and began to go away to college. She had more time to look at her life and at how she and Jeffrey were getting along. By 1985, she was pretty sure her husband was an alcoholic. He "knew" he wasn't. She went to Alanon, AA's organization for family members of alcoholics, and decided that she had two problems—her husband's drinking and her own.

Jane stopped drinking, and her world came into sharper focus. Looking back, she saw that over the years she had allowed her life to dissolve into Jeffrey's. She discovered she had needs and a point of view and a personal history that were quite independent of his. She realized that she had been traumatized by a stepfather who used to beat her with a belt and a mother she now came to think of as emotionally abusive. She also discovered that her husband was having an affair, that he'd been having them continually, and that she'd been ignoring them, as she had his alcoholism and her own.

A year later, Jane was diagnosed with breast cancer. "I felt then, and I feel now," she told my students and me, "that the emotional blows I received had something to do with my getting cancer. When I found out about Jeffrey's affairs, I felt so betrayed, devastated really. It was the worst feeling in my life, far worse than being told I had cancer. I had devoted my whole life to my marriage, and it had blown up in my face. I didn't know who I was or what I was supposed to do."

Jane began a long round of surgery, radiation, and chemotherapy. As she continued to go to AA and Alanon, she began to discover she had a wider range of emotions than she had ever imagined. Beneath her placid exterior, concealed within the cheerful activity of the suburban matron, were fear, confusion, and rage. "What really changed me was getting desperate. Before I went to Alanon, I thought you were supposed to be self-sufficient, not to have any problems or at least not to admit to any. When I began to realize what was going on in my house, I saw that I had many more problems than I had ever imagined. Still, it wasn't easy to share them. After the cancer diagnosis, I felt like I had to let other people know something about me or I was going to die. I don't know why I felt that way, but I knew it was true."

Jane joined a counseling group and began to feel the shell of her personality cracking. She was opening and softening, reaching out to other people, talking about and sharing her vulnerability for the first time in her life. The cancer returned, and she underwent more chemotherapy. She told her children about her fears, and their love and support, and her willingness to ask for it, made her feel stronger.

Still, things at home didn't change. She couldn't trust Jeffrey. His protestations of concern and fidelity were unconvincing. It seemed to her that she was still the follower, still less than a person in her husband's and, too often, her own eyes. The rounds of duties and parties went on.

Late one night, after an evening spent caring for her husband's dying mother, Jane arrived home. "I heard Jeffrey on the phone, and there was something about the way he was talking. A light went on. I asked him who it was, and he told me it was Debbie, and I knew that he was seeing her. In that moment everything that I'd suppressed for years came out. I was angrier than I'd ever been. 'How long, Jane,' I said to myself, 'how long will you tolerate his behavior?' I took this huge bottle of single malt Scotch, that was his favorite, and I threw it, and it broke against the wall. That was it. Oh God, I felt great! I knew it was over, and I've never wavered for one second from that decision. That was four years ago this June.

"I changed everything in my life. I'd always lived in the suburbs, and I moved to the city. I'd been a Protestant, and I became a Catholic. I started traveling and taking theology classes here at Georgetown and working at the Church. I thought, 'I've got to live now. This is all I've got.' When you have cancer you realize these things. If not now, when? After I'm dead? There's a certain urgency about doing what you feel is right.

"I went on a mission to El Salvador, visited with the poor people there. I lived like they did. I felt a tremendous anger at our government for the lies they told us. We kept that war going. The most valuable experience was seeing the story of Christ being lived out over again. I met a mother whose five sons had all been murdered, and I couldn't help thinking of Mary and her sons."

A year ago, as the cancer spread to her lungs—"it looks like lacework," Jane informs us—she began to think about how she had dealt with her illness. She tells us, turning from me, to make sure my students get the point, that she knows her cancer has been the motivating force behind all the changes she has made. It has allowed her "to say yes to my own life and to say yes to anything that comes along that can teach me and help me to grow. Before, I'd just been going along. Now I was involved in creating my own life, finding my own truth. But recently I realized that I still wasn't involved in my own treatment. I wanted to know if there was anything else I could do."

She began to do some reading on her own. She came to understand that cancer is a condition that occurs when the immune system is compromised, when it no longer fulfills its function of monitoring and destroying the cancer cells that each of us inevitably produces. The immune system is, she learned, adversely affected by stress and feelings of powerlessness. Meditation, relaxation, and guided imagery are, she read, capable of improving immune functioning.

She went on to read and hear about some of the many unconventional therapies that well over half of all cancer patients are currently using. She spoke with friends with cancer who had made forays into the vast and labyrinthine "cancer underground." She heard rumors about psychological blocks that may contribute to immune dysfunction, and special visual images that are supposed to be particularly useful in destroying cancer cells. She heard stories about herbal therapies and special diets, acupuncture and homeopathy, and a variety of unorthodox chemical treatments. All seemed to hold out the promise of cure or at least longer life, and none were practiced or discussed by any of the doctors she knew.

Jane was hopeful but also confused. Was there anything more she needed to learn about herself, any emotional binds that were still inhibiting the functioning of her immune system? How could she possibly sort out the bewildering array of unconventional therapies, since the physician she relied on, her oncologist, categorically dismissed them all as nonsense? Did any of them really have anything to offer, or was it all wishful thinking?

If she wanted information on the smallest part of her conventional medical treatment—say, the way her oncologist determined dosages of chemotherapy—it was available. But there was no way to find out anything reliable about any of these alternatives. She believed that the route she took into this unknown territory might well determine how long she lived, yet there didn't seem to be anyone around to offer the kind of guidance she needed. It was at this point that her friend, David, suggested she call me.

When Jane finishes, I tell her how moved I am by her courage, by the way she has used her illness as a catalyst to transform her life. She seems, I say, to have used her own deepening understanding to explore the binds she was in. She is experiencing fully many of the unlived parts of herself. Her willingness to take an active part in her treatment seems to me, as to her, to be the next logical step.

We spend the better part of the next hour discussing the possible use of alternative and complementary therapies. I suggest that Jane read Michael Lerner's *Choices in Healing*, a comprehensive, reasoned overview of alternative cancer treatments. I advise her to contact either Ralph Moss or Mike McGrady, one in New York the other in Seattle, each of whom keeps an up-to-date data bank on which alternatives seem most useful for what kinds of cancer. I tell her that their information is largely anecdotal—with none of the carefully controlled studies for which either her oncologist or I would hope. Still, it's all there is; it's what I would check out if I had cancer. At our next meetings we'll take a careful look at the information she receives.

In the meantime I talk with her about a basic regimen that she can follow while she takes her tamoxifen. It will support her immune system and perhaps slow or even halt the spread of her cancer. I tell her that some foods, particularly soy products and the cruciferous vegetables like broccoli and cabbage, seem to be anticarcinogenic; and that vitamins E and C and beta carotene and selenium—the antioxidants—have in some studies been shown to be useful in preventing or slowing the growth of cancer. I suggest she discontinue eating sugar, caffeine, and red meat, decrease her intake of fat, and begin to exercise for at least forty minutes a day.

I tell Jane that regular acupuncture will support her immune system and generally balance her emotional and physical functioning; and that I will recommend combinations of Chinese herbs that have immune-stimulating and cancer-fighting activity. The next time we meet, after I have a chance to look at her tongue and feel her pulses, I will come up with a prescription tailored to her particular needs.

We speak then about using visual images to mobilize her immune system. I explain that a clear connection between using images and living longer has not been made, but that studies have repeatedly shown that imagery and relaxation can reduce stress and make a real and measurable difference in the immune functioning of both cancer patients and people without the disease.

Jane says this makes sense to her but that she is disturbed by all the images that she thinks cancer patients are supposed to use. She just doesn't like the idea of Pac-Man white cells gobbling up cancer cells or Star Wars gunners shooting them down: "it just isn't me." I tell her we will work to find images that feel right to her.

All of these efforts, I tell Jane, are important, but I feel, as she does, that attitude is just as important. "You've done such a beautiful job of self-exploration, of changing through and in the midst of crisis. It's really inspiring. There's not much I have to add, but I do think,"—the thought comes to me just as I say it—"you're a little too serious. You need to celebrate as well as plumb the depths of life. Even Jesus," I go on, hoping, I suppose, that it will tickle rather than offend her, "even Jesus used to just hang out and drink some wine. What would you think about dancing, putting on fast music and losing yourself in it for thirty minutes every morning?"

"Yes," she says, still earnest but now smiling and nodding. "I think you're right. I've almost forgotten what it is to dance, and I've always loved it. I really do need"—the next words sound foreign in her mouth, as if bracketed by quotation marks—"to lighten up."

I meet with Jane and the students every week for the next few months. I look at her tongue, and feel her belly, and take her pulses, and give her a prescription for Chinese herbs, and do acupuncture. We work together on her visual imagery—eventually her white cells appear as ushers, gently coaxing the cancer from her body, as if at the end of a show. And we talk.

Perhaps I wouldn't see Jane as often if the students weren't with me. There's no pressing "medical" justification for it—probably nothing that would satisfy a hardnosed insurance auditor—but spending time with her reminds me once again of how important those hours can be. It reminds me also of how we physicians too easily narrow our definition of what is and is not properly medical—and in the process devalue the personal contact that may be the most valuable therapeutic thing most of us do most of the time.

Each meeting feels like a privilege for me and my students. It often seems that we are all on a journey together. I am the guide, but just as often, it is Jane who is leading me. Each week I feel us moving toward an understanding and a wisdom that my students and I have not yet been able to, or not yet been forced to, arrive at on our own. Many times, sitting with her, I have the sense that she and I are simply companions, each of us with skills to share and help to offer.

This sense of a shared journey, of the physician as participant and guide as well as observer and technician, has always been integral to the work of indigenous healers. These men and women were often chosen because, as children, they had undergone and survived the journey through life-threatening illness. The community's shaman, or healer, had watched these children draw strength from within and grow under his guidance. Their own experience was the precondition and preparation for them becoming healers, for learning how to help others to make this same healing journey.

The great classical medical traditions—the Hippocratic, Chinese, and Ayurvedic—also recognize the power of the healing ordeal. Their physicians' education also balanced the accumulation of technical knowledge with an emphasis on self-awareness and self-knowledge. Apprentice-physicians had to become aware of their psychological armor, anxiety, fear, and arrogance. As they experienced their own wounds and let these defenses go, they were able to experience the healing force, the spirit, that is the source of all their therapeutic work and the root of their own and their patients' health.

The education of modern physicians, though rich in technical mastery, is poor in personal and spiritual growth. The youth and health of medical students give them a feeling of invulnerability. The emphasis on technical mastery and the intolerance of uncertainty only intensifies the students' need to appear strong and in control.

This has had very real and very dangerous consequences for medical practice. Unschooled in our own thoughts, feelings, and reactions, we come to see ourselves as fundamentally different from those for whom we care. Simulating competence, fearful, defensive, and unbowed by humility, we can be grossly unaware of our own moods and motivations and insensitive to the power of our words to heal or harm.

Meeting with Jane and my students, week after week, I have the sense that we are reclaiming our birthright as healers. We are also healing some of the divisions between doctors and patients, and participating in a shared journey of discovery that is larger than all of us.

Jane tells us how difficult it is, at first, to do the visualizations and take the time to dance—she is so used to being available to others—but of how rewarding she soon finds it to be. "I can't tell you how important those forty minutes a day are, closed off in a room by myself. I do the visualizations, and I feel such a sense of satisfaction: I'm helping to take care of myself. Then I dance, and my body feels free, and I hear songs in my head, and the answers to my problems just present themselves. I feel if I just remain open and willing, everything I need will come to me."

On her sixth visit, Jane is visibly upset. She reports that twice she awoke at night and had to rush to the bathroom to vomit. That hasn't happened since she last had chemotherapy. What, she wonders, is going on? Could it be the herbs? I'm not sure, but I've never heard of this reaction. I ask if there were other symptoms. She says there weren't. Then it occurs to me to ask what went on in the previous week. Was there any physical or emotional trauma?

Jane pauses for a moment, sighs, and says she guesses there was. She had an appointment with her oncologist and told him that she was trying some of the alternative therapies she'd asked him about. His response shocked her. He said they were all a "waste of time." Anything that might have been useful, he blithely assured her, would have already been included in the conventional treatments he prescribed. She heard ignorance compounded by arrogance. His words and the way he said them reminded her of her marriage and even of the U.S. intervention in El Salvador. These were people in power intimidating and abusing those who were vulnerable to them.

"I started to think about it," she tells us. "I wasn't so disturbed by his ignorance as I was by his arrogance. It was as if I were seeing it for the first time. I guess up until a few weeks ago I had just expected it. I thought it was the way things had to be. Because you know, in all my fifty-four years, there's only been one other doctor who ever really treated me with respect. All the rest, the so-called 'best doctors' in this city, acted as if they were up there and I was down here, and there was no reciprocity. It seems like I say, 'These are my symptoms,' and they look in the computer or wherever, and they say, 'Here's a prescription and that's the appointment.' And then it got worse.

"I thought, 'I'm trying to learn as much as I can about the herbs and acupuncture, but I really ought to ask him about the tamoxifen because a friend told me she'd heard it sometimes causes uterine cancer.' So I asked him very politely, and he snapped back at me, 'Well, if it causes cancer, we'll just have to yank it out.' I didn't say anything then. I was so shocked and hurt, and I still have that lifelong habit of keeping my anger in.

"What," I ask, almost as shocked as she, "would you like to have said?"

"I wanted to tell him that I wished he had a uterus so I could 'yank it out.' And I wanted to say that if you have authority over people's lives, you have to use it wisely." Here she turns again to my students. "You have a huge responsibility," she tells them. "We put our trust in you, and we need to be able to feel that you are open and willing to listen to us, that we are free to say the things we can't say in other places. When I come here, I leave feeling empowered and hopeful, ready to take responsibility for myself. Leaving that man's office, I felt terrible and ashamed. I think I'm going to write to him. He needs to know what he does."

I tell Jane that I think it's a very good idea. She needs to tell him what he's done, and he needs to hear how hurtful his words were. I suggest that Jane also ask her oncologist for the research studies on tamoxifen and that we look at them together.

After going over the studies he sends, Jane agrees that the possible benefits of suppressing the spread of the breast cancer outweigh the risk of tamoxifen causing uterine cancer. She resumes taking the drug.

Her oncologist never acknowledges Jane's hurt and anger, but his attitude seems to change, and she begins to feel better about her dealings with him. She is still sad that she can't confide in him, but she now feels strong and at ease in his office.

Over the next weeks, I begin to help Jane evaluate and choose among alternative cancer treatments. She takes most of the Chinese herbs I've prescribed but can't stomach the taste of one often-used combination. She's changed her diet but has not embraced, as some of my patients have, either the raw foods and juices of the Gerson diet or macrobiotics. She is impressed with what she reads about essiac tea, an American Indian cancer remedy about which there are many miraculous stories (but unfortunately no good studies), and decides to use it. She also participates in healing retreats and prayer circles and shares her experience with others who are suffering from cancer and other chronic illnesses.

About a year after I first met Jane, I mention a new book I've read. Called *Remarkable Recovery,* it is a follow-up to a project on spontaneous remission that California's Institute of Noetic Sciences undertook. The researchers found many hundreds of cases in the medical literature of people with cancer, AIDS, and other life-threatening illnesses who lived far longer than their physicians had imagined possible. The book takes a close look at what some of these people are like and what they did to help themselves.

The stories, I tell Jane, reveal some important commonalities among the people. They all had a strong will to live, and all staunchly refused, often in the face of overwhelming evidence and impressive statistics, to accept pessimistic medical predictions. Most energetically embraced dietary and exercise regimens. They had at least one close and supportive person in their lives, as well as a physician or healer in whom they had faith. They had a feeling that they were being transformed through their illness, put in touch with some sense of their authentic selves that they had not known or had lost long before. And they were finding in themselves an extraordinary capacity for love and a connection to some belief or force or purpose beyond their individual humanity.

Jane reads the book. It all rings true for her, and much of it sounds like her own experience. Still, she wonders if such a miracle can happen to her. "You know, it's not easy. Sometimes I worry that if I really wanted to get cured, I would have to try to manipulate God's plan, and that would be really dangerous.

"Then I think that's just superstitious and grandiose too: how could I manipulate God? And sometimes I think that it's just a matter of my not wanting to give up my old belief system. I've experienced so much change and have surrendered so much, but there's still this stubborn rational way of thinking I have. It's almost as if to be well, I have to give up all the expert information that says I'm not going to get well, the whole Western medical way of looking at and treating my kind of cancer.

"Then there are moments when I look at my infant grand-daughter, crying and flopping around, and I think how small our science is, how little the doctors know, and how limited their power is. And I say to myself, 'I'm no more in control and all those doctors are no more in control of what happens than she is.'

"In the Catholic Church they talk a lot about pride. I think that's what I have to work on now, the pride I have in knowing, and the desire I have to be sure, and the difficulty I have of letting go and really allowing God's will to be done. It would be a shame"—and here Jane smiles—"to die because of pride."

Early on, Jane told us about her children's lives. Six months into her visits with me, she is marveling at their concern, feeling it soften her rigidity, and melt her reserve. "I cannot believe how much they love me. They're coming in from all over the country. They say they want to be around me so that they can learn 'everything' from me, and that they want *their* children to get to know me better. I realize, in retrospect, that I had years of really deep depression. Then I could only let a little love in. I didn't believe it, didn't think I was worth it. Now, since my cancer, I'm willing to consider things from another angle, to feel their love, to be open to everything that life has to give me."

Over the two years I've known her, Jane has continued to try to get the benefits of conventional cancer treatment without being overwhelmed by the pessimism of the prognosis. She has had to deal with the ups and downs of physical symptoms—colds and coughs—that come and go, pains in her back and hips, suggesting now spread of the cancer, now false alarms; and with laboratory tests that lurch between menace and promise. "Cancer is a chronic disease," she told me a year ago. "At first I thought I would either get over it or die right away, but now I know that it's a part of my life. Sometimes I grieve for my innocence, for the place in life where

FIFTEEN

Creating the New Medicine ∾

T HE NEW MEDICINE is an evolutionary advance on the biomedicine of the last three hundred years. It includes biomedicine's belief in analysis and observation and its understanding of illness as a physical and chemical phenomenon. It also makes use of its powerful genetic and biochemical observations and its pharmacologic and surgical treatments, but it is not limited to or defined by them. It puts all of these into a context in which they are aspects of a broader view of medicine and healing and indeed being human. It offers a larger, more generous approach, and a more relevant, and more effective practice.

In the practice of the new medicine, the drugs and surgery that are currently central to biomedicine are peripheral, highly prized but seldom and carefully used. Approaches that have been regarded as peripheral—self-awareness, relaxation, meditation, nutrition, exercise—are its vital center. Self-care is understood to be the true primary care. Health promotion is a way of life.

At the heart of the new medicine is an approach to physical and psychological functioning that is at once scientific and celebratory. The new medicine fosters an optimistic and hopeful attitude toward the experience of illness. It is based on a therapeutic relationship that is more egalitarian than authoritarian. And it creates a new synthesis of ancient and modern, conventional and unconventional techniques, the best of modern science and the most enduring aspects of perennial medical wisdom.

Each aspect of this approach, every opening of the mind and heart that I have described, enriches and enlarges all the others. David Donne began his journey toward healing because he was dissatisfied with a system of care and a worldview that condemned him to chronic pain and disability, to drugs and their side effects. He had hope that there could be another way and was willing to follow that way.

Once he took the first steps, he saw for himself that what he thought and ate and how he exercised could affect his arthritis. He trusted his experience and continued to act on it. He was willing to take charge of his own health, to decrease and then eliminate his dependence on medication. Though his hands still bear the bony deformities of ten years of conventionally treated arthritis, he is now essentially well. Because Ty and Leslie and Jane began to see for themselves that their physical symptoms were connected to how they lived and thought and felt, they were willing to critically evaluate their lives, then to do something about them.

Increasing numbers of us are offering this new medicine of self-care, partnership, and transformation to patients whose desperation or discernment has driven them to search for it. The challenge now is to create the conditions that will enable this kind of practice to grow. We must find out which aspects of it work best, when to use them, and how to combine them most intelligently. We need to ensure that this new synthesis that we are jointly creating is available to everyone.

The new medicine begins with each of us. In the final chapter I will discuss some of the ways we can use our intelligence, our insight, and our passion to get the kind of health care we want and deserve. Here I want to describe some of the attitudinal and structural changes, as well as the professional, social, and economic restructuring that must support this new medicine.

There are, to my way of thinking, five areas that need to be addressed and transformed, five elements that are essential to the growth and development of the new medicine: how we take care of people; how we pay for that care; how we hold caregivers accountable; the research that determines the kind of care we offer; and the education we give those who will provide care. Put briefly: service delivery, financing, malpractice, research, and medical education. Each of these is intimately connected to and dependent on all the others, ideologically and practically. Changes in one can reinforce and multiply the effects of changes in the others. Resistance to change in one area can slow the development of the others.

Medical practice must address the causes, not just the symptoms, of illness and the felt needs of patients as well as their diagnostic entities. Methods of financing should reflect and extend, not constrict, the range of therapeutic options. Malpractice must be totally dismantled and restructured, to reward real injury, reeducate ignorant physicians, and punish malefactors rather than line the pockets of insurance companies and lawyers. Research has to be willing to explore entirely new territory, as well as to make small advances in present directions. Education in medicine—and in the other health professions—must be animated most of all by love and service, curiosity and courage, not hope of financial gain or career advancement or even the accumulation of expertise.

SERVICE DELIVERY

Here is a little-known and infrequently admitted secret: serving others is a blessing for the one who serves. I remember the day I received my first paycheck as an intern. Our yearly salary was $3,800 plus all we could eat in the hospital cafeteria, so I must have been paid about $150, minus taxes, for my two weeks work. Even in 1967 that wasn't a princely sum, yet I was so pleased, so awed. "You mean," I remember thinking to myself, "I'm actually getting money for doing this work? For having the privilege of learning about and sharing the lives of other people, for extending a little bit of loving care to them?" It boggled my mind.

It wasn't that internship was without difficulties or anxieties, but they seemed to pale in the light of the knowledge that every morning when I walked into the hospital, I knew that I was going to be doing interesting things; and that every time I ended a shift, I had done or at least tried to do something to make others' lives a bit better. I might be tired, even at times intimidated or irritated by what had happened in the hospital, but I felt good.

In medical school I had sometimes envied my non-medical student friends' freedom. As an intern, that envy disappeared. In the hospital, figuring out how to write orders for IVs, delivering babies, taking care of Jermayne and Jerome in the ER, visiting with home-bound patients in the farthest reaches of San Francisco, I had a sense of pride and satisfaction. Within the constraints of the hours and demands, I felt an incredible freedom. What I was doing meant something, both to my patients and to me.

Any attempt to describe what health services should be must begin with this sense of service as a privilege, this appreciation for the meaning it gives our lives. Any health services that want to be more than pit stops must encourage and, indeed, insist on this attitude. Everything else—the quality of the relationships we have with our patients, the kinds of services we offer, the way we structure those services, the nature of the environment in which we work, even the very information on which we base all of our decisions—will be shaped by it.

Service begins with the way we approach our patients. Often this is through a process of question and answer, taking a "medical history." We all learn in medical school to proceed slowly and respectfully, to ask about our patient's psychological and developmental history, to find out about family, work, and social lives. In most practices, however, this respectful, comprehensive understanding is reduced to a hurried frontal assault on the biochemical and physiological facts.

Even though a huge number of people—the majority, I would say, of those who come to see me—suffer greatly from frustration and dissatisfaction on their jobs, their work life is reduced to a line on a form about occupation. Concern with the family, which so profoundly shapes our emotional and mental lives, dwindles to a few questions, angling for genetic causation, about parents' and siblings' fatal and most significant illnesses.

The exclusive focus is too often on the "chief complaint" and the "present illness." Physicians are there to get the essential information so that they can formulate a treatment plan, order the tests and procedures necessary to make a definitive diagnosis, and prescribe the appropriate drugs and the necessary surgery. The whole range of people's lives and histories, save for their previous surgeries, major diseases, and allergies to medication, is cropped from the picture.

Just about everything in the current medical system—from the narrowness of the biomedical perspective, to the time pressures on interns and residents, to the partially self-generated and endlessly justified economic pressures—encourages this way of seeing and doing things.

It all has to change.

Once we understand that our work is to serve others, we will do our best to find out who they are and what their needs are. All our learning and all *our* need to define and definitively treat will be put in the larger context of serving *their* good. To do this, we have to find out, not assume we know, what that good is.

Runaway kids don't want or need to be told that their behavior constitutes a psychiatric disorder. Diagnosis, drugs, and "therapy" are irrelevant to their real and immediate needs—for a place to rest for a while, and for people who are open to hearing their side of the story. People with chronic illnesses, like David, Ty, Leslie, and Jane, don't want more of what hasn't served them well, or admonitions to learn to "live with" their illness, or bland reassurance. They are asking to be heard and understood. They are hoping to find someone who can care for them and help them care for themselves in a different, more respectful, and hopefully more effective way.

All this takes time. There has to be time during each person's first visit to take the complete history that all of us were taught in medical school—a history of family interactions as well as illnesses, of social class and ethnic background and their meanings and problems. We need not only to note their "occupation," but also to learn the story of our patients' work lives and life's work. What gratifies and what frustrates them?

We need to learn how people eat and exercise, to observe how they walk and talk and breathe. We need to take the time to respond, without defensiveness or impatience, to anxieties or challenges about who we doctors are and why we do things the way we do, and time to just plain get to know one another. I set aside an hour and a half for that first visit and feel that this is just about adequate.

Our patients sit in front of us in a state of great hope and fear, as vulnerable to our words and attitudes as one might expect of people who are often quite literally putting their lives into our hands. We have to respect this trust, to respond to its concerns. Primary care physicians have to remember that this is the beginning of a relationship that might well last a lifetime. Specialists should understand that a procedure that is routine to them is often a terrifying turning point to their patients.

Subsequent visits can, of course, be shorter. But here again time is vital. Ten minutes—the average length of current office visits, more than the average time most physicians spend per patient on their hospital rounds—may occasionally be enough, but often it is not. What if someone is trying to make a vital decision about a treatment, or needs to ask questions about the effects and side effects of a medication, or wants to explore the way anxiety or depression may be contributing to an illness, or just needs to talk or cry?

Sometimes patients, overcome by fear and suffering, begin to weep in my office, then quickly apologize, as if they have committed a social blunder. They have come to believe that the place of healing is inappropriate for feeling. We need quite consciously to alter this belief. We need to let them know that we have created a safe place for them and have established a sacred time—when those who come for help can actually receive it, in the ways that they need to.

Doctors are not mechanics, responsible simply for repairing broken parts. We shouldn't act that way, or if we want to, we should do the perfectly honorable work of tending to machines. The work we've chosen, the promise our position holds out to suffering people, is different. We are there to be present for and serve people with real and complex lives and with thoughts and feelings about every aspect of those lives.

If we respectfully listen to our patients, we will come to see them not simply as objects of our interest and ministrations but as whole people capable of exploring all aspects of their lives and of interacting with us as equals. If we indicate to them that we want to reverse the passivity or rebelliousness with which so many of them have previously approached medical care, they will respond. If we say we want to create a healing partnership with them, they will likely be surprised and very pleased.

Our job is to ask the questions that help them see themselves and their problems more clearly. We can do this by giving them the sense that they are whole and unique, especially when illness or anxiety has robbed them of their confidence and threatened to reduce them to the sum of their pathological findings. We can offer information and expert opinions, while guiding and teaching them.

There are, of course, times for authoritative medical intervention, of both the conventional and the unconventional kind. Someone with an overwhelming infection is in need of an expert to select and administer the most appropriate antibiotic, just as Ty needed "the maestro" to crack his chest and open and repair his heart. Jacob was perhaps saved from years of suffering and inappropriate medication by my manipulation of his neck. But these are relatively rare instances. For the kinds of chronic problems with which David and Ty and Leslie and the vast majority of people must daily deal, teaching, not treatment, is primary. And teaching, the respectful sharing of perspectives and knowledge, depends on a therapeutic partnership.

Patients appreciate hearing that there are other ways to understand and approach illnesses than those advanced by conventional medicine, that there are things they can do for themselves that can have a powerful effect on every system in their body and every kind of illness. They respond well when they are told that most anyone who is willing can change his attitude and mobilize his mind—through biofeedback, meditation, hypnosis, and visual imagery—to positively affect virtually every physiological process in his body. They are encouraged to learn that we can alter our diets and our patterns of exercise and often affect our physiology as profoundly as if we were using the most powerful drugs. And it is reassuring to them to know that if they share their feelings with others, they may find emotional relief and support, and in the bargain perhaps improve their immune and cardiovascular functioning.

As they come to understand that considering options is more than an intellectual exercise, they will begin to regain a sense of control. This, in turn, will make them feel better and may well contribute to a better outcome, no matter which options, conventional or alternative, they choose.

We can show our patients ways they can learn about themselves and what makes them feel better or worse. We can suggest ways that they can take care of themselves. We can provide them with names of books or workshops and physicians or other teachers who will further their education. And we can, most important of all, convey our faith that they *can* learn and do for themselves, that such investigation and action is itself a vital part of the healing process.

In this context it is perfectly natural that a fundamental reordering of therapeutic priorities takes place. We will inevitably reaffirm and really abide by the wonderful Hippocratic injunction to "first do no harm." Except in life- or disability-threatening situations, or ones of overwhelming pain and discomfort, our therapeutic work will be based firmly on approaches and techniques that patients can learn and do for themselves. These include exercises to promote self-awareness; relaxation, meditation, guided imagery, biofeedback, and self-hypnosis; changes in diet and the use of herbal therapies; physical exercise, the meditative movements of yoga and t'ai chi, breathing techniques, and postural reeducation. These will be both the heart of healing practice and the central elements of a lifelong process of health education and promotion.

When actual treatment—the doing of something to one person by another—is necessary, physicians will preferentially employ means that aim at restoring the body to its natural state of balance rather than those that interfere with normal as well as abnormal biological processes, produce side effects, and reduce symptoms without addressing the causes of illness. This should be our approach to all the chronic illnesses from which the vast majority of people suffer.

For example, we will insist on manipulation, acupuncture, massage, and baths for an injured back prior to even considering long-term use of anti-inflammatories or back surgery. Homeopathy, dietary changes, and herbal remedies—not antibiotics, antihistamines, or decongestants—will be the initial treatment for such common ailments as sinus and middle ear infections, diarrhea, hay fever, and other allergies. For asthma, we would no longer routinely prescribe inhalers, bronchodilators, and steroids—substances that combat the inflammation and constriction of the bronchi but create dependence and do not significantly alter the course of the illness or address its causes. These have their place, but as last resorts, not as primary treatments. Instead, we would preferentially, and wherever possible, begin therapy with acupuncture and herbs, as well as family discussions, self-awareness, and relaxation techniques, breathing exercises, dietary and environmental change, and yoga.

This new medicine of self-care and nontoxic intervention is already being practiced by many hundreds, perhaps several thousands of physicians. Some, like me, work individually, using a number of modalities themselves and, when appropriate, referring to conventional and nonconventional practitioners— Jane's oncologist, David's yoga teacher. Increasingly, physicians are working in groups with nurses, acupuncturists, biofeedback technicians, nutritionists, massage therapists, chiropractors, and other practitioners. Some of these function as the private practices of M.D.'s, in which nurses and other professionals are ancillary; others are holistic health centers, more or less close confederations of professionals who work collaboratively and refer patients to one another.

This kind of perspective and practice is also emerging in hospitals: psychological aspects of illness are being addressed by psychiatric consultation-liaison services. Long skeptical cancer specialists like Jane's are asking psychotherapists to use relaxation and guided imagery techniques with their patients. Orthopedists and physiatrists—physicians concerned with rehabilitation—are introducing manipulative therapies and massage into their wards and clinics. Nurses in intensive care units are providing therapeutic touch along with high-tech medical interventions. Acupuncture is already a primary treatment for addiction; and biofeedback has become a staple of pain control. In multidisciplinary units of "behavioral," "mind-body," "complementary," and "alternative" medicine, these modalities and others are being combined to address such stubborn problems as chronic pain, hypertension, and insomnia.

This kind of practice initially seemed most appropriate for adults with chronic illness. Indeed, it is in this area, in the outpatient programs I have described at Harvard, Stanford, the University of Massachusetts, and the Preventive Medicine Research Institute, that its benefits have so far been most clearly demonstrated.

This approach is, however, equally relevant in every specialty and at every stage of life, in all health care settings, and with people with every kind of illness. The challenge now is to bring together the most relevant and effective therapeutic modalities in the most thoughtful way to create a new healing synthesis.

All patients can be taught what they need to know—about self-awareness, relaxation, visual imagery, meditation, nutrition, and exercise—to help themselves in illness and to stay well. They can be encouraged to look with an equally critical eye and open mind at conventional and nonconventional alternatives and to work collaboratively with their physicians to make decisions about treatment. Combinations of therapies can be offered. These may draw on different healing traditions and the talents of a variety of practitioners, but all will be designed to maximize the patient's capacity for self-healing and to minimize harmful side effects. Groups can and should be used for instruction, for support, and for their power to transform attitudes and enhance any individual treatment.

This perspective and process is relevant to every part of the health care system. For convenience, I'll begin in emergency rooms, where all of us may appear for the treatment of trauma or heart attacks and many poor Americans come for routine care. In these settings overworked physicians and nurses are often wonderful at acute care but are neither prepared nor encouraged to deal with the true causes of the problems many patients bring to them. More than one quarter of all visits by women to ERs are related to physical abuse, yet the focus of care is too often simply on suturing their wounds.

ERs need to be places that address the relationships in which the wounding occurs. The physicians, nurses, and social workers who staff them need to pay attention not only to the breathing capacity and medication levels of asthmatic children like Jermayne and Jerome but to the social and family circumstances that precipitate their attacks. Since patients rarely keep follow-up appointments, provisions have to be made for those who are seen in the ER to continue to work with the professionals who are initially helpful to them, people in whom they may have developed some trust.

Hospital wards are even more in need of renewal. For most people they are grim, unfriendly places where patients feel objectified by a harried staff. Often the pain and fear of their illness and dissatisfaction with the way they are being treated seem to overwhelm the possibility of healing. Recognizing this, the Planetree Project (so named for the tree under which Hippocrates sat while he met with his patients) has been bringing the human and indeed the aesthetic element to hospital settings. On units designed by Planetree, libraries of books on medical care and self-care are available, as are music tapes and videos. There may be paintings by local artists and activity rooms for ceramics or games or watercolors. There is even an effort to make the customarily abominable hospital food tasty and healthy.

Instead of permitting or even contributing to the isolation that terrifies so many patients, Planetree encourages a sense of continuity with their life outside. Family members are regarded not as impediments to medical efficiency but as "care partners," guardians of the patient's rights, representatives of his needs and interests to the staff, and participants in his care. They and the patients are invited to read the medical charts, ask questions, change bandages, and make home-cooked meals in the ward kitchen. Family members are encouraged, not grudgingly allowed, to sleep overnight in their loved ones' rooms, in chairs that are designed for that purpose.

The spirit of collaboration and of service is everywhere. Once you see it or hear about it, it is so obvious. It still seems "experimental" to many hospital administrators, but to me and to many others who've seen it in action, it's quite simply the way all hospitals should be.

If we were to include in this supportive setting a variety of specific life-enhancing therapeutic approaches, we would have some idea of what the new medicine could look like in hospital practice. We know, for example, that the briefest of psychotherapeutic interventions, some questions about and discussion of fears and concerns, can reduce by two days the time of hospitalization for elderly patients who have fractured their hips. Studies have shown that a few preoperative minutes learning relaxation and breathing techniques from an anesthesiologist decrease the amount of anesthesia patients require, as well as their doses of postoperative medication and their rate of complications. I would hope that in the very near future these kinds of approaches will be considered part of a truly comprehensive medical approach, as vital to good hospital care as drugs and surgery.

Massage—desperately needed by people lying lonely and worried in hospital beds and wonderfully effective for improving mood and reducing anxiety—will be universal. Acupuncture, which relieves pain and nausea and insomnia, producing a feeling of calm, even euphoria, without sedation or side effects, will, wherever possible, be used in preference to anti-nausea and analgesic drugs and sleeping pills. Visual imagery will be taught to patients by nurses, physicians, and psychotherapists, to help them anticipate and move more easily through the pain and violation of procedures. Meetings with couples and families, to help husbands and wives and children work together to deal with the challenge of illness, not quarrel and fragment under its strain, will be an integral part of every hospitalized person's treatment plan.

This approach is necessary at every stage of life, particularly at its beginning and end. Childbirth cries out for it. This most natural of all human processes has, in the United States, become a medical procedure, immersed in technology and saturated with fear. The anxiety of laboring mothers as they enter the hospital often decreases the force and effectiveness of their contractions. Pain medication and anesthetics, promiscuously prescribed in many settings, further slow labor and present potential risks to babies. The electronic fetal monitors to which laboring women are routinely attached have never been shown to improve outcome for either low-risk newborns or mothers, but they do tend to provoke anxious obstetricians to hurry labor. And if their labor doesn't "progress" to their doctor's satisfaction, these mothers are, with alarming frequency told they must have cesarean sections. The rate, for all causes, is over 25 percent in a number of hospitals.

The new medicine suggests another approach, one in which vigilance for possible complications is balanced by enthusiasm for the mother's capacity to facilitate and enjoy the process of childbirth, in which the fear and isolation of hospital birth is overcome. In this approach, self-hypnosis and yoga would be as much staples of prenatal care as periodic blood pressure checks and daily vitamins. The former has been shown to reduce pain and anxiety and to contribute to a sense of confidence and control in labor as well as pregnancy. Yoga facilitates muscular stength and flexibility and appears to encourage pelvic relaxation.

Early in pregnancy, every expectant mother would be assigned to a birth attendant, a sympathetic and experienced woman who would be available during pregnancy and continually present during labor and delivery. We know from several studies, first in Guatemala and then in the United States, that the presence of these *doulas* during labor significantly decreases the incidence of complications for mothers and newborns. It shortens the time of labor, drastically reduces the need for medication and anesthesia, cuts hospital stays, and diminishes the rate of C-sections by as much as 50 percent. If, in spite of these measures, labor slows or falters, we might, instead of rushing to drugs or surgery, use acupuncture, which works to stimulate labor gently, decreases pain, and may even reverse the position of breech babies.

We also need a new understanding of and a new approach to the last stages of life. This is, potentially, a period of possibility and adventure, a time for addressing unfinished business and developing wisdom and a spiritual perspective, rather than simply protesting against death or fighting resignation and despair. Older people should be offered the same kinds of comprehensive programs as patients with chronic illness. They need opportunities to explore the meaning of this time of life, to review the past and to address their concerns about death. And everything should be done—in doctors' offices, at home, and in extended care facilities—to maintain and even improve their functioning.

Efforts can be made to encourage old people to keep control over the choices in their lives, and to be involved in the lives of others. Medications—the elderly are notoriously and toxicly overmedicated—should be reviewed regularly by a single physician who is responsble for their care. Self-help techniques can be taught to reduce or eliminate the need for many of the drugs that are routinely prescribed: exercise and deep breathing improve muscle tone, increase oxygenation to the brain, and seem to contribute to improved physical and mental functioning and better sleep; yoga helps preserve or restore flexibility; and t'ai chi seems to enhance balance and help forestall injuries from falls.

Death, the very last stage of life, also needs to be addressed differently. If we did not fear it quite so irrationally or regard it as our sworn enemy, we would be unlikely to reflexively mobilize extraordinary and extraordinarily dehumanizing and debilitating technological measures to prolong the lives of patients who are clearly dying. In spite of the wishes of patients and their families, people whose brains are all but nonfunctional are left for days or weeks on artificial life-support systems. Long-demented nursing home patients are rushed to the hospital to aggressively treat acute urinary infections instead of being allowed to recover, or peacefully expire, where they are. Instead of acting out of a blind instinct to preserve life, any kind of life, at all costs, we ought, as many hospices are currently doing, to devote our time, energies, and resources to spending time with dying people and their families; to helping them accept death; and to holding and talking to them as they make the transition out of this life.

Nor should service or health care be restricted to medical settings or times of extraordinary change. The same kind of approach that we are successfully using for people with chronic illness and that I am advocating for in hospitals is, with slight modifications, completely appropriate for schools and workplaces. "Worksite wellness programs," which are far less comprehensive than the ones I'm describing, have already been shown in a variety of settings to improve health, encourage weight loss and smoking cessation, and reduce absenteeism.

School programs have even greater promise. Youth is the time when health habits are learned and formed, but our schools teach our young about themselves and their health in only the most perfunctory and abstract way. Some information may be presented about smoking, drinking, drugs, and sexuality, but there is no experience of our extraordinary power to use our minds to affect our feelings and our bodily functions. The health and well-being of teachers, who communicate attitudes and set limits on what students will learn, are completely ignored. We need comprehensive programs of self-awareness and self-care, presented in an interesting and engaging way—dance as well as didactics, the experience of massage as well as the medical facts—for both teachers and students.

Herbert Benson and his group from the Deaconess Hospital have successfully used instruction in relaxation techniques to decrease stress levels and to improve classroom performance in public and private schools. At the Center for Mind-Body Medicine we're developing a comprehensive program of self-awareness, movement, meditation, massage, yoga, dietary education, and breathing exercises in the Washington, D.C., schools.

We know that what we've done so far has encouraged teachers and students to learn about the psychology and biology of stress; that it's helped them deal better with difficult situations. A few deep breaths can sometimes head off a self-defeating burst of temper or, in inner-city schools, an episode of lethal violence. We're also seeing its power to help young people experience their competence and move slowly over and beyond significant psychological blocks. It is so moving to watch as adolescents who have been physically and sexually abused reach out, at first fearfully and tentatively, then with real joy, to massage one another's hands and backs.

We suspect, too, that in time our program will help decrease rates of chronic illness, anxiety, and violence and increase school performance among students, that it will improve the health and well-being and decrease the rate of burnout among teachers. We expect to create groups of high school and junior high school students who, having learned to help themselves, are eager to teach younger children to take care of themselves. Our hope is to make self-awareness, self-care, mutual help, and respect for and joy in our bodies an integral part of the entire educational process.

FINANCING

In 1990 one third of the American people were spending some $13.7 billion on "unconventional" medical care, $10.3 billion of which they paid out of their own pockets. There is little doubt that since then, all these figures have increased significantly. There are times when the National Institutes of Health's tiny Office of Alternative Medicine receives almost as many calls for information as the entire NIH. Hardly a week goes by that there isn't a lead story in the nation's major newspapers and magazines and on TV news programs about one or another "alternative" or "mind-body" treatment. Almost every issue of every women's magazine contains a piece on "Herbs for Weight Loss," "Acupressure for Pain" or "What PNI (Psychoneuroimmunology) Can Mean to You."

Every aspect of the new medicine is more visible and more widely accepted now than it was six years ago. There are far more health food stores than there were in 1990, and many carry complete lines of herbal products, food supplements, and homeopathic remedies. Even conventional pharmacies and chain drugstores have set aside whole sections for "natural remedies." Comprehensive training in acupuncture, homeopathy, massage, and naturopathy, or natural medicine, is widely available, and most major cities have introductory courses in these and other alternative approaches.

Ten or even five years ago, when I appeared on radio or television to discuss "holistic" or "alternative" or "mind-body" medicine, I was looked at more as an anthropologist than as a physician, an explorer of some exotic culture reporting his curious and provocative findings back to the home country. Today I'm treated like the family doctor, a trusted expert providing the answers to questions that informed listeners and viewers feel are vitally important. It's no longer "How could herbs possibly be any good?" or "Do you really believe the mind can affect the body?" but "Which herbs should I use for my sinus problems?" and "Is there evidence that visualization is more effective then simple relaxation?"

This ever-increasing consumer and professional interest and demand, coupled with the inadequacies and prohibitive expense of the current system, have already had an impact on the financing of health care. Some of this effect is not easily visible. When physicians who practice the new medicine charge a patient for an office visit, the bills don't specify whether they are doing hypnotherapy or psychotherapy, discussing MRIs or changes in lifestyle, the dosage of prescription drugs or the benefits of dietary change and herbal therapies. When the Mind/Body Medical Institute at Harvard or the Stress Management Clinic at the University of Massachusetts bills, they call their work "office visits" and "mental health services" and are reimbursed accordingly.

There are, however, changes and charges that are visible on the forms we send to insurance companies. Many of these are dismissed and returned to us as "uncovered," but others are, for the first time, being reimbursed. This is certainly promising, but these liberalizations of benefits have not been, as one might hope, based primarily on the scientific evidence for a procedure or its demonstrated benefits to patients. These therapeutic concerns aren't wholly irrelevant, but so far they have been far less important than legal and political pressure and economic self-interest.

The most striking change in insurance reimbursement, for example, has been for chiropractic care. Some savvy companies recognized early on that manipulation of the back, particularly of the injury-prone lower back, could conceivably forestall the need for surgery and help return a number of people to work sooner. There were workmen's compensation studies that suggested this as early as the mid-1970s. It wasn't, however, until an antitrust suit forced physicians to recognize the legitimacy of chiropractors that such coverage became mandatory.

Similarly, patients of mine who belong to Blue Cross/Blue Shield of Maryland are reimbursed for my acupuncture treatments, but Washington, D.C., residents who are members of Blue Cross/Blue Shield of the National Capital Area are usually not. The reason: there is a large, well-organized, and powerful lobby on behalf of acupuncturists and their patients in the state of Maryland.

In the last few years some insurance companies and HMOs have become aware that providing coverage for aspects of the new medicine may be good business. The original impetus for this change probably came from business itself, from organizations that, over the last fifteen years, have established "worksite wellness" and "health promotion" programs. In study after study, corporations like General Motors, Johnson & Johnson, Prudential Life, and AT&T have demonstrated that physical exercise, smoking cessation, and weight management classes, along with counseling and stress management sessions, decreased the number of employees who smoked, encouraged weight loss, reduced the number of days employees spent in the hospital and off the job, and saved the corporation money.

More recently studies on the "alternative" or "mindbody" approach to specific disease conditions have demonstrated comparable "cost-benefits." Work with people with chronic pain at Harvard's Mind/Body Medical Institute showed that ten classroom sessions—covering information on the mind-body connection, problem-solving skills, relaxation training, and yoga—not only decreased the depression and anxiety that ordinarily accompany this condition but saved $100 per person per year in physician visits and other medical costs. Stanford's Arthritis Self-Help Program recorded even larger savings for its patients: as much as $648 per person over a four-year period for people with rheumatoid arthritis. Since as many as seventy million Americans have chronic pain and two million have rheumatoid arthritis, the potential savings for these two conditions alone is enormous.

The economic benefits of bringing this new medicine into high-cost hospital settings are even greater. One simple intervention, the use of regular therapeutic massage for low-birth-weight babies, not only produced more normal growth and development and strengthened the maternal-infant bond, but saved a great deal of money. These babies were able to leave the hospital on an average of six days earlier than those who were not massaged, at an average saving of some $3,000 per child.

Pairing every laboring mother with a *doula* could produce even more dramatic results and savings. In the studies done so far, the reduction in C-section rates (by as much as 67 percent), the markedly decreased use of oxytocin to induce labor, and of anesthesia and forceps for delivery combined to reduce significantly both the rate of complications and the length of hospital stay by as much as 50 percent. It has been estimated that if every woman in the United States had a *doula* with her throughout labor, we might be able to reduce the costs of childbirth by as much as two billion dollars per year.

So far, the most striking and influential cost-benefit analysis has been done on Dean Ornish's Lifestyle Heart Trial, a comprehensive program that addresses the number one killer in the United States and embodies the spirit of the new medicine and several of the techniques that are most frequently used by its practitioners.

In 1993, after Ornish published his results, Mutual of Omaha decided to finance a two-year study of its subscribers. Ninety-five percent of the two hundred people who began Ornish's program completed it. Only one of these prime candidates for angioplasties and bypasses has subsequently required heart surgery. Mutual estimates that it saved $6.50 for each dollar it invested.

Impressed by the results, fifteen other carriers subsequently agreed to underwrite the program. Now hospitals from around the country are paying Ornish and his colleagues to train their staffs to offer it.

At the same time, several insurance companies and HMOs have begun to offer benefit plans that cover alternative approaches to all illness and to health maintenance as well. American Western Life, Blue Cross/Blue Shield of Washington and Alaska, and U.S. Health Care are all signing up new policyholders for comprehensive plans that include massage therapists, naturopaths, acupuncturists, and physicians who practice homeopathy. The Sharp Health Plan, a 16,000-member HMO in southern California, now offers all its members an eight-session "wellness program" designed by Deepak Chopra. In the last year alone, I've been contacted by a dozen other managed care companies and hospital chains that are eager to attract new subscribers with alternative or complementary care programs.

All these developments indicate that these new approaches to health care are potentially profitable as well as useful and popular. They are, however, only hints of what should be happening, not blueprints for the deep and pervasive change that is necessary. We need a system that not only makes available but mandates a more comprehensive approach to health and illness; one that makes prevention and teaching, not treatment, the cornerstone of care; one that offers care to all, not options for a fortunate few; one that is based on serving people, not on maximizing profits.

Such a system could well be based on the development of a program of government-administered national health care like the single-payer plan, supported by the five thousand members of Physicians for a National Health Plan and proposed in Congress in 1993 by Representative Jim McDermott. The need for this kind of plan is so obvious that only the power and money of huge corporations and appeals to the most primitive fears of the American people have been able to keep it from happening. In fact, a national system of health care, with the government as its single payer, would be most likely not only to guarantee services to the forty million Amercians who are now uninsured by our private system but to allay the fears of intrusion, control, impersonality, and scarcity that have been raised about changes in health care.

A plan like McDermott's would begin by cutting in half the single most wasteful component of health care system, its administrative costs. Currently 25 percent of our hospital costs and as much as 20 percent of the entire health care budget is spent on administration. Much of this goes to satisfying the endless demands of the insurance companies and to insuring that these companies make a substantial profit. Under a single-payer plan, the costs of government administration would likely approximate the Canadian figure of 11 percent, a savings of close to *$100 billion a year* at our current rate of expenditure!

Creating such a plan would also set the stage for a different kind of service. Curently more and more Americans and their physicians are being pressured to participate in managed care programs, which are often owned and operated by the profit-making insurance companies. Though some people are pleased with the care they receive from HMOs and PPOs, the levels of satisfaction are far higher for patients who continue to see physicians who practice on their own.

During the 1993–94 debates on health care reform, insurance companies repeatedly raised the specter of lost freedom under government administration. In fact, precisely the opposite would be true. Under a single-payer plan, Americans, like Canadians, would once again have the freedom to be cared for by any physican they might choose or any managed care program they might select, and physicians would have the freedom to practice as they choose.

Organization and monitoring of the system could take place at a single state agency, eliminating the incredible and time-consuming confusion and frustration of having to deal with a number of insurers with differing demands and expectations. This same agency could help establish a more rational, collaborative, and cost-saving approach to allocating hospital beds and such expensive high-tech enterprises and equipment as coronary bypass units and MRIs.

A comprehensive single-payer plan that covered *all* Americans would, according to most estimates, be unlikely to be much more expensive than the present inadequate and inequable system. The highest estimate suggests that it would cost perhaps 4 to 8 percent more. And one authoritative report, issued in 1991 by the U.S. government's General Accounting Office, suggested that even if we were to cover all Americans fully and continue to perform all of the *unnecessary* tests and procedures that we currently use, we might expect, under a single-payer plan, to *decrease* our health budget by 0.4 percent.

In fact, a single-payer system could result in a far more significant decrease in health care costs. This is because such a program would permit major changes in emphasis and in the kind of health care we give and receive. A pure fee-for-service practice puts all the economic incentives on the side of providing more, and more expensive, care. Doctors are paid only when patients are sick, and they are reimbursed at a far higher rate for doing procedures—electrocardiograms and echocardigrams to check on the heart, sigmoidoscopies to examine the large intestine, blood tests, X rays, and CT scans in their own laboratories—than for using their eyes and ears and common clinical sense. Managed care errs in the other direction: the less service provided, the more the company profits; the fewer referrals to specialists that a primary care physician makes, the more money he or she gets to keep. One system tends to overtreat, the other to undertreat or ignore patients. Under both, the poor and the uninsured, to whom services are usually provided grudgingly and less profitably, suffer.

A single-payer system, administered by the government and responsive to the people, not to the economic aspirations of physicians or the greed of stockholders, is at least potentially, free from these sometimes overwhelming and distorting pressures. It could routinely provide to everyone the kind of comprehensive cost-effective new medicine that is now available only to the well-to-do. It could create the conditions for this new medicine to develop and flourish in different ways, in a variety of environments. It could encourage innovative individual and small group practices as well as managed care settings, each designed to make the most of practitioners' talents and to meet the needs of particular groups of people.

What follows are some of the ways in which the power of the purse could be used to help shape a more responsive, effective, and cost-effective medicine. This medicine would be, in turn, more helpful to and respectful of patients, and more rewarding and encouraging to physicians who want to care for patients and help them to care for themselves:

1. *Physicians could be reimbursed for the time they spend with patients, not for the particular procedures they perform on patients.* Surgery and specialized diagnostic procedures require significant skill and painstaking attention, but they do not, in fact, require any greater professional expertise than caring for a chronically ill child, dealing with a seriously dysfunctional or poverty-stricken family, or addressing the multiple physical, emotional, and spiritual issues that an aging person faces. There is no intrinsic reason why an hour in the operating room should be rewarded at twenty or thirty times the rate of an hour of sensitive history-taking and thoughtful counseling and treatment.

Significantly reducing fees for surgical and diagnostic procedures and increasing those for office visits would discourage the promiscuous use of expensive high-technology procedures. It would put the therapeutic emphasis where it belongs, on the doctor-patient relationship, and could save a significant amount of money. It would send a clear message that subspecialties are no more important than primary care, and subspecialists no more highly regarded than generalists. It would encourage physicians to enter the severely understaffed primary care fields and discourage those who see the already overpopulated specialties and subspecialties as paths to great riches. People who want to become surgeons or radiologists or anesthesiologists should do so because they love the science and art of these crafts, not because they hope to make half a million dollars or more a year.

Similarly, nurses and others who provide health care services would be offered financial incentives to continue to provide direct patient care, not rewarded disproportionately for becoming administrators.

2. *Except in emergency situations, physicians would be expected to make preferential use of low-technology, nontoxic therapies that have been shown to be effective.* Patients with back pain would receive a course of manipulation, acupuncture, and massage, as well as instruction about diet and exercise and education about posture — before surgery or long-term use of anti-inflammatories is even considered. Bypass surgery would be reserved for those for whom an Ornish-style educational program has not proved effective. Depressed people would be discouraged from using antidepressants and encouraged first to combine dietary change, meditation, and an intensive program of physical exercise with psychotherapy.

In situations where hospital care is required, these kinds of approaches and extensive social support would be combined with any necessary conventional medical or surgical treatment — and reimbursed. So, for example, all patients would be taught relaxation and breathing exercises and self-hypnosis for pain control prior to surgery; laboring mothers would have *doulas* assigned to them; acupuncture would be available to control nausea and pain and improve bowel functioning; massage would be an accepted part of all nursing care; and counseling sessions with hospitalized patients and their families would be routine.

3. *Practice guidelines would be developed that require that everyone who comes to see a physician be helped to understand the emotional, environmental, work, and social stresses that may contribute to illness; advised about proper nutrition and exercise; and taught relaxation techniques, self-hypnosis, and other appropriate strategies for self-awareness and self-regulation.* These approaches could be taught in a series of cost-effective classes that would be regarded as an integral part of health care. This would help to shift the

emphasis from treating to teaching and from intervention to prevention and would encourage both physicians and patients to value self-care as the true primary care.

4. *Licensed "alternative" practitioners and the services they offer would be regarded as an integral part of the health care system and reimbursed accordingly.* This kind of inclusion would be based on the demonstrated merit of the practice. It would encourage collaboration between conventional and alternative practitioners and the continual development of a variety of different kinds of comprehensive and effective services, designed to meet the needs of all who would use them.

MALPRACTICE

It is hard to overestimate the profoundly deforming effect that the fact and threat of malpractice suits exert on American medicine. A story my students tell is illustrative. Because of the overwhelming costs of medical education, many of them have elected to exchange future military service for scholarships. During the summer they work at army, navy, and air force hospitals around the world. On morning rounds, they tell me, a chief resident, after reviewing a patient's chart, will write on a blackboard a dozen different and very expensive laboratory, radiologic, and clinical diagnostic procedures. "These," he will announce, "are the tests we would order if we were in a civilian hospital." Then he will pause for dramatic effect. "But since we are here at Fort X and do not have to worry about malpractice suits"—and here he begins to erase one after the other of the CT scans, twenty-four hour urine collections, and fiberoptic procedures—"we will order only the two tests that are *really* necessary."

The story is funny and horrifying, but the style of practice it mocks is pervasive, expensive, and dangerous. A study undertaken in 1989 by the American Medical Association estimated that in that year some $15.1 billion was expended on tests and procedures *designed to* ward off malpractice suits. When this figure is added to the cost that physicians paid for malpractice insurance — $5.0 billion in 1990 — and to the esti mated costs of insurance and defensive medicine for hospitals, the total sum for unnecessary defensive medicine came to $24.9 billion. And since then both premiums and self-protectiveness have increased.

Nor do these figures include the true cost of the medical profession's anxiety about malpractice litigation, or the public's, especially its lawyers', preoccupation with it. Because malpractice insurance costs so much money, physicians charge more for all the work they do. Obstetricians in some states may pay up to $75,000 a year for their premium. The unnecessary tests and procedures they order to "protect" themselves may produce substantial injury—directly, through the harm they may cause, and indirectly, by creating anxiety about findings that may or may not be significant but that still have to be exhaustively investigated. There are other problems as well.

Worries about malpractice suits stifle creativity, stall innovation, and even stunt intellectual curiosity. Many physicians shy away from exploring and using even the most promising alternative therapies because they know they are not part of the "standard of care" in their community. If they use these therapies, they fear they will be vulnerable to malpractice suits and judgments. Why learn about something you know you're going to be afraid to use?

Finally, the concern with malpractice contributes to a climate of distrust that devalues clinical judgment in favor of "objective" tests and lends a counterproductive, adversarial atmosphere to medical practice. More than half of the malpractice suits are said to be the result of poor physician-patient communication, and disabling fears of malpractice only contribute to this difficulty.

This peculiarly American preoccupation with malpractice litigation—we have, for example, thirty times as many suits as the Japanese—not only costs large sums of money, causes harm, and inhibits change, it does little or nothing for patients who have actually been injured.

A 1991 study of 31,000 hospital records in New York State revealed that one percent of these patients had legitimate claims for injury and compensation, but only two percent of those three hundred patients ever even filed a claim. Of the malpractice suits that were actually brought by the 31,000 patients in the study, fewer than half were instituted by people who were independently judged to have justifiable claims to injury. The conclusions: the majority of those who are bringing suits have no reason to do so; those who are actually injured are rarely compensated.

Under the current system physicians are intimidated and punished by malpractice suits whether or not they've actually done anything harmful to their patients. On the other hand, if they've been at fault, they are neither encouraged nor helped to practice better medicine nor even adequately punished. If a judgment is made against them, the insurance company, not the doctor, pays most if not all of the damages. Meanwhile, physicians who have been sued tend to become even more suspicious of and distant from their patients and to practice a more defensive medicine.

Current efforts to improve the malpractice situation center on "tort reform," attempts to limit the amount of money awarded in lawsuits and to decrease or eliminate the practice of contingency fees—in which lawyers base their fees on a percentage of the award their clients may eventually receive. This kind of reform, which is designed to weed out exorbitant judgments and to discourage the filing of "frivolous" suits (lawyers and their clients will sometimes ask for money even when their case is weak, because they expect that the malpractice insurer would rather pay something than incur prohibitive court costs) seems reasonable to almost everyone, except malpractice lawyers who profit both from patients' injuries and physicians' need to defend themselves. It is, however, a poor compromise.

We need a system that is fair and effective, one that makes appropriate compensation easy and affordable for all who have been injured; one that eliminates adversarial proceedings and third-party self-interest; one that serves to improve, not further burden, medical care; and one that strengthens, rather than sabotages, the physician-patient partnership. The current system doesn't need reform. It should be eliminated.

The first step is to create a fund for compensation and a "no-fault" procedure. Under a single-payer health plan this fund would be subsidized as part of the overall health system. Patients who believe they have been injured would make claims that would be adjudicated by citizen boards including some, but by no means a majority of, health care professionals. This kind of approach is similar to the current systems of workmen's compensation and no-fault auto insurance in the United States. It is a plan that works well in Sweden and New Zealand, where it is currently in effect. In these countries physicians, freed from having to defend themselves, may testify on behalf of their patients. Their concern is, as it should be, with the welfare of those for whom they are caring.

Awards would be based on injury and lost time at work. Such a system would undoubtedly elicit more, and more justifiable, claims, but it probably wouldn't cost more money. An analysis of the New York State study I mentioned earlier suggests that all the awards made would not cost more than the sum total of the malpractice premiums that physicians are currently paying.

Physican responsibility would be considered entirely separately, by a board concerned with both patient and physican welfare. The aim would be to help physicians remedy educational or emotional shortcomings that may have led to poor judgment or practice. Those few who were repeatedly or willfully negligent would have their licenses suspended or revoked and could be referred for criminal prosecution.

This kind of re-creation of the malpractice system would eliminate a shadow that is currently cast over all medical practice, a shadow that constrains and intimidates young people even in their first years of medical school. It would foster a renewed reliance on sound clinical judgment and help diminish the excessive use of diagnostic tests and procedures. It would go a long way to eliminating fears that keep some physicians from establishing therapeutic partnerships. It would also foster diversity and creativity in practice by encouraging all physicians to explore promising but so far unconventional approaches.

RESEARCH

Research is the means by which medicine extends its boundaries and deepens its understanding. It is highly valued for both the information and perspectives it produces and also as a sign of medicine's status as a science as well as an art. Medical students are taught in their first two years almost exclusively by men and women who are primarily laboratory scientists, researchers into the "basic" biological processes and mechanisms, rather than clinicians. From their first day in school, students are impressed with the certitude and power of the findings of these researchers, with the necessity of appealing, as their final authority, to the studies that their research produces. Later, on rounds in the hospital, clinical research—studies of the causes, course, and treatment of illness, chronicled in hundreds of "peer-reviewed" journals—serves to shape decisions about patient care and to distinguish among therapeutic options.

Research is not, however, a pure enterprise. What is valued and accepted as truth at one time and place depends on many factors, including the prevailing worldview and economic interests of those who define truth and control the research enterprise that produces it. Currently, the randomized controlled trial (RCT) is the clinical research design of choice. This is a procedure in which research "subjects," matched for similar disease states and demographic characteristics, are randomly assigned to two or more groups; one group receives the "intervention"—for example, a drug presumed to be useful for their condition, a surgical procedure, or a course of psychotherapy—while the other, "untreated" group serves as the "control." In drug studies those who haven't been treated are most often given a placebo so that they too will believe they are being treated.

The results of the study are "significant" if the treated group on the average does markedly better (as determined by statistical procedures) than the control or placebo group. Wherever possible, those who administer the treatment and those who evaluate the results of these studies are "blinded"; that is, they are unaware of which people have received the treatment and which haven't.

This approach is particularly useful in assessing the effectiveness of new drugs, but it has some limitations when it comes to other therapies. How can a surgeon be "blinded" to what he is doing? And what is an appropriate and ethical placebo control for surgery? Similar problems arise with psychotherapy, with hands-on healing techniques like acupuncture and chiropractic, and with approaches like exercise and visual imagery, which depend for their effectiveness on active patient participation and commitment.

The problems with the RCT are, however, political and economic as well as methodological. Because of its utility and because the results are easily quantified, it has become the "gold standard" of clinical research, the one by which all other studies are judged. This has real consequences, because many new approaches have been ignored or dismissed by the medical establishment because their efficacy has not been demonstrated by RCTs. It is also important because the structure of the RCT helps to determine what can be most definitively judged to be effective. RCTs work best for simple interventions with easily definable disease states. Here the complexity of the individual and the variability among individuals—our uniqueness—are ignored in favor of statistically averaged outcomes: intervention X lowers blood pressure in 50 percent of patients with hypertension.

The RCT is important in another way. It is the central element of "clinical trials," the complex series of studies that must be undertaken before any new drug can be approved for use by the Food and Drug Administration. These trials, which begin with animal studies of the safety of the drug and go on to large and several-years-long RCTs of its efficacy in human beings, cost tens, often hundreds of millions of dollars. This enormously expensive process shapes the U.S. medical research agenda in a variety of ways.

Since clinical trials are so expensive, they can be undertaken only by pharmaceutical companies with enormous resources or, much more rarely, by the government. The drug companies are likely to expend their money on developing products that have a high likelihood of both clinical success and profitability. This usually means they will develop new drugs for conditions that are prevalent. It often leads them to experiment with compounds that are in many ways similar to drugs that have already proved successful, often altering only a single chemical bond here or there. It also means that once developed and approved, these drugs, on which the company holds an exclusive patent for seventeen years, will be marketed incredibly aggressively and sold at a very high price.

Physicians, medical schools, and hospitals are handsomely paid by drug companies to study and use their products. Researchers publish articles on the usefulness of these drugs and build careers based on those studies. Drug companies devote hundreds of millions of dollars to advertising, marketing, and distributing free samples of drugs that have been approved.

This system is inherently restrictive. The financial incentives are simply not there to launch similar investigations of substances and devices that cannot be patented—including herbs, vitamins, homeopathic remedies, dietary regimens, and other food supplements. There will inevitably be far fewer and far less elaborate clinical investigations of them, as well as of acupuncture, chiropractic, and all of the mind-body therapies. This imbalance has nothing to do with which approaches are more promising, only with which ones might be most profitable

Equally important, the economic resources and journal space devoted to this particular model of investigation tend to make physicians and the general public less interested in and confident about other kinds of research. Studies that focus on individual responses to therapeutic regimens or on complex psychological and social interventions or responses are often described as "soft" and have less authority in the medical marketplace. If anyone had come up with a new drug that doubled the life of women with metastatic breast cancer, every oncologist in America would have had his or her prescription pad ready; when David Spiegel demonstrated that support groups could make this kind of difference, his work hardly made a wave on the surface of orthodox medical practice.

Nor has this same standard of proof been applied equally to all therapeutic interventions. Very few surgical procedures—which are not, as drugs are, subject to FDA approval— have ever been through large-scale clinical trials. This is also true of many long-used conventional diagnostic techniques and drugs: a 1978 study by the U.S. Congress' Office of Technology Assessment indicated that approximately 85 percent of all therapies and procedures that were commonly used by physicians and in hospitals had never received any kind of rigorous evaluation.

The answer is not to apply RCTs and clinical trials to all tests, drugs, and procedures but to take an inventory of what we know and what we don't, to open up the process to other kinds of research and other ways of knowing.

At present, medical research and practice are entwined in a tight tango—exciting and energizing to the investigators and physicans who dance, gratifying to the pharmaceutical houses, manufacturers, hospitals, and medical schools who play the tunes; occasionally fascinating but largely irrelevant to the rest of us who watch.

The therapies that are at the center of the new medicine, therapies that hold out real hope for chronic illness and for some aspects of acute illness—biofeedback, nutrition, exercise, hypnosis, visualization, acupuncture, herbal therapies, manipulation, massage, attitudinal change, and group support—are for the most part still waiting at the edge of the dance floor, ignored or avoided by the drug companies, only barely acknowledged by the government: the National Institutes of Health has a budget of $11 billion, its Office of Alternative Medicine (OAM) only $7.5 million.

The rhythms need to change. Generous invitations should be extended. A significant portion of the public research budget needs to be devoted to these therapies, which over one third of the population are now using. The NIH prides itself on spending $8 million dollars, in addition to the OAM's $7.5 million, on these approaches. Eighty million or even $800 million would make more sense. The potential health benefits and economic payoffs are enormous.

We need to begin by making the results of the excellent studies that have already been published—for example, on meditation, relaxation, hypnosis, guided imagery, homeopathy, chiropractic, acupuncture, and herbal therapies—far more widely available. I've presented a number of them in this book. More are noted in the 1995 report to the OAM, *Alternative Medicine: Expanding Medical Horizons,* which two hundred clinicians and researchers spent two years writing and editing. The report provides an impressive amount of authoritative information about the effectiveness of these and other practices and possible directions for future research. It's a good start and needs to be far better known.

We also need the comprehensive database that the OAM is beginning to develop—all the articles on all the alternative approaches gathered in one place, and easily accessible to researchers, clinicians, and consumers. We need to make sure that the information in the report and the database actually exercises some effect on medical practice and research. Drug companies expend hundreds of millions of dollars to make sure the research findings on their products are presented, over and over, to every physician and medical student. We should, in the public interest, spend a portion of the NIH's money to do the same for all the promising, nonpatentable, nonpharmacological therapies.

Once we're a bit clearer about what we already know, we can create a national medical research agenda that reflects the needs of the American people and the concepts and practices of the new medicine. We should sponsor follow-up studies of regimens—for example, homeopathy in the treatment of allergies and diarrhea, *doulas* attending laboring women, massage for low-birth-weight infants, and support groups for patients with cancer. These regimens produced results that seem impressive but are not as yet powerful enough to produce widespread changes in medical practice. Perhaps the weight of other positive research findings will help tip the scales of practice toward a more humane and effective care. We also need to take longer and harder looks at some of the therapies that so many millions of people use and believe are effective but that have not been carefully studied: chiropractic, exercise, vitamins, food supplements, and herbs.

We need to be courageous enough to look at highly unconventional treatments that small numbers of people believe have cured life-threatening illnesses—for example, essiac tea, the American Indian herbal brew that Jane uses and that some say is effective in treating cancer; intravenous ozone therapy, which has been claimed to reverse HIV infection; chelation therapy, the intravenous infusions which many believe remove plaque from arteries and forestall aging; intercessory prayer, which has been reported to make a life saving difference in every conceivable condition.

We need to scientifically address the whole question of "energy medicine." What are the biological and physical mechanisms by which therapies like homeopathy, acupuncture, prayer, laying-on-of-hands, and psychic healing accomplish the results that have been recorded? Do they have—as the Chinese and Indians have maintained for thousands of years—something to do with the circulation of energy in the body and the transmission of energy from one person to another? If so, what is this energy? How can we measure and influence it? We ought to devote some of our resources to understanding the fundamental biological and physical principles that may underlie their action and effectiveness. Such innovative "basic" research may yield not only the mechanisms of specific therapies but a larger understanding of healing and what it means to be human.

Too many researchers are like Mulla Nasruddin, the fool in the old Sufi story. When his friend found him late at night, Mulla was crawling on his hands and knees under a streetlight. "What are you doing there?" the friend asked. "I'm looking for my keys," Mulla replied. "Did you lose them there?" "No," he answered, "but I'm looking here because this is where the light is." The glory of research is shining light into *new* places, taking chances to find something genuinely valuable.

Instead of being satisfied with statistical averages, we need to ask questions that help us identify the conditions that are most conducive to healing and to learn from the exceptions that have something vital to teach us: What are the unique factors that enable one person to recover—to experience a "spontaneous remission"—from a metastatic cancer to which all others succumb? If placebos produce effective results 30 or 40 or sometimes 70 percent of the time, what can we do to maximize the positive belief on which the placebo response is based—and to minimize the negative expectations that may undermine it? If physician-patient relationships have an effect on outcome in illness, what are the factors that go into producing this effect, and how do we make sure our physicans—and our patients—make the best use of them?

It's not a matter of discarding the randomized controlled trial but of respecting and using other methodologies as well. "Outcomes studies," examinations of clinical practice in its natural setting, are, for example, far less expensive and far simpler to perform than RCTs. They are often perfectly adequate to answer questions about what works: Dean Ornish's Lifestyle Heart Trial, in which patients' progress was monitored, was such a study. Also descriptive, "qualitative" methods are necessary to help us understand why some people get better and others worse from a particular regimen. These methods could assess how and why, as well as whether, a support group might improve physical and emotional health.

We need to use methods that respect the integrity of the systems or techniques that are under study. So for example, if we are looking at the effectiveness of a Chinese medical approach, we may need to assess it according to its ability to affect conditions that are defined and described according to Chinese, not Western categories. If we are evaluating a complex, synergistic approach like Ornish's, we may need to be content with seeing that the approach works, without feeling desperate to know whether it is the diet, the relaxation, or the group support that *really* does the job.

Finally, we need to widen the concerns of our research, from its too exclusive focus on magic bullets—which one set of experts will design and manufacture and another will fire— to the human being whose illness is being targeted. What we have so far learned about our ability to use hypnosis and biofeedback, visual imagery and prayer, exercise and postural reeducation, attitudinal change and group support, to affect our physical and emotional functioning and well-being, are, I feel, just hints of our true capacity. Research should not only help us see what we can do to and for others but help us realize what we all are capable of doing for ourselves and give us the confidence to do it.

MEDICAL EDUCATION

Each spring I give an eight-week-long seminar on "The Healing Partnership" to first-year Georgetown medical students. Each student keeps a journal, practices a simple meditative technique daily, and commits to a regular program of exercise. We talk about the connections between our own self-awareness and understanding our patients. We also discuss the central importance of self-care to medical care; and the integration of a variety of unconventional therapies into primary care and specialty practice. We review some of the literature on psychoneuroimmunology, biofeedback, self-hypnosis, acupuncture, and group support. We meet regularly with a new patient who shares with us her ongoing experience of the medicine I practice. At the end of the course the students write a research paper on some aspect of the new medicine.

Each year in the first class, I ask the students to draw pictures; the first is of "yourself," the second of "yourself in medical school." The results are very interesting to all of us and provide the starting point for a valuable discussion.

There are some students whose two pictures closely resemble one another. One young woman pictured herself standing outside, circled by a flower, a sailboat, a tree, and a tennis racquet. In her second picture the same smiling woman is still outside, only this time she is surrounded by open medical books. Often, however, there are striking differences. Facial expressions regularly change from smiles to frowns; hands are missing from the medical school figures; clocks are prominent; faces are turned from the viewer; profanity is scrawled on the page; huge piles of books crowd small figures; prison bars obscure our view of obviously suffering students.

The pages of their journals and our classroom discussions repeat these themes. Where did *I* go, they wonder. Where is that curious person who loved life and was always up for some new challenge or learning experience? What happened to my interest in art or music? What about the desire I had to help people? It's there, but it feels—and these are their words— "stifled," "crowded out," "buried." Instead there is an uncomfortable preoccupation with learning more and more, a reliance on rote memory, a competitiveness, and a concern for grades that seems alternately embarrassing and desperately necessary.

Many of the students feel they are holding their breath until the third year, when they will surface onto the medical and surgical wards and learn what it's like to be a "real doctor." Many find that though they enjoy patient care and the challenges of the hospital, they are still holding their breath when they emerge into the open space of fourth-year electives.

Somehow the rich air of undergraduate life is still absent, and the ideals that drew many of them into medical school are still on hold.

By the fourth year, many want to take a look at other systems of healing, to respond to the needs of the poor, to learn about their own feelings and reactions to patients and to becoming a doctor, but so much else lays claim on their attention and their time. There is internship to think about, and getting the right residency; huge student loans or armed forces obligations; worries about malpractice; and dire warnings from teachers about the decline in freedom that managed care spells for physicians. It's not just at Georgetown. I hear the same themes when I talk to students at Harvard and Johns Hopkins and Columbia and at state medical schools around the country.

The new medicine demands a new kind of medical education, at once more personal and experiential and more thoughtful. It's not that what students are learning is destructive or even incorrect, or that progressive deans aren't aware of and moving to address some of its problems. It's rather that medical education is limited in its perspective and is less than what it can and should be. We need constantly to recall that the scientific knowledge and technical expertise that we venerate take their true meaning from the purpose of our profession, the service we offer to others, and that our habits of critical thinking need to be applied to all that we teach and the way we teach and learn it. Finally, we need to continually remind our students that what we do with and for other people depends on who we are.

Changes in medical education can begin with changes in its financing and its school admissions policies. We should publicly fund the education of all students—not just those who are willing to enter the armed forces—and in return require that all graduates devote three years to the chronically underserved in the inner cities and rural areas. This would establish the value we, as a society, place on service to all, and discourage those who see medicine as a vehicle primarily for technical mastery or monetary gain. It would encourage students who are interested in primary care and eliminate barriers to medical school for those, largely poor, who cannot imagine incurring debts of as much as $150,000 to $200,000. It would also eliminate one of the obvious and unpleasant rationalizations that doctors advance to justify the inflated incomes that many of us achieve. Admissions policies should be changed to reflect this perspective, with commitment to service, open-mindedness, life experience, and intellectual curiosity weighed equally with high scores in science classes and on the Medical College Admissions Test.

There also need to be major changes in medical education. Medical schools tend to be parochial, often more like high schools or trade schools than universities. There is a lot of hard work, but it is often neither intellectually challenging nor stimulating to the imagination.

We need to teach our students to examine biomedicine, the experimental methods on which it is based, and the social system in which it is practiced from an historical and a cross-cultural perspective. They ought to know that our medicine is one among many; that healing systems that have been ignored or dismissed as "primitive" have a long and successful history, can be scientifically investigated and validated, and are more and more widely used by their patients.

Medical students need this breadth and depth to help them challenge prevailing opinions and to encourage them to remain open to learning about whatever best serves their patients. They need an education which helps to temper the arrogance to which high status and the power of their interventions will urge them.

We must show medical students from the first day that each of us is unique and that all of us are far more than the sum of our diseased organs, that we are whole people living in rich and complex environments. This can happen only if we ground medical education in specific human perspectives and experiences as well as facts and diagrams. A renewed emphasis on the primacy of the physician-patient relationship is most essential as is an appreciation of the world in which their patients live. Students need to visit with patients in their homes and at the places where they work, to interview whole families, not just the patient. They need to thoughtfully observe the effects of hospitalization and, indeed, all medical treatment on patients' physical and emotional states, to appreciate the negative as well as the positive effects of medical technology (for example, the rise of antibiotic-resistant bacteria and the unnecessary prolongation of life of the demented elderly). And always they should be encouraged to engage in dialogue as well as inquiry.

In most aspects of the medical curriculum, we tend to divide knowledge into convenient and somewhat arbitrary categories, disciplines, and specialties. There is biochemistry and bacteriology as well as internal medicine and preventive medicine, otolaryngology and pulmonology. We need to balance this sharp focus with broader, more integrated perspectives. When students learn gross anatomy, they shouldn't learn only where each muscle originates and ends but how they work together. They should experience their own anatomy in action, through the stretches of yoga and the hands-on work of massage. Lectures on respiratory physiology should be paired with a variety of breathing exercises; talks on the mechanics of digestion, with experiences of the qualities of foods and the many ways to combine and prepare them.

The physiology of stress, which is usually only touched on, is one comprehensive and coherent way of looking at the effects of our environment, our thoughts, and our feelings on our biological being. It also represents a wonderful opportunity for experiential teaching. Instead of monitoring a dog's physiology, students can observe how stress raises *their own* blood pressure, alters their own blood chemistry and changes their own moods. Similarly, the new discipline of psychoneuroimmunology, which is almost never mentioned in required medical school curricula, would help students to see the reciprocal connections among—indeed the inseparability of—the mind, the brain, and the rest of the body.

From the first day of school, we need to balance the necessity for analytic study and expertise with introspection and personal experience, the acquisition of knowledge with the necessity of wisdom. Several schools make sure their students know the names and life stories of the cadavers they dissect and hold a ceremony of appreciation for those whose bodies serve our learning. A few ask their students to experience at first hand the dehumanizing potential of medical care: a visit, as a patient, to an overwhelmed ER; a simulated pelvic examination with their legs in stirrups for males; a brief ward admission, complete with unclosable hospital gown, for all.

In some schools, students are already working together in small groups. This is a beginning. In these groups, however, they should attend not only to "problem-based learning" about patients, but to understanding and helping themselves. If they pay attention to the influence of their own family, class, race, and environment, students will be far more likely to be sensitive to the power of these dimensions of their patients' lives. If they are willing explore their own stresses and attitudes and discover their own ability to deal with them through awareness, relaxation, meditation, exercise, and diet, they will find it natural, once they are on the wards and in the clinics, to teach this approach and these therapeutic modalities to their patients.

If students share their thoughts and feelings with one another, they will realize the power of this process to ease anxiety, break down interpersonal barriers, and create bonds of trust. Later, on wards and in clinics, they will feel more comfortable inviting their patients to do the same with them. If they begin to explore their own need for meaning and purpose—if they address the role of the spiritual in their lives—they will be open to understanding the vital importance of this dimension to those who are passing through terrifying and life-threatening crises.

Medical students who learn in this deeply personal and mutually respectful way will be far less vulnerable to the isolation and self-protectiveness of unhealthy competition.

They'll be less inclined to be passive recipients or dogmatic purveyors of information, and more likely to formulate and create together their own versions of a more comprehensive and responsive new medicine. As they continue to explore their own capacity for self-awareness, self-care, and mutual help, they will be far more likely to value and encourage these possibilities in their patients. If they are treated and learn to regard one another with love and respect, they may well come to treat their patients the same way.

SIXTEEN

Next Steps ᵔᵔᵔ

T HIS BOOK is a manifesto for and a guidebook to a new
medicine. I hope it has made that medicine come alive
for you. I've traced its roots to their origins in ancient
healing systems and in our contemporary need to transcend
the limits of a powerful but incomplete biomedical approach.
I've shared stories of how I and others include alternative
therapies in our work with people whose problems have
resisted the best efforts of biomedicine and its physicians. I've
tried to show how we—patients, physicians, and other health
professionals—are together creating a more comprehensive,
compassionate, and effective model of care, a larger synthesis
that includes both the precision and power of biomedicine
and the wisdom of other healing traditions. I've given you a
glimpse of how this new medicine is beginning to, and some-
day may, transform the way we practice and learn in all our
hospitals, clinics, and medical schools. This is a book of my
hope and my vision as well as my experience.

I hope, too, that what I've written, the map I've drawn, will
encourage you to take the next steps on your own healing
journey. Here in this last chapter, I want to remind you of

some strategies for making that journey easier and more ful-filling and to suggest some ground rules for finding guides and companions along the way.

I want to begin with desperation and despair because these states are the ones in which we often find ourselves just before we finally decide that change is necessary. Some people, in increasing numbers now, are freely embracing the principles and practices of the new medicine when they're feeling well. This is very hopeful, and I only wish more of us could learn with less pain. However, most of us are ready for a profound change only when we're at the end of our rope. We've tried everything that has worked before—anti-depres-sants and tranquilizers, analgesics and alcohol, protests and denial, drugs and surgery—and it hasn't done the trick. We don't feel better. We haven't found the physical, emotional, or spiritual change we know we need. It is then that we feel desperate or despairing. And this empty, endless-seeming despair, accepted, is paradoxically the beginning of our heal-ing. Having hit bottom, we have nowhere to look but up.

Sometimes despair kills us or prompts us to kill ourselves. But in throwing us deep inside, despair can also put us in touch with what is left when all else is, or seems, gone. We find the core of who we are, a vitality, a spirit that resists disability, death, and self-destruction. This spirit is the engine that moved David and Leslie and Ty and Jane and me and all the people in ARRIVE to take one more chance. It is what we need to be open to, and listen to and trust, when we feel there is nothing more to do.

Hope is a part of that vitality and the name we give to the feeling that things might somehow work out. Research sug-gests that hope stimulates our immune functioning and helps protect us against the onset of illness of all kinds. Hope is the voice that suggests that the glass might be not half empty but half full. Hope and the expectation that goes with it, are active ingredients in the powerful placebo response. Hope is the energy that encourages us to try once more and that allows us to participate in the healing partnership and to reach out to one another. Hope, like some basic force of nature, seems to live stubbornly, if barely perceptibly, inside even the most depressed of us, waiting like some sleeping beauty for the faintest glimmer of light, the slightest sympathetic touch, to awaken it. We should cherish hope.

Self-awareness tells us where we are and how we got there, and it allows us to consider where we might be going. There is a story about the Russian mathematician Peter Ouspensky. Eighty years ago, after a long workshop with the spiritual teacher George Gurdjieff, he returned from the country to St. Petersburg. As he walked on the familiar streets of that beautiful city, he found himself becoming more and more agitated. Carriages were careening down the boulevards, motorcars, new to Russia, were weaving in and out of traffic, pedestrians were hurrying every which way. Ouspensky felt terrified that the cars and carriages would crash or run down the pedestrians. How could they keep going the way they were and not collide? To him, newly alert after weeks of meditation, all the drivers, all the people on foot, looked as if they were asleep!

Most of us spend much of our lives in this state of psychological sleep. We have habits of behavior and thought, ideas and beliefs about ourselves to which we are devoted, routines that protect us from surprises and hedge us against change. When life, in the form of another person or an event or an illness, challenges us and our habits or even holds a mirror up to them, we rise to their defense with arguments as skillful as those of the highest-priced lawyers and with the demented passion of a two-year-old in a tantrum.

Waking up, self-awareness, is the beginning of wisdom and the prerequisite for self-care. Once we see what we are doing and thinking and how we are feeling, we can do something about it. And seeing is really not so hard. All you have to do is close your eyes and breathe slowly and deeply for a few minutes, letting thoughts come and go as they will, bringing your attention gently back to your breath. After you feel a bit relaxed, noticing where your feet rest on the floor and your back touches your chair, you can ask yourself a question—

"What is going on?" or "Why am I tense or sick?" will work perfectly well—and then wait for the answer. Very soon your unconscious, which is a rich repository of healing wisdom, will respond.

We—and this includes everybody, from the most highly educated to the illiterate—know much of what is good for us, even though we may not yet know that we know. If you just assume that something will come—it may be a direct verbal response or a visual image or a joke—and that it will be informative, you will get useful information. It happens nine out of ten times with my patients. It's usually not technical—most people don't have that information available to them—but it can be highly specific: "Your stomach is upset because you're swallowing your anger" or "Your back keeps bothering you because you're carrying around other people's loads." Then we can ask "What should I do about it?" and again, almost always, a useful answer comes.

When you receive answers, pay attention. There are certainly times when our unconscious produces nonsense or reflects our fears or fantasies. Still, in my experience these exercises yield unexpected nuggets of therapeutic wisdom. Don't dismiss the answers you get because they seem unconventional, or contrary to what you've always believed, or "silly." If the "sensible" conventional answers were working, you wouldn't have had to ask the question.

Each of us is always changing and unique and may require an approach that is not only different from the one we've used before but different from the one appropriate to someone else whose situation seems similar. And don't be dismayed if no answer comes the first time you try this exercise. Do it again later. When your unconscious is ready, it will communicate.

Interrupting our activities to periodically ask ourselves these questions is a way of maintaining self-awareness, of being continually informed about what is going on inside and around us. Keeping a journal, as Leslie did, works too. It's a bit awkward at first, because most of us believe that somewhere there's an audience that's going to read and judge what we've written and who we are. However, once we realize that the journal is just for us, that we can be as vulnerable or ungrammatical, as pretentious or naughty as we want, it begins to flow more freely.

This is such a good, simple way to find out what's going on with you. There you are out there on the page: that's what you think. Journal keeping also *feels* good. It's a relief, a catharsis, to express yourself. In fact, there are studies that show that keeping a journal relieves stress. And as we write, we grow: unaccustomed thoughts and feelings and happy turns of phrase enlarge the boundaries of who we thought we were.

Meditation is another good way to observe and get some perspective on the contents of our minds. Sitting every day and saying a mantra or paying attention to the breath or walking slowly, we watch as thoughts, feelings, and sensations arise. We see how our minds work, and how obsessive or petty or fearful we are. And as we watch, day after day, our watching creates a bit of space between the contents of our minds, the intensity of our feelings, and ourselves. Increasingly they seem to be "just thoughts," "just feelings," palpable and powerful to be sure but no longer quite so enveloping and overpowering, so intrinsic to who we are, so inevitable. They now seem different from us, from the "I" that is observing them come and go. Sometimes we find ourselves laughing at them. There is space around us. Change is possible.

Working with the body is the natural complement to working with the mind, but body-oriented therapies are even less likely to be a part of conventional health care. Many mental health professionals, themselves victims of the mind body split and of sanctions against "practicing medicine," feel uncomfortable prescribing physical changes of any kind. Doctors, who should know better, are often ignorant of or underestimate the power of movement, food, touch and breathing, and rarely pay enough attention to these approaches. The moral is: don't wait for health professionals to suggest what you should do with your body; they may be experiencing limitations of their own.

Begin by moving. Everyone I work with does it. You may want to read books, or talk with teachers, or go to a few classes to figure out if you should start a program of aerobics, swimming, yoga, or t'ai chi. But while you're waiting, just begin with what feels good to you. Dancing worked wonders for Leslie and Jane, and it does for most people's moods. So do long walks. If you're craving a challenge, find one, and if you're concerned about your physical limitations, work within them. The less you feel like moving, the more likely you probably are to benefit from it.

There are a bewildering array of opinions and books about food. I've listed some of the books I like best in the Books section on page 329. But books can only be guides or resources. They don't have the persuasive power of personal experience. You need to discover for yourself what's good, or not good, for you.

One way to begin is to simplify your diet for several weeks or a month. Eliminate or cut way down on foods that put unnecessary stress on your system—sugar, caffeine, red meat, sodas, artificial sweeteners, preservatives, and colorings—and eat primarily raw foods, brown rice, vegetables, and fish. To encourage good bowel function, drink more water, especially when you first get up, and have three or four tablespoons of unprocessed bran each morning. Unless you're already a really slow eater, eat at half the speed you normally do. Check in with yourself after several weeks. Then if you want, try some of the foods you've eliminated. See how they taste and how they make you feel. Once you've broken your eating habits, you'll be able to see how you react to those foods you've grown accustomed to and whether or not you really want to eat them. The goal is not to be on a permanent diet or to eat what some expert says is correct for everybody, but to know what's right for you.

Breathe. And breathe some more. Slow deep breathing is, with the possible exception of exercise, probably the single best antistress medicine we have. Choose any of the breathing practices I've suggested to people in this book—"soft belly," or counting breaths, or chaotic breathing, or alternate-nostril breathing—or any other that suits you, and see how it works for you. Use it for as long as you like, whenever you feel under stress, and any other time you see fit—the more the better. Change if you get tired of a technique. Put up signs to remind yourself. Breathe!

Remember that hands—and the rest of our bodies—were made for touching. You can begin to get to know your own body as I did, taking hot relaxing baths. Get a massage too. If you can't afford one, call a massage school and go to the school clinic, where a student will work on you free or at low cost. Learn how to do massage yourself—there are many good books, some of which are listed at the end of this book—and trade massages with a friend who's interested. Doing this kind of work, on yourself and friends, helps overcome the fears that so many of us have about touching our own and others' bodies. Working on someone else will make you feel wonderfully helpful and competent. Having someone you like work on you will make you feel great.

Change is always possible. The cells in all the organs in our body are continually being replaced. Our physical and emotional capacities, our life span, our capacity to recover even from devastating illnesses are rarely completely determined. David Donne was crippled and dependent on medication for ten years; Ty had had ulcers most of his life; Leslie was looking forward to a wheelchair; Jane and many of the people in ARRIVE "should have" been dead some time ago. Remember, there are thousands of recorded cases of spontaneous remission—remarkable recoveries—from ordinarily fatal illnesses. Nature's way is one of change, adaptation, and regeneration. Only our ideas and our habits are fixed. Miracles can happen, particularly if we don't compound our problems by expecting the most dismal outcome.

Learn from everything. Attitude, as we know from a number of the studies I've cited, is extraordinarily important in maintaining health and recovering from illness. I like approaching life as a student, and so do most of my patients.

So do the people who are in our groups and workshops. It's dignified, and it dignifies everything that happens to us.

No matter how trying or terrifying an experience is, there is always something that can be learned from it, clues about the ways we were living or feeling that may have contributed to the situation, hints about how we might see or do things differently in the future. Looking at it as a learning experience actually changes the nature of the experience. Because you're learning something from it, it's no longer unrelievedly bad, no longer so likely to debilitate you. In fact, learning gives you a different relationship to the experience, a sense of mastery. There is nothing to lose from looking at your life this way, and everything to gain.

Remember too that understanding why something is afflicting you, or what your reactions are to it, is different from blaming yourself. Most of us are likely to do that anyway—we do, after all, live in a puritanical culture. We have to learn to accept responsibility that is our due without wallowing in blame. If others are inclined to blame us—"you've caused your cancer"—that is, as the saying goes, their problem.

Speaking of other people, help is almost always available. This doesn't mean that health care for the people in this country is adequate: the best care money can buy is, as some of my patients' stories show, too often useless or even dangerous; and poor people or those without insurance are much worse off. It does mean, on a personal level, that if we are open to it and willing to look hard for it, we can find some kind of help, people who are really there for us and, increasingly often, professionals who believe in and practice the new medicine.

The best place to start is with your friends. I mean this in several ways. Friends, along with family, are an incredible source of support and wisdom. When you are ill or deeply troubled, many will welcome the opportunity to be there for you. It gives them a feeling that who they are and what they have to offer matters to someone else, a feeling that is rare for most of us outside the narrow circle of our families. Having someone with you when you go for a medical appointment may make the difference between an experience of terror and confusion and one of reassurance and clarity.

Knowing you can ask for help outside the family spreads the burden of dealing with a protracted illness and decreases the inevitable stress on the family. This kind of crisis situation often turns out to be a way of deepening a friendship too, of discovering commonalities and an intimacy that otherwise would never have been possible. It's simply a matter of asking in a direct but undemanding way, for a little time, a little advice, or some intelligent feedback about one's situation.

Ask your friends about support groups too. Chances are someone will have had some experience with them. Some of these groups have professionals who are leaders and require a fee; others, like AA, are leaderless "peer" groups. Some, like the ones Jon Kabat-Zinn runs in Massachusetts and ours in Washington, are for people with any kind of condition; others are exclusively for people with cancer or asthma or MS or intestinal disorders. Like physicians and other health professionals, these groups vary greatly. If the atmosphere is heavy with self-pity or the air weighted with resignation, keep looking. If the group seems too heavily invested in a particular therapy—alternative or conventional—be wary. If a group isn't right for you, it doesn't mean there's anything wrong with you. And a support group that may seem obnoxious on one visit may look like a lifesaver two weeks or six months later.

Friends are also the best place to start looking for people who practice the new medicine. Since over a third of the people in this country are currently using one or another alternative health practice, it's quite likely that several people you know have experience and contacts with physicians or other practitioners who could help you. The great advantage of asking friends for referrals is that because they know you as well as the people they might suggest, they'll have a sense of who would be right for you. Also, you'll be able to hear about and evaluate your friend's experience with a practitioner and to ask the frank questions that matter to you. As you listen to your friend and question her, you'll start having feelings about whether this practitioner is right for you. My own experience, as I mentioned when I told Jane's story, is that referrals to me from my patients—people who know my peculiarities as well as my strengths—usually work out wonderfully well.

What kind of person are you looking for? Ideally, it would be a physician (M.D. or D.O.) or nurse-practitioner who practices the new medicine. This person would be at home with and competent in conventional biomedicine, committed to a healing partnership, open to and conversant with a variety of alternative therapies, and dedicated to creating a larger synthesis that includes both biomedicine and the alternatives. It would be best if that person used some of these approaches—at a minimum, he or she should be experienced in strategies for self-awareness, relaxation therapies and meditation, nutritional interventions, and physical exercise—and could intelligently refer you to other practitioners.

There are people like this in every large city, most smaller ones, and a number of rural areas. They have the knowledge to make a good overall assessment of your situation and to help you evaluate and put together the various elements of your health care. Some of these men and women call themselves holistic—and some are members of the American Holistic Medical Association or American Holistic Nurses Association. Others may be described as practicing behavioral or preventive, nutritional, environmental, or psychosomatic medicine, while still others are known for their use of one or another nonconventional approach—for example, homeopathy or acupuncture.

There are some physicians, an increasing number, who do not themselves use any of these alternatives but are intelligent, well-informed, and modest enough to make referrals to appropriate alternative practitioners. And in many conventional medical settings there are nurses and physicians' assistants who are knowledgeable about the new medicine and familiar with local practitioners. They can be an excellent source of referrals as well as care.

Nonphysicians who specialize in one or another modality—chiropractors, acupuncturists, nutritionists, massage therapists, and psychotherapists, among others—lack formal medical training but generally know enough about conventional medicine to know the limits of their expertise and refer to others. If they seem in any way grandiose, promising cures or assuring you that if you would only sign up for so-and-so-many sessions, all would be well—be wary. One of the major pitfalls for all healers is arrogance. In those practicing outside of the mainstream, it can be compounded by insecurity and the grandiosity that insecurity often produces.

You might choose alternative practitioners for the fit between what's troubling you and what they have to offer. For example, the chiropractor's office would be the logical first stop for a back injury, a massage therapist for muscle pain and general relaxation, and an acupuncturist or nutritionist for an evaluation of most any chronic problem. Chiropractors in particular are generally well trained to deal with a wide range of health problems and to refer when necessary. Naturopaths (N.D.'s) are trained in a number of non-pharmacological approaches including nutrition, herbalism, mind-body techniques, and massage, and function, in some states, as primary care providers.

You're often better off if you can find a situation where several alternative practitioners work together in collaboration with an M.D. or D.O. This helps to ensure a more integrated and comprehensive perspective and easier referrals. In any case, whoever you visit should be open to communicating with your other physicians and therapists. Sometimes it's vitally important that your acupuncturist and internist can talk, and talk respectfully to one another. Don't hesitate to tell them so. If they have a problem with each other's perspective and practices they can get over it. It's not their professional egos but you that they're supposed to be concerned about.

Licensure by an official state body generally guarantees a certain level of competence, whether the practitioner is conventional or alternative. For example, here in Washington, D.C., where I sit on the Acupuncture Board, we require that every candidate have a long and thorough education in acupuncture and pass a theoretical and practical exam. But neither licensure, nor competence in a profession, nor even recommendations from a satisfied patient or trusted physician can guarantee that you'll feel good about or comfortable with a given practitioner, whether holistic, alternative, or conventional.

Finally, only you can be sure who is appropriate for you. There will be moments when you will be desperate for help. You have a bad infection and will accept antibiotics from anyone licensed to prescribe them. Your back is killing you and just about any chiropractor or osteopath is welcomed. In the long run, however, it's very important to find someone you can rely on when you need them, a man or woman with whom you can fully participate in a healing partnership. It's here, in your choice of a true healing partner, that you really need to use your intuition as well as your intelligence.

Over the years I've found that certain qualities and a certain kind of chemistry are necessary for a healing partnership. It begins with a feeling that there's a fit between your needs and what your partner has to give, both as a person and as a clinician. The practice of medicine is a kind of dance, a continual and shifting play between partners. Your physician should be able to be there for you in different ways at different times—now quiet and reflective, now decisive, now inquiring, now instructional. You should be as comfortable with him or her as with any human being, and be able to discuss your deepest fears and share those secrets that are most shameful to you. You should have the sense that he or she understands the connection between your emotional life and your physical symptoms, and is open to the possibility that illness may represent a spiritual crisis as well as a biological problem.

Your physician's familiarity with your body should be a reflection of and a metaphor for his or her familiarity with your whole being. Every question and procedure, the whole atmosphere of his or her office, should convey the sense that you are respected, understood, and accepted.

One of the reasons many people feel so uneasy about going to doctors is that the visits often entail pain or discomfort, and that the most they can hope for is a reprieve: their tests are normal. This is sad. It is also a major reason why so many people are seeking out alternative medical prationers. The techniques that we use, like meditation, guided imagery, manipulation, acupuncture, and massage are not only therapeutic, they also have very direct, immediate beneficial effects. Even when you're quite ill or discouraged, they make you feel better. Ideally, every physician—or someone in her office—should be able to offer this kind of help and relief.

Even more important, your physician should relate to you in a way that is itself healing. One of the main problems people have with their doctors is the way they act when there's no easy medical answer, their tendency to avoid their patients physically, and to back away emotionally, just when they're most needed. A good physician will schedule a longer session at times like this, be more available. You should feel comfortable enough to ask for more time if he hasn't arranged it. And he should be intelligent and sensitive enough to readily agree to it.

Your physician should be optimistic, thoughtful, and careful, as well as available. It is possible that doctors do more harm with their attitudes and their words than they do with any procedures they may misuse. I have seen hundreds of people who, like Leslie and Jane, feel insulted and diminished by the condescension or indifference of those who are supposed to help them. Even more people feel imperiled and condemned by their physicians' gloominess and fears. You would not want to use a surgeon who didn't believe that your body could heal the incision he must make. You should have a physician who appreciates, encourages, and trusts—as well as stimulates—your innate capacity for physical and emotional healing.

Finding a healing partner is enormously gratifying. So is being one. The experience of illness can be a bridge to others. I see this most clearly in a program like ARRIVE or in AA, or in our own and others' support groups. Infection with the HIV virus or the impending destruction of our lives by alcohol, cancer, or chronic pain forces us to feel the limitations of our unaided power and brings us face-to-face with our mortality. Our mortality, in turn, allows us to see through the illusion of our separateness, makes us aware of the life and death we have in common with every living thing.

Wounded, we are vulnerable, and in this vulnerability and humility we can open ourselves to others. All of us who are ill have the opportunity to see and feel how much family, friends, and even acquaintances may care about us. Depending on, literally leaning on them, can bring us closer in every way. It may occur to us, too, that just as they are helping us, so we could help others.

If you are or have been needy, you know what a long way a little bit of caring can go. Extend that caring to others. Every day in my practice I see people whom illness has made more generous. Their husbands or wives or children will often comment on it to me. A program like ARRIVE or AA, or the support groups that our Center and many others run, provides a chance for people to help others turn the pain of illness into an opportunity for growth, for giving as well as receiving.

As we continue to grow and change, some of us find that we want to share what we're learning more widely. Often, this generosity surprises us. Sometimes it gives a new shape to our lives. Sometimes, it may also give birth to new programs, like the one ARRIVE has started for the prisoners at Riker's Island or many of the new self-help groups.

Take the opportunities for sharing when they arise. Listen to the inner voice that urges you, in the midst of suffering, to reach out to someone else who is also suffering. It is one of the great antidotes to the self-absorption that physical illness and emotional pain can bring and, I am sure, one of the powerful individual and collective healing mechanisms that Nature has programmed into us. People who value relationships highly seem to suffer from fewer illnesses than the rest of us. Studies of people with AIDS suggest a definite correlation between helping others who also have the virus and long-term survival.

We are far wiser than we know. When, through meditation or grace, our mind's chatter quiets down and everyone else's ideas about who we are or what we should do fall away like clothes at the end of the day, then we are ready to observe and learn, to be self-aware. Then it is easier to follow the rhythms that breathe and move in us. We can listen to the inner voice that tells us to reach out or hold back, to act or be patient. Then we can know what to eat and whom to touch and how, and what we must say and do.

Illness, physical and emotional, is for many of us the great teacher. We struggle against it, looking to the old authorities, mobilizing the old ways. We have all the tests and take all the drugs, and maybe we have our bodies opened. We plead and bargain and scream and protest. Some of us are quickly helped and cured. We may do our best to forget that we have been so intimately threatened, and move on. Some of us, at some point, drop to our knees. Nothing has worked, or all the old things that have worked no longer do. We say "okay," or "I surrender," or "uncle." Then, as we begin to let go of what hasn't worked, something else may appear to us, an opening to another way, a promise of change that is far deeper than the relief of symptoms, a reassurance, against all the odds of our illness and our suffering, that somehow all will be well.

The new medicine values help and curing, whatever their origins: antibiotics and acupuncture, surgery and group support are all blessings. The new medicine is based on a healing partnership in which loving help is given and received and knowledge shared. It is a work of teaching as well as treating.

The lessons are those of the wise use of food and drugs, our minds and our hearts, movement and breath, massage and manipulation.

And beyond all this, the new medicine is a path. It reminds us in the most intimate way possible—in the book of our bodies and our minds—that when illness comes, it is, or can be, an invitation to move more deeply into our own lives.

The guides, the healing partners we meet on this path, help us to become aware of, and clear away, the physical, mental, and spiritual blocks that may have contributed to our suffering, and to uncover the place from which, once again, growth can begin. They encourage us to learn the lessons that illness offers us. They remind us that, if we care to listen closely enough, we will remember that we are here to learn about and care for ourselves, and to help one another.

NOTES

CHAPTER 1: *Time for a Change*

p. 2, **sixty million Americans who each year use "unconventional therapies"**: David M. Eisenberg et al., "Unconventional Medicine in the United States: Prevalence, Costs, and Patterns of Use." *New England Journal of Medicine,* Jan. 28, 1993; 328(4); 246–52.

p. 2, **arthritis statistics:** Arthritis Foundation (Atlanta, Ga.), personal communication.

p. 5, **the statistics cited are taken from the following sources:** U. S. Department of Health and Human Services, *Healthy People 2000: National Health Promotion and Disease Prevention Objectives,* DHHS pub. no. PHS-91-50212 (Washington, D.C., 1990).
Merck Manual, 16th ed. (Rahway, N.J.: Merck Research Laboratories, 1992).
G. B. J. Andersson, "Epidemiologic Aspects of Low Back Pain," *Spine,* 1981; 6; 53–59.
Charles P. Cozic, ed., *The AIDS Crisis* (San Diego, Calif.: Greenhaven Press, 1991).
American Council for Headache Education, *Migraine: The Complete Guide* (New York: Dell, 1994).
Donald Klein and Paul Wender, *Understanding Depression* (New York: Oxford, 1993).
Arthritis Foundation, "People With Arthritis, United States (Projected)," Graph based on U.S. Centers for Disease Control and Prevention, *Morbidity and Mortality Weekly Report,* June 24, 1994.

American Cancer Society, *Cancer Facts and Figures—1995* (Atlanta, Ga., 1995).

p. 5, **cancer statistics:** National Cancer Institute, *SEER Cancer Statistics Review, 1973–1991: Tables and Graphs,* NIH pub. no. 94-2789 (Bethesda, Md., 1994), Figure I–3, p. 40; and Table I–10, p. 25.

p. 5, **asthma statistics:** K. B. Weiss, P. J. Gergen, and D. K. Wagner, "Breathing Easier or Wheezing Worse? The Changing Epidemiology of Asthma Morbidity and Mortality," *Annual Review of Public Health,* 1993; 14; 491–513.

p. 5, **Mayo Clinic study on MS:** A. D. Sadovnick and G. C. Ebers, "Epidemiology of Multiple Sclerosis: A Critical Overview," *Canadian Journal of Neurological Sciences,* 1993; 20; 17–29.

p. 6, **survey of "Unconventional Medicine in the United States":** David M. Eisenberg et al., "Unconventional Medicine in the United States: Prevalence, Costs, and Patterns of Use," *New England Journal of Medicine,* Jan. 28, 1993; 328(4); 246–52.

p. 9, **costs of medical procedures:** Georgetown University Hospital billing office, personal communication.

p. 9, **routine electronic fetal monitoring has never been shown to improve the health of low-risk newborns:** Mindy A. Smith, Mack T. Ruffin, and Lee A. Green, "The Rational Management of Labor," *American Family Physician,* May 1, 1993; 47(6); 1471–81.

p. 9, **1993 poll:** Lynn K. Harvey, *Physician Opinion on Health Care Issues* (report). (Chicago, Ill.: American Medical Association, May 1993), p. 21.

CHAPTER 2: *Biomedicine and Beyond*

p. 22, **annual cost of biomedicine at almost one trillion dollars and close to 15 percent of GNP:** Kevin Grumbach and Thomas Bodenheimer, "Painful vs. Painless Cost Control," *Journal of the American Medical Association,* Nov. 0, 1004; 272(18); 1458 61.

pp. 23ff., **helpful resources on the history of medicine include:** Erwin H. Ackerknecht, *A Short History of Medicine,* (rev. ed.) (Baltimore: Johns Hopkins University Press, 1982).
James H. Cassedy, *Medicine in America: A Short History* (Baltimore: Johns Hopkins University Press, 1991).
F. H. Garrison, *Contributions to the History of Medicine* (New York and London: Hafner, 1966).
Albert S. Lyons and R. Joseph Petrucelli, *Medicine: An Illustrated History* (New York: Abradale Press, Harry N. Abrams, 1987).
Henry E. Sigerist, *A History of Medicine* (New York: Oxford University Press, 1987; originally published in 1951).

pp. 25ff., **useful resources include:** Edward S. Golub, *The Limits of Medicine: How Science Shapes Our Hope for the Cure* (New York: Times Books, 1994).

Jeffrey A. Fisher, *The Plague Makers: How We Are Creating Catastrophic New Epidemics and What We Must Do to Avert Them* (New York: Simon and Schuster, 1994).

p. 27, **the work of William Castle:** Lawrence Kass, "William B. Castle and Intrinsic Factor," *Annals of Internal Medicine,* 1978; 89; 983–91.

CHAPTER 4: *Physician Heal Thyself*

p. 48, **books mentioned include:** Jethro Kloss, *Back to Eden* (Coalmont, Tenn.: Longview, 1968; originally published in 1939).
Maude Grieve, *A Modern Herbal* (Darien, Conn.: Hafner, 1970; originally published in 1931; also, New York: Dover, 1971).

p. 50, **the fundamental text of Chinese medicine:** Ilza Veith, trans., *The Yellow Emperor's Classic of Internal Medicine* (Berkeley: University of California Press, 1972).

pp. 50–51, **books mentioned include:** René Dubos, *Mirage of Health* (New York: Harper and Row, 1959). Ivan Illich, *Medical Nemesis: The Expropriation of Health* (New York: Pantheon Books, 1982; originally published in 1976).

p. 51, **drug overuse and overprescription:** Edward M. Brecher and the *Consumer Reports* editors, *Licit and Illicit Drugs: The Consumer's Union Report on Narcotics, Stimulants, Depressants, Inhalants, Hallucinogens, and Marijuana, Including Caffeine, Nicotine, and Alcohol* (Boston: Little, Brown, 1973).

p. 51, **U.S. House of Representatives report on unnecessary surgery:** U.S. House of Representatives, Committee on Interstate and Foreign Commerce, *Cost and Quality of Health Care: Unnecessary Surgery* (Washington, D.C.: U.S. Government Printing Office, 1976).

p. 51, **Rockefeller Institute conference proceedings:** John H. Knowles, ed., *Doing Better and Feeling Worse: Health in the United States* (New York: Norton, 1977).

CHAPTER 5: *We Are All Unique*

pp. 60–62, **the work of Dr. Roger Williams:** McGraw-Hill Encyclopedia of Science and Technology, *McGraw-Hill Modern Men of Science,* volume 2 (New York: McGraw-Hill, 1968).
Roger John Williams, *Biochemical Individuality* (Austin, Tex.: University of Texas Press, 1980).
Roger John Williams, *Nutrition Against Disease* (New York: Pitman, 1971).

p. 62, **articles on functional deficiencies and supplementation of vitamin B12:** Hans J. Naurath et al., "Effects of Vitamin B12, Folate, and Vitamin B6 Supplements in Elderly People with Normal Serum Vitamin Concentrations," *Lancet,* 1995; 345(8967); 85–89.

J. Lindenbaum et al., "Diagnosis of Cobalamin Deficiency II: Relative Sensitivities of Serum Cobalamin, Methylmalonic Acid, and Total Homocysteine Concentrations," *American Journal of Hematology,* 1990; 34; 99–107.

CHAPTER 6: *Whole People in Their Total Environments*

p. 66, **Minuchin's studies on children and adolescents with serious physical illnesses:** Salvador Minuchin, Bernice Rosman, and Lester Baker, *Psychosomatic Families* (Cambridge, Mass.: Harvard University Press, 1978).

p. 67, **Hoebel's work with men with coronary artery disease:** F. C. Hoebel, "Coronary Artery Disease and Family Interaction: A Study of Risk Modification," in Paul Watzlawick and John Weakland, eds. *The Interactional View* (New York: W. W. Norton, 1977), pp. 362–75.

p. 68, **asthma has been increasing steadily:** K. B. Weiss, P. J. Gergen, and D. K. Wagner, "Breathing Easier or Wheezing Worse? The Changing Epidemiology of Asthma Morbidity and Mortality," *Annual Review of Public Health,* 1993; 14; 491–513.

p. 68, **discrepancies between blacks and whites:** Colin McCord and Harold Freeman, "Excess Mortality in Harlem," *New England Journal of Medicine,* 1990; 322; 173–77.

p. 68, **articles on the Roseto study include:** J. G. Bruhn, "An Epidemiological Study of Myocardial Infarction in an Italian-American Community," *Journal of Chronic Diseases,* 1965; 18; 352–65.
J. G. Bruhn et al., "Social Aspects of Coronary Heart Disease in Two Adjacent, Ethnically Different Communities," *American Journal of Public Health,* 1966; 56(9); 1493–1506.
C. Stout et al., "Unusually Low Incidence of Death from Myocardial Infarction: Study of an Italian American Community in Pennsylvania," *Journal of the American Medical Association,* 1064; 188; 845–49.
S. Wolf, "Protective Social Forces that Counterbalance Stress," *Journal of the South Carolina Medical Association,* 1976; 72(2); 57–59.

p. 68, **studies on Japanese immigrants:** Michael G. Marmot and S. Leonard Syme, "Acculturation and Coronary Heart Disease in Japanese-Americans," *American Journal of Epidemiology,* 1976; 104(3): 225–247.
Lisa F. Berkman, "The Relationship of Social Networks and Social Support to Morbidity and Mortality," in Sheldon Cohen and S. Leonard Syme, eds., *Social Support and Health* (Orlando, Fla.: Academic Press, 1985).

p. 69, **Department of Health, Education and Welfare survey:** *Work in America: Report of a Special Task Force to the Secretary of Health, Education, and Welfare* (Cambridge, Mass.: MIT Press, 1973).

p. 69, **"high strain" jobs:** R. A. Karasek et al., "Job, Psychosocial Factors, and Coronary Heart Disease," *Advances in Cardiology,* 1982; 29; 62–67.

R. A. Karasek et al., "Job Characteristics in Relation to the Prevalence of Myocardial Infarction in the U.S. Health Examination Survey (HES) and the Health and Nutrition Examination Survey (HANES)," *American Journal of Public Health,* 1988; 78(8); 910–18.

p. 69, **heart attacks in the United States occurring on Monday mornings:** S. W. Rabkin, F. A. L. Mathewson, and R. B. Tate, "Chronobiology of Cardiac Sudden Death in Men," *Journal of the American Medical Association,* 1980; 244; 1357–58.

D. R. Thompson, J. E. F. Pohl, and T. W. Sutton, "Acute Myocardial Infarction and Day of the Week," *American Journal of Cardiology,* 1992; 69; 266–67.

p. 69, **Jan Christian Smuts:** Jan Christian Smuts, *Holism and Evolution* (New York: Macmillan, 1926).

CHAPTER 7: *The Healing Partnership*

p. 85, **literature survey by Sackett:** D. L. Sackett and J. C. Snow, "The Magnitude of Compliance and Noncompliance," in R. B. Haynes, D. W. Taylor, and D. L. Sackett, eds., *Compliance in Health Care* (Baltimore: Johns Hopkins University Press, 1979).

p. 85, **22 percent of patients' prescriptions were being consumed properly:** J. Boyd, T. Covington, W. Stanaszek, and R. Coussons, "Drug Defaulting Part II: Analysis of Noncompliance Problems," *American Journal of Hospital Pharmacy,* 1974; 31; 485–94.

p. 87, **clinical research on "stress hardy" individuals:** S. Kobasa, "Stressful Life Events, Personality, and Health: An Inquiry into Hardiness," *Journal of Personality and Social Psychology,* 1979; 37(1); 1–11.

p. 88, **Langer and Rodin's clinical research on nursing home patients:** E. J. Langer and J. Rodin, "The Effects of Choice and Enhanced Personal Responsibility for the Aged: A Field Experiment in an Institutional Setting," *Journal of Personality and Social Psychology,* 1976; 34; 191–98.

p. 88, **use of relaxation techniques with skiers:** R. Swearingen, "The Physician as the Basic Instrument," in J. Gordon, D. Jaffe, and D. Bresler, eds. *Mind, Body, and Health: Toward an Integral Medicine* (New York: Human Sciences Press, 1984).

p. 88, **study on surgical patients:** L. D. Egbert et al., "Reduction of Postoperative Pain by Encouragement and Instruction of Patients: A Study of Doctor-Patient Rapport," *New England Journal of Medicine,* 1964; 270; 825–27.

CHAPTER 8: *Self-Care as Primary Care: The Power of the Mind (I)*

p. 95, **the work of Claude Bernard:** Claude Bernard, *La Science Expérimentale* (Paris: Librairie J.-B. Baillière et Fils, 1878).

Claude Bernard, *An Introduction to the Study of Experimental Medicine,* trans. Henry Copley Greene (Henry Schuman, 1949).

p. 96, **the work of Walter Bradford Cannon:** Walter B. Cannon, *The Wisdom of the Body* (New York: W. W. Norton, 1926).

p. 96, **Hans Selye's definition of stress:** Hans Selye, *The Stress of Life* (New York: McGraw-Hill, 1956).

p. 96, **the work of Helen Flanders Dunbar and Franz Alexander:** Harold Kaplan and Helen Kaplan, "An Historical Survey of Psychosomatic Medicine," *Journal of Nervous and Mental Disease,* 1956; 124; 546–68.

p. 99, **type A executive:** Meyer Friedman and Ray H. Rosenman, *Type A Behavior and Your Heart* (New York: Knopf, 1974).

p. 99, **the hypothalamus as "headquarters" of immune regulation:** George F. Solomon and Alfred A. Amkraut, "Emotions, Immunity, and Disease," in Lydia Temoshok, Craig Van Dyke, and Leonard S. Zegans, eds., *Emotions in Health and Illness: Theoretical and Research Foundations* (New York: Grune and Stratton, 1983).

p. 99, **cells of the immune system can be "conditioned":** Robert Ader, ed., *Psychoneuroimmunology* (New York: Academic Press, 1981).

p. 99, **receptors for peptides exist in both the brain and the immune system:** Candace Pert and Harris Dienstfrey, "The Neuropeptide Network," *Annals of the New York Academy of Sciences,* 1988; 521.

p. 102, **George Engel's correlation of "giving up" with onset of illness and relapses:** G. Engel, "A Life Setting Conducive to Illness: The Giving Up—Given Up Complex," *Bulletin of the Menninger Clinic,* 1968; 32; 355–65.

pp. 104—105, **Herbert Benson and the "relaxation response":** Herbert Benson and Miriam Klipper, *The Relaxation Response* (New York: Avon, 1976).
H. Benson, J. F. Beary, and M. P. Carol, "The Relaxation Response," *Psychiatry,* 1974; 37; 37–46.

p. 105, **relaxation can decrease levels of stress hormones:** J. W. Hoffman et al., "Reduced Sympathetic Nervous System Responsivity Associated with the Relaxation Response," *Science,* 1982; 215; 100–02.

p. 105, **improve immune functioning:** J. K. Kiecolt-Glaser and R. Glaser, "Stress and the Immune System: Human Studies," in A. Tasman and M. B. Riba, eds., *Annual Review of Psychiatry,* 1991; 11; 169–80. (Washington, D.C.: American Psychiatric Press).
J. K. Kiecolt-Glaser and R. Glaser, "Psychoneuroimmunology: Can Psychological Interventions Modulate Immunity?" *Journal of Consulting and Clinical Psychology,* 1992; 60; 569–75.

p. 105, **diminish chronic pain:** M. Caudill et al., "Decreased Clinic Use by Chronic Pain Patients: Response to Behavioral Medicine Intervention," *Journal of Chronic Pain,* 1991; 7; 305–310.
K. A. Holroyd et al., "A Comparison of Pharmacological (Amitriptyline HCL) and Nonpharmacological Therapies for Chronic Tension Headaches," *Journal of Consulting and Clinical Psychology,* 1991; 59; 387–93.

K. A. Holroyd and D. B. Penzien, "Pharmacological versus Non-pharmacological Prophylaxis of Recurrent Migraine Headache: A Meta-Analytic Review of Clinical Trials," *Pain,* 1990; 42; 1–13.

p. 105, **improve mood:** H. Benson et al., "Treatment of Anxiety: A Comparison of the Usefulness of Self-Hypnosis and a Meditational Relaxation Technique," *Psychotherapy and Psychosomatics,* 1978; 30; 229–42.

p. 105, **enhance fertility:** A. D. Domar, M. M. Seibel, and H. Benson, "The Mind/Body Program for Infertility: A New Behavioral Treatment Approach for Women with Infertility," *Fertility and Sterility,* 1990; 53; 246–49.

p. 109, **the use of placebos:** H. Benson and M. Epstein, "The Placebo Effect: A Neglected Asset in the Care of Patients," *Journal of the American Medical Association,* 1975; 232; 1225–27.

p. 110, **placebos on average 35 percent as powerful as drugs:** H. K. Beecher, "The Powerful Placebo," *Journal of the American Medical Association,* 1955; 159; 1602–06.

p. 110, **70 percent of patients given "ineffective" treatments had good outcomes:** Alan H. Roberts et al., "The Power of Nonspecific Effects in Healing: Implications for Psychosocial and Biological Treatments," *Clinical Psychology Review,* 1993; 13; 375–91.

p. 110, **patients receiving placebos experienced negative side effects of active treatment:** S. Wolf and R. Pinsky, "Effects of Placebo Administration and Occurrence of Toxic Reactions," *Journal of the American Medical Association,* 1954; 155; 339–41.
R. Aznar-Ramos et al., "Incidence of Side Effects with Contraceptive Placebo," *American Journal of Obstetrics and Gynecology,* 1969; 105; 1144–49.

p. 114, **psychological difference between sisters who developed rheumatoid arthritis symptoms and those who did not:** G. F. Solomon and R. H. Moos, "Psychologic Comparisons Between Women With Rheumatoid Arthritis and Their Non-Arthritic Sisters: I. Personality Test and Interview Rating Data," *Psychosomatic Medicine,* 1965; 27; 135–49.
G. F. Solomon and R. H. Moos, "Psychologic Comparisons Between Women With Rheumatoid Arthritis and their Non-Arthritic Sisters: II. Content Analysis of Interviews," *Psychosomatic Medicine,* 1965; 27; 150–64.

CHAPTER 9: *Self-Care as Primary Care: The Power of the Mind (II)*

p. 116, **Edmund Jacobson's "progressive muscular relaxation":** E. Jacobson, *Progressive Relaxation* (Chicago: University of Chicago Press, 1974).

p. 118, **work of Neal Miller:** "Neal Miller, the Dumb Autonomic Nervous System, and Biofeedback" in Harris Dienstfrey, ed., *Where the Mind Meets the Body* (New York: HarperCollins, 1991).

p. 119, **useful references on biofeedback include:** J. V. Basmajian, ed., *Biofeedback: Principles and Practice for Clinicians,* 3d ed. (Baltimore: Williams and Wilkins, 1989).

> J. P. Hatch et al., *Biofeedback: Studies in Clinical Efficacy* (New York: Plenum, 1987).

pp. 119ff., **useful references on the history of hypnosis include:** Michael Murphy, *The Future of the Body: Explorations into the Further Evolution of Human Nature* (Los Angeles: Jeremy P. Tarcher / Perigee Books, 1993).

> Henri F. Ellenberger, *The Discovery of the Unconscious: The History and Evolution of Dynamic Psychiatry* (New York: Basic Books, 1970).

p. 122, **hypnosis has been shown to:** J. Achterberg, L. Dossey, and J. S. Gordon (cochairs), et al., "Mind-Body Interventions," in *Alternative Medicine: Expanding Medical Horizons.* A Report to the National Institutes of Health on Alternative Medical Systems and Practices in the United States, NIH pub. no. 94-066 (Washington, D.C.: U.S. Government Printing Office, 1994).

p. 125, **Johannes Schultz and autogenic training:** Johannes Schultz and Wolfgang Luthe, *Autogenic Training* (Grune and Stratton, 1959).

pp. 125ff., **work on therapeutic imagery:** "Mind-Body Interventions," in *Alternative Medicine: Expanding Medical Horizons.* A Report to the National Institutes of Health on Alternative Medical Systems and Practices in the United States, NIH pub. no. 94-066 (Washington, D.C.: U.S. Government Printing Office, 1994).

> J. Achterberg, *Imagery in Healing: Shamanism and Modern Science.* (Shambhala, 1985).

> J. Achterberg and G. F. Lawlis, *Imagery and Disease: Diagnostic Tools?* (Champaign, Ill.: Institute for Personality and Ability Testing, 1984).

p. 129, **Achterberg and imagery's effects on white blood cells:** J. Achterberg and M. S. Rider, "The Effect of Music-Mediated Imagery on Neutrophils and Lymphocytes," *Biofeedback and Self Regulation,* 1989; 14; 247–57.

CHAPTER 10: *Self-Care as Primary Care: Touch, Movement, and Breathing*

p. 131, **books on René Spitz:** H. Colton, *The Gift of Touch* (New York: Harper and Row, 1987).

> R. Emde, ed., *René A. Spitz, Dialogues from Infancy* (New York: International Universities Press, 1983).

p. 132, **Harry Harlow:** H. A. Harlow and C. Mears, *The Human Model: Primate Perspectives* (Washington, D.C.: V. H. Winston and Sons, 1979).

p. 132, **contact between mother and infant in the hours after birth:** M. Klaus and J. Kennell, *Maternal and Infant Bonding* (St. Louis: C. V. Mosby, 1976).

p. 132, **newborn rat pups removed from their mother:** M. J. Meaney et al., "Effects of Neonatal Handling on Age-Related Impairments Associated with the Hippocampus," *Science,* 1988; 239; 766–68.

p. 132, **rat pups removed early from mothers showed decreases in growth hormone and delays in development:** S. M. Schanberg and T. M. Field, "Sensory Deprivation Stress and Supplemental Stimulation in the Rat Pup and Preterm Human Neonate," *Child Development,* 1987; 58; 1431–47.

p. 134, **general reference on Swedish massage:** Lucinda Lidell, Sara Thomas, et al., *The Book of Massage: The Complete Step-by-Step Guide to Eastern and Western Techniques* (New York: Fireside/Gaia Books, 1984).

p. 135, **studies on the beneficial effects of massage to relieve cancer distress:** S. Sims, "Slow Stroke Back Massage for Cancer Patients," *Nursing Times,* 1986; 82(47); 47–50.

A. T. Ferrell-Torry and O. J. Glick, "The Use of Therapeutic Massage as a Nursing Intervention to Modify Anxiety and the Perception of Cancer Pain," *Cancer Nursing,* April 1993; 16(2); 93–101.

p. 135, **to relieve pain of back injuries:** M. Weintraub, "Alternative Medical Care: Shiatsu, Swedish Muscle Massage, and Trigger Point Suppression in Spinal Pain Syndrome," *American Journal of Pain Management,* 1992; 2(2); 74–78.

p. 135, **to lower blood pressure and heart rate in the elderly:** C. Fakouri and P. Jones, "Relaxation Rx: Slow Stroke Back Rub," *Gerontological Nursing,* 1987; 13; 32–35.

p. 135, **to relieve depression and anxiety in adults on coronary care units:** P. Heidt, "Effect of Therapeutic Touch on Anxiety Level of Hospitalized Patients," *Nursing Research,* 1981; 30(1); 32–37.

p. 135, **to alleviate depression and anxiety of adolescents in psychiatric wards:** T. Field et al., "Massage Reduces Anxiety in Child and Adolescent Psychiatric Patients," *Journal of the American Academy of Child and Adolescent Psychiatry,* 1992; 31; 125–31.

p. 135, **popular accounts of the benefits of therapeutic massage:** R. Byass, "Soothing Body and Soul," *Nursing Times,* 1988; 84(24); 39–41.

P. Turton, "Touch Me, Feel Me, Heal Me," *Nursing Times,* 1989; 85(19); 42–44.

p. 135, **premature infants massaged several times a day:** T. M. Field et al., "Tactile/Kinesthetic Stimulation Effects on Preterm Neonates," *Pediatrics,* 1986; 77(5); 654–58.

p. 135, **effects of massage on preterm babies of cocaine-using mothers:** A. Wheeden et al., "Massage Effects on Cocaine-Exposed Preterm Neonates," *Journal of Developmental and Behavioral Pediatrics,* 1993; 14; 318–22.

p. 136, **elderly people massaging babies:** T. Field, "Massage Therapy for Infants and Children," *Developmental and Behavioral Pediatrics,* 1995; 16(2); 105–111.

p. 136, **Alexander technique:** F. M. Alexander, *The Resurrection of the Body* (New York: University Books, 1969).

p. 137, **Feldenkrais method:** M. Feldenkrais, *Awareness Through Movement: Health Exercises for Personal Growth* (New York: Harper and Row, 1972).

p. 137, **Rolfing:** Don Johnson, *The Protean Body* (New York: Harper Colophon, 1977).

p. 138, **work of Wilhelm Reich:** Wilhelm Reich, *The Function of the Orgasm* (New York: Orgone Institute, 1942).

Wilhelm Reich, *Character Analysis*, trans. V. Carfagno (New York: Farrar, Straus and Giroux, 1972).

p. 141, **aerobic exercise decreases high blood pressure, lowers heart rate:** Claude Bouchard et al., eds., *Exercise, Fitness, and Health: A Consensus of Current Knowledge* (Champaign, Ill.: Human Kinetics Books, 1990).

William D. McArdle, Frank I. Katch, and Victor L. Katch, *Exercise Physiology: Energy, Nutrition, and Human Performance.* 3d ed. (Philadelphia: Lea and Febiger, 1991).

p. 141, **increases HDL:** T. C. Rotkis et al., "Increased High-Density Lipoprotein Cholesterol and Lean Weight in Endurance-Trained Women Runners," *Journal of Cardiac Rehabilitation,* 1984; 4; 62–66.

A. Lehtonen et al., "Serum Triglycerides and Cholesterol and Serum High-Density Lipoprotein Cholesterol in Physically Active Men," *Acta Med. Scand.,* 1978; 204; 111–14.

p. 141, **helps smokers cut down or stop:** Bess H. Marcus et al., "Usefulness of Physical Exercise for Maintaining Smoking Cessation in Women," *American Journal of Cardiology,* 1991; 68; 406–407.

Bess H. Marcus et al., "Exercise Enhances the Maintenance of Smoking Cessation in Women," *Addictive Behaviors,* 1995; 20(1); 87–92.

p. 141, **weight-bearing exercise in menopausal women protects against cardiovascular disease, decreases rate of osteoporosis:** Mona M. Shangold, "Exercise in the Menopausal Woman," *Obstetrics and Gynecology,* April 1990; 75(4) (Suppl.); 53S–58S.

Arthur C. Santora, "The Role of Nutrition and Exercise in Osteoporosis," *American Journal of Medicine,* 1987; 82, Suppl. 1B; 73–78.

p. 141, **studies on the beneficial effects of aerobic exercise on immune status:** S. L. Nehlsen-Cannarella et al., "The Effects of Moderate Exercise Training on Immune Response," *Medicine and Science in Sports and Exercise,* 1991; 23(1); 64–70.

J. M. Weiss, "Effects of Exercise on the Immune System: Relationship to Stress," in *Biological Effects of Physical Activity* (Champaign, Ill.: Human Kinetics Books, 1989), 71–83.

Arthur R. LaPerriere et al., "Exercise Intervention Attenuates Emotional Distress and Natural Killer Cell Decrements Following Notification of Positive Serologic Status for HIV-1," *Biofeedback and Self-Regulation,* 1990; 15(3); 229–42.

p. 141, **aerobic exercise releases endorphins:** Daniel B. Carr et al., "Physical Conditioning Facilitates the Exercise-Induced Secretion of

Beta-Endorphin and Beta-Lipotropin in Women," *New England Journal of Medicine*, 1981; 305(10); 560–63.

William D. McArdle, Frank I. Katch, and Victor L. Katch, *Exercise Physiology: Energy, Nutrition, and Human Performance*. 3d ed. (Philadelphia: Lea and Febiger, 1991).

J. Soares et al., "Increased Serotonin Levels in Physically Trained Men." *Brazilian Journal of Medical and Biological Research*, 1994; 27(7); 1635–38.

p. 142, **exercisers less likely to exhibit stress response:** Michael H. Sacks, "Exercise for Stress Control," in Daniel Goleman and Joel Gurin, eds., *Mind-Body Medicine: How to Use Your Mind for Better Health* (Yonkers, N.Y.: Consumer Reports Books, 1993).

p. 142, **exercise and anxiety and depression:** John H. Griest et al., "Running as Treatment for Depression," *Comprehensive Psychiatry,* Jan.–Feb. 1979; 20(1); 41–54.

Robert E. Hales and Thomas V. Travis, "Exercise as a Treatment Option for Anxiety and Depressive Disorders," *Military Medicine,* June 1987; 152; 299–302.

Anne D. Simons et al., "Exercise as a Treatment for Depression: An Update," *Clinical Psychology Review,* 1985; 5; 553–68.

International Society of Sport Psychology, "Physical Activity and Psychological Benefits: A Position Statement," *Sport Psychologist,* June 1992; 6; 199–203.

E. W. Martinsen et al., "Comparing Aerobic with Nonaerobic Forms of Exercise in the Treatment of Clinical Depression: A Randomized Trial," *Comprehensive Psychiatry,* July–Aug., 1989; 4; 324–31.

J. Fremont and L. W. Craighead, "Aerobic Exercise and Cognitive Therapy in the Treatment of Dysphoric Moods," *Cognitive Therapy Research,* 1987; 11(2); 241–51.

E. J. Doyne et al., "Aerobic Exercise as a Treatment for Depression in Women," *Behavior Therapy,* 1983; 14; 434–40.

p. 142, **yoga:** B. Blackwell et al., "Effects of Transcendental Meditation on Blood Pressure: A Controlled Pilot Experiment (abstract)," *Psychosomatic Medicine,* 1975; 37; 86.

M. M. Gore, "Effect of Yogic Treatment on Some Pulmonary Functions in Asthmatics," *Yoga Mimamsa,* 1982; 20; 51–58.

R. Monroe, A. K. Ghosh, and D. Kalish, *Yoga Research Bibliography: Scientific Studies on Yoga and Meditation* (Cambridge, England: Yoga Biomedical Trust, 1989).

R. E. Monroe and L. Fitzgerald, "Follow-up Survey on Yoga and Diabetes," *Yoga Biomedical Bulletin,* 1986; 1(4); 61.

D. Ornish et al., "Effects of Stress Management Training and Dietary Changes in Treating Ischemic Heart Disease," *Journal of the American Medical Association,* 1983; 249; 54–59.

p. 142, **t'ai chi:** D. Zhuo et al., "Cardiorespiratory and Metabolic Responses During Tai Chi Chuan Exercise," *Canadian Journal of Applied Sports Sciences,* 1984; 9(1); 7–10.

P. Jin, "Efficacy of T'ai Chi, Brisk Walking, Meditation, and Reading in Reducing Mental and Emotional Stress," *Journal of Psychosomatic Research*, 1992; 36(4); 361–70.

L. B. Downs, "T'ai Chi," *Modern Maturity*, 1992; 35; 60–64.

S. K. Tse et al., "T'ai Chi and Postural Control in the Well Elderly," *American Journal of Occupational Therapy*, 1992; 46; 295–300.

p. 146, **physiological effects of the "complete breath":** James E. Loehr and Jeffrey Migdow. *Take a Deep Breath*. Random House, 1986.

Swami Rama, Rudolph Ballentine, and Alan Hymes. *Science of Breath: A Practical Guide*. Himalayan Publications, 1979.

CHAPTER 11: *Self Care as Primary Care: "When I Eat, I Eat"*

p. 150, **statistics on overweight:** R. J. Kuczmarski et al., "Increasing Prevalence of Overweight Among U.S. Adults: The National Health and Nutrition Examination Surveys, 1960 to 1991," *Journal of the American Medical Association*, 1994; 272; 205–211.

p. 150, **evidence that obesity predisposes us to illnesses, and weighing less may contribute to longevity:** J. E. Manson et al., "Body Weight and Mortality Among Women," *New England Journal of Medicine*, Sept. 14, 1995; 333(11); 677–85.

C. Iribarren et al., "Association of Weight Loss and Weight Fluctuation with Mortality among Japanese American Men," *New England Journal of Medicine*, Sept. 14, 1995; 333(11); 686–92.

T. Byers, "Body Weight and Mortality," *New England Journal of Medicine*, Sept. 14, 1995; 333(11); 723–24.

p. 150, **Paleolithic diet:** S. Boyd Eaton and Melvin Konner, "Paleolithic Nutrition: A Consideration of Its Nature and Current Implications," *New England Journal of Medicine*, Jan. 31, 1985; 312(5); 283–89.

p. 152, **health-promoting utility of regimens based on consumption of large amounts of grains, fruits, and vegetables and very small quantities of fat and/or animal products:** Gar Hildenbrand (Chair) et al., "Diet and Nutrition in the Prevention and Treatment of Chronic Disease," in *Alternative Medicine: Expanding Medical Horizons*, A Report to the National Institutes of Health on Alternative Medical Systems and Practices in the United States. NIH pub. no. 94-066 (Washington, D.C.: U.S. Government Printing Office, 1994).

p. 152, **studies on Seventh-Day Adventists:** B. Armstrong, A. J. van Merwyk, and H. Coates, "Blood Pressure in Seventh-Day Adventist Vegetarians," *American Journal of Epidemiology*, 1977; 105; 444–49.

R. L. Phillips et al., "Mortality among California Seventh-Day Adventists for Selected Cancer Sites," *Journal of the National Cancer Institute*, 1980; 65; 1097–1107.

R. L. Phillips and D. A. Snowden, "Association of Meat and Coffee Use with Cancers of the Large Bowel, Breast, and Prostate among Seventh-Day Adventists: Preliminary Results," *Cancer Research*, 1983; 43(Suppl.); 2403–2408.

U. D. Register and L. M. Sonnenberg, "The Vegetarian Diet," *Journal of the American Dietetic Association*, 1973; 62; 253–61.

p. 152, **macrobiotic diet:** F. M. Sacks, B. Rosner, and E. H. Kass, "Blood Pressure in Vegetarians," *American Journal of Epidemiology*, 1974; 100; 390–98.

p. 152, **Mediterranean diet:** M. S. de Lorgeril et al., "Mediterranean Alpha-Linolenic Acid-Rich Diet in Secondary Prevention of Coronary Heart Disease," *Lancet*, 1994; 343; 1454–59.
W. C. Willett et al., "Relation of Meat, Fat, and Fiber Intake to the Risk of Colon Cancer in a Prospective Study among Women," *New England Journal of Medicine*, 1990; 323; 1664–72.

p. 153, **high-fiber diets may diminish risk of gallstones:** K. C. Hayes et al., "Dietary Impact on Biliary Lipids and Gallstones," *Annual Review of Nutrition*, 1992; 12; 299–326.

p. 153, **may diminish risk of kidney stones:** J. Hughes, "Diet and Calcium Stones," *Canadian Medical Association Journal*, 1992; 146(2); 137–43.
H. J. Schneider, "Preventing the Recurrence of Kidney Stones with Farnolith Bran Preparation," in V. R. Walker et al., eds., *Urolithiasis* (New York: Plenum Press, 1989), 871.
S. Ebisuno et al., "Results of Long-Term Rice Bran Treatment on Stone Recurrence in Hypercalciuric Patients," *British Journal of Urology*, 1991; 67(3); 237–40.

p. 153, **oat bran fiber decreases LDL and total cholesterol:** M. H. Davidson, "The Hypocholesterolemic Effects of B-glucan in Oatmeal and Oat Bran," *Journal of the American Medical Association*, 1991; 265(14); 1833–39.
C. M. Ripsin, "Oat Products and Lipid Lowering: A Meta-Analysis," *Journal of the American Medical Association*, 1992; 267(24); 3317–27.

p. 153, **wheat bran reduces chances of colon cancer:** J. J. DeCosse, "Effect of Wheat Fiber and Vitamins C and E on Rectal Polyps in Patients with Familial Adenomatous Polyposis," *Journal of the National Cancer Institute*, 1989; 81(17); 1290–97.
D. S. Alberts, "Effects of Dietary Wheat Bran Fiber on Rectal Epithelial Cell Proliferation in Patients with Resection for Colorectal Cancers," *Journal of the National Cancer Institute*, 1990; 82; 1280–85.

p. 153, **beans decrease LDL and total cholesterol:** J. W. Anderson et al., "Serum Lipid Response of Hypercholesterolemic Men to Single and Divided Doses of Canned Beans," *American Journal of Clinical Nutrition*, 1990; 51(6); 1013–19.

p. 153, **soy decreases LDL and total cholesterol:** James W. Anderson et al., "Meta-Analysis of the Effects of Soy Protein Intake on Serum Lipids," *New England Journal of Medicine*, 1995; 333; 276–82.
John W. Erdman, "Control of Serum Lipids with Soy Protein," *New England Journal of Medicine*, 1995; 333; 313–15.

p. 153, **soy as an anticancer food:** M. Messina, "The Role of Soy Products in Reducing Risk of Cancer," *Journal of the National Cancer Institute*, 1991; 83(8); 541–46.

S. Barnes, "Soybeans Inhibit Mammary Tumors in Models of Breast Cancer," *Progress in Clinical and Biological Research,* 1990; 347; 239–53.

p. 153, **fish and omega-3 fatty acids dilate blood vessels, decrease platelet clumping, prevent arterial plaques:** Alexander Leaf and Peter C. Weber, "Cardiovascular Effects of n-3 Fatty Acids," *New England Journal of Medicine,* 1988; 318; 549–57.

W. Hermann, "The Influence of Dietary Supplementation with Omega-3 Fatty Acids on Serum Lipids, Apolipoproteins, Coagulation, and Fibrinolytic Parameters," *Zeitschrift für Klinische Medizin,* 1991; 46; 1363–69.

Isabelle Bairati et al., "Double Blind, Randomized, Controlled Trial of Fish Oil Supplements in Prevention of Recurrence of Stenosis after Coronary Angioplasty," *Circulation,* 1992; 85; 950–56.

M. R. Milner, "Usefulness of Fish Oil Supplements in Preventing Clinical Evidence of Restenosis after Percutaneous Transluminal Coronary Angioplasty," *American Journal of Cardiology,* 1989; 64(5); 294–99.

p. 153, **damp down inflammatory response:** J. M. Kremer, "Clinical Studies of Omega-3 Fatty Acid Supplementation in Patients Who Have Rheumatoid Arthritis," *Rheumatic Disease Clinics of North America,* 1991; 17; 391–402.

p. 153, **anticancer properties of onions:** W. C. Yu et al., "Allium Vegetables and Reduced Risk of Stomach Cancer," *Journal of the National Cancer Institute,* 1989; 81(2); 162–64.

S. Belman, "Onion and Garlic Oils Inhibit Tumor Promotion," *Carcinogenesis,* 1983; 4(8); 1063–65.

p. 153, **onions increase HDL:** Victor Gurewich, personal communication.

p. 153, **onions decrease risk of blood clots:** A. N. Makheja et al., "Effects of Onion Extract on Platelet Aggregation and Thromboxane Synthesis," *Prostaglandins,* 1979; 2(6); 413–24.

A. N. Makheja et al., "Altered Arachidonic Acid Metabolism in Platelets Inhibited by Onion or Garlic Extracts," *Advances in Prostaglandin Thromboxane Leukotriene Research,* 1980; 6; 309–12.

p. 153, **onions prevent allergies and asthma attacks:** W. Dorsch and J. Ring, "Suppression of Immediate and Late Cutaneous Anti-IgE-Induced Skin Reactions by Topically Applied Alcohol/Onion Extract," *Allergy,* 1984; 39; 43–49.

W. Dorsch and J. Weber, "Prevention of Allergen-Induced Bronchial Obstruction in Sensitized Guinea Pigs by Crude Alcoholic Onion Extract," *Agents and Actions,* 1984; 14; 626–29.

W. Dorsch, "Antiasthmatic Effects of Onions," *International Archives of Allergy and Applied Immunology,* 1989; 88; 228–30.

W. Dorsch and H. Wagner, "New Antiasthmatic Drugs from Traditional Medicine?" *International Archives of Allergy and Applied Immunology,* 1991; 94; 262–65.

p. 153, **garlic controls infections:** Tariq H. Abdullah et al., "Garlic Revisited: Therapeutic for the Major Diseases of Our Times?" *Journal of the National Medical Association,* 1988; 80(4); 439–45.

MANIFESTO FOR A NEW MEDICINE

pp. 153–154, **garlic reduces cholesterol levels, decreases elevated blood pressure:** N. D. Barrie, "Effects of Garlic Oil on Platelet Aggregation, Serum Lipids, and Blood Pressure in Humans," *Journal of Orthomolecular Medicine,* 1987; 2(1); 15–21.

J. V. Gadkari, "The Effect of Ingestion of Raw Garlic on Serum Cholesterol Level, Clotting Time and Fibrinolytic Activity in Normal Subjects," *Journal of Postgraduate Medicine,* 1991; 37(3); 128–31.

S. Warshafsky et al., "Effect of Garlic on Total Serum Cholesterol: A Meta-Analysis," *Annals of Internal Medicine,* 1993; 119; 599–605.

W. Auer, "Hypertension and Hyperlipidaemia: Garlic Helps in Mild Cases," *British Journal of Clinical Practice Symposium Supplement,* Aug. 1990; 69; 3–6.

p. 154, **garlic enhances immune functioning:** Benjamin H. S. Lau, "Garlic Compounds Modulate Macrophage and T-lymphocyte Functions," *Molecular Biotherapy,* 1991; 3; 103–107.

T. H. Abdullah et al., "Enhancement of Natural Killer Cell Activity in AIDS with Garlic," *Deutsche Zeitschrift für Onkologie,* 1989; 24; 52–53.

p. 154, **garlic may improve mood:** G. Vorberg and B. Schneider, "Therapy with Garlic: Results of a Placebo-Controlled, Double-Blind Study," *British Journal of Clinical Practice Symposium Supplement,* Aug. 1990; 69; 7–11.

p. 154, **ginger to control nausea and vomiting:** Daniel B. Mowrey and Dennis E. Clayson, "Motion Sickness, Ginger, and Psychophysics," *Lancet,* Mar. 20, 1982; 655–57.

p. 154, **olive oil lowers LDL:** Giovannella Baggio et al., "Olive-Oil-Enriched Diet: Effect on Serum Lipoprotein Levels and Biliary Cholesterol Saturation," *American Journal of Clinical Nutrition,* 1988; 47; 960–64.

p. 154, **olive oil raises HDL:** Pedro Mata et al., "Effects of Long-Term Monounsaturated- vs Polyunsaturated-Enriched Diets on Lipoproteins in Healthy Men and Women," *American Journal of Clinical Nutrition,* 1992; 55; 846–50.

p. 154, **olive oil's protective effect against LDL damage to arteries:** M. Aviram and K. Eias, "Dietary Olive Oil Reduces Low-Density Lipoprotein Uptake by Macrophages and Decreases the Susceptibility of the Lipoprotein to Undergo Lipid Peroxidation," *Annals of Nutrition and Metabolism,* 1995; 37; 75–84.

p. 154, **sugar does indeed produce hyperactivity in some children:** T. W. Jones et al., "Enhanced Adrenomedullary Response and Increased Susceptibility to Neuroglycopenia: Mechanisms Underlying the Adverse Effects of Sugar Ingestion in Healthy Children," *Journal of Pediatrics,* 1995; 126(2); 171–77.

p. 155, **caffeine is highly addictive, causes withdrawal symptoms:** R. R. Griffiths, "Low-Dose Caffeine Physical Dependence in Humans," *Journal of Pharmacology and Experimental Therapeutics,* 1990; 255(3); 1123–32.

R. Smith, "Caffeine Withdrawal Headache," *Journal of Clinical Pharmacy and Therapeutics*, 1987; 12; 53–57.

K. Silverman et al., "Withdrawal Syndrome After the Double-Blind Cessation of Caffeine Consumption," *New England Journal of Medicine*, 1992; 327(16); 1109.

p. 155, **caffeine causes anxiety:** M. S. Bruce, "The Anxiogenic Effects of Caffeine," *Postgraduate Medical Journal*, 1990; 66 (Suppl. 2); S18–24.

p. 155, **coffee irritates the stomach:** G. H. Elta, "Comparison of Coffee Intake and Coffee-Induced Symptoms in Patients with Duodenal Ulcer, Nonulcer Dyspepsia, and Normal Controls," *American Journal of Gastroenterology*, 1990; 85(10); 1339–42.
S. Cohen, "Pathogenesis of Coffee-Induced Gastrointestinal Symptoms," *New England Journal of Medicine*, 1980; 303; 122–24.

p. 155, **caffeine may promote cysts in breasts:** J. P. Minton et al., "Response of Fibrocystic Disease to Caffeine Withdrawal and Correlation of Cyclic Nucleotides with Breast Disease," *American Journal of Obstetrics and Gynecology*, Sept. 1979; 135(1); 157–58.

p. 155, **lactose intolerance:** P.G. Bianchi, "Lactose Intolerance in Adults with Chronic Unspecified Abdominal Complaints," *Hepatogastroenterology*, 1983; 30(6); 254–57.

p. 155, **milk protein hard for infants to digest:** J. P. Campbell, "Dietary Treatment of Infant Colic: A Double Blind Study," *Journal of the Royal College of General Practitioners*, 1989; 39(318); 11–14.
I. Jakobsson, "Food Antigens in Human Milk," *European Journal of Clinical Nutrition*, 1991; 45 (Suppl. 1); 29–33.
P. S. Clyne and A. Kulczycki, "Human Breast Milk Contains Bovine IgG. Relationship to Infant Colic?" *Pediatrics*, 1991; 87; 439–44.

p. 155, **milk may produce allergic reactions, including arthritic flares:** J. Rodriquez, "Allergy to Cow's Milk with Onset in Adult Life," *Annals of Allergy*, 1989; 62(3); 185a–b.
R. S. Panush, "Food Induced (Allergic) Arthritis: Inflammatory Arthritis Exacerbated by Milk," *Arthritis and Rheumatism*, 1986; 29(2); 220–25.

p. 155, **headaches and flushing from MSG:** A. L. Scopp, "MSG and Hydrolyzed Vegetable Protein Induced Headache: Review and Case Studies," *Headache*, 1991; 31(2); 107–10.

p. 155, **asthma and allergic reactions from sulfites:** *Reexamination of the GRAS Status of Sulfiting Agents* (Springfield, Va.: National Technical Information Service, U. S. Department of Commerce, 1985).

p. 155, **headaches caused by aspartame:** R. B. Lipton, "Aspartame as a Dietary Trigger of Headache," *Headache*, 1989; 29(2); 90–92.
S. M. Koehler, "The Effect of Aspartame on Migraine Headache," *Headache*, 1988; 28(1); 10–14.

p. 156, **Japanese study on fasting for chronic illness:** J. Suzuki et al., "Fasting Therapy for Psychosomatic Diseases in Japan," *Psychotherapy and Psychosomatics,* 1979; 31; 307–14.
Y. Yamauchi et al., "Fasting Therapy for Psychosomatic Diseases with Special Reference to Its Indication and Therapeutic Mechanism," *Tohoku Journal of Experimental Medicine,* 1979; 118(S); 307–14.

p. 158, **ginkgo biloba and rehmannia:** Dan Bensky and Andrew Gamble, *Chinese Herbal Medicine: Materia Medica,* rev. ed. (Seattle: Eastland Press, 1993).

p. 158, **Saint-John's-wort:** D. Laudahn, "High Dosed Saint-John's-Wort Extract for Treatment of Mild and Moderate Depressions." *Acta Horticulturae,* 1993; 332; 265–72.

p. 158, **ginseng root:** X. J. Cheng et al., "Comparison of Action of Panax Ginsenosides and Panax Quinquonosides on Anti-Warm Stress in Mice," *Journal of Shenyang College of Pharmacy,* 1986; 3(3); 170–72.
W. X. Yuan et al., "Effects of Ginseng Root Saponins on Brain Monoamine and Serum Corticosterone in Heat Stressed Mice," Presented at the 5th Southeast Asian and Western Pacific regional meeting of pharmacologists, Chinese Pharmacological Association, Beijing, 1988.

p. 158, **echinacea:** B. Braunig et al., "Echinacea purpureae radix for Strengthening the Immune Response in Flu-like Infections," *Zeitschrift für Phytotherapie,* 1992; 13; 7–13.

p. 159, **saw palmetto:** G. Champpault, J. D. Patel, and A. M. Bonnard, "A Double-Blind Trial of an Extract of the Plant *Serenoa repens* in Benign Prostatic Hyperplasia," *British Journal of Clinical Pharmacology,* 1984; 18(3); 461–62.

p. 160, **the work of Roger Williams:** R. Williams, *Biochemical Individuality* (Austin, Tex.: University of Texas Press, 1980).

Significant vitamin and mineral deficiencies in major portions of the population: Melvyn H. Werbach, "Common Nutritional Deficiencies— Part 2," *Townsend Letter for Doctors,* Feb.-Mar. 1995, 24.
Ashima K. Kant, and Gladys Block, "Dietary Vitamin B-6 Intake and Food Sources in the U.S. Population: NHANES II, 1976-1980," *American Journal of Clinical Nutrition,* 1990; 52; 707-716.
Adrianne Bendich, and Lillian Langseth, "Safety of Vitamin A," *American Journal of Clinical Nutrition,* 1989; 49; 358–371.
Suzanne P. Murphy, Amy F. Subar, and Gladys Block, "Vitamin E Intakes and Sources in the United States," *American Journal of Clinical Nutrition,* 1990; 52; 361–67.
Amy F. Subar, Gladys Block, and L. Denise James, "Folate Intake and Food Sources in the U.S. Population," *American Journal of Clinical Nutrition,* 1989; 50; 508–516.
"NIH Consensus Conference: Osteoporosis," *Journal of the American Medical Association,* 1984; 252(6); 799–802.

R.A. Anderson, "Chromium and Its Role in Lean Body Mass and Weight Reduction," *Nutrition Report*, 1993; 11(6).

M. Seelig, *Magnesium Deficiency in the Pathogenesis of Disease*, (New York: Plenum Press, 1980).

p. 161, **vitamin E to prevent thromboses:** J. D. Kanofsky and P. B. Kanofsky, "Prevention of Thromboembolic Disease by Vitamin E," *New England Journal of Medicine*, 1981; 305; 173–74.

p. 161, **magnesium as a treatment for asthma:** H. Okayama et al., "Bronchodilating Effect of Magnesium Sulfate in Bronchial Asthma," *Journal of the American Medical Association*, 1988; 257; 1076–78.

S. P. Hauser and P. H. Braun, "Intravenous Magnesium in Asthmatic Patients. A Clinical Trial and Review of the Literature," in B. Lassere and J. Durlach, eds., *Magnesium—A Relevant Ion* (London: John Libbey, 1991).

R. M. McNamara et al., "Intravenous Magnesium Sulfate in the Management of Acute Respiratory Failure Complicating Asthma," *Annals of Emergency Medicine*, 1989; 18; 197–99.

p. 161, **magnesium as a treatment for cardiovascular disease:** K. L. Woods and S. Fletcher, "Long-Term Outcome After Intravenous Magnesium Sulphate in Suspected Acute Myocardial Infarction: The Second Leicester Intravenous Magnesium Intervention Trial (LIMIT-2)," *Lancet*, 1994; 343; 816–19.

K. L. Woods et al., "Intravenous Magnesium Sulphate in Suspected Acute Myocardial Infarction: Results of the Second Leicester Intravenous Magnesium Intervention Trial (LIMIT-2)," *Lancet*, 1992; 339; 1553–58.

p. 161, **folic acid helpful in preventing cardiovascular disease:** Johan B. Ubbink et al., "Vitamin Requirements for the Treatment of Hyperhomocysteinemia in Humans," *Journal of Nutrition*, 1994; 124; 1927–33.

p. 161, **folic acid and neural tube defects in fetuses:** Andrew E. Czeizel and István Dudás, "Prevention of the First Occurrence of Neural-tube Defects by Periconceptional Vitamin Supplementation," *New England Journal of Medicine*, 1992; 327; 1832–35.

Irwin H. Rosenberg, "Folic Acid and Neural-tube Defects—Time for Action?" *New England Journal of Medicine*, 1992; 327; 1875–77.

p. 161, **free radical production as major source of cardiovascular disease, cancer, and chronic illness in industrial societies:** Denham Harman, "Free Radical Theory of Aging: Role of Free Radicals in the Origination and Evolution of Life, Aging, and Disease Processes," in John E. Johnson, Jr. et al., eds., *Free Radicals, Aging, and Degenerative Diseases* (New York: Alan R. Liss, 1986).

Byung Pal Yu, ed., *Free Radicals in Aging* (Boca Raton, Fla.: CRC Press, 1993).

Denham Harman, "Free Radical Theory of Aging: The 'Free Radical' Diseases," *Age*, 1984; 7; 111–31.

p. 162, **antioxidants' protective effect against several kinds of cancer:** William J. Blot et al., "Nutrition Intervention Trials in Linxian, China:

Supplementation with Specific Vitamin/Mineral Combinations, Cancer Incidence, and Disease-Specific Mortality in the General Population," *Journal of the National Cancer Institute*, 1993; 85(18); 1483–92.

Paul Knekt et al., "Vitamin E and Cancer Prevention," *American Journal of Clinical Nutrition*, 1991; 53 (Suppl.); 283S–286S.

Gladys Block, "Vitamin C and Cancer Prevention: The Epidemiologic Evidence," *American Journal of Clinical Nutrition*, 1991; 53 (Suppl.); 270S–282S.

p. 162, **antioxidants against cardiovascular disease:** Meir J. Stampfer et al., "Vitamin E Consumption and the Risk of Coronary Disease in Women," *New England Journal of Medicine*, 1993; 328; 1444–49.

Eric B. Rimm et al., "Vitamin E Consumption and the Risk of Coronary Disease in Men," *New England Journal of Medicine*, 1993; 328; 1450–56.

p. 162, **antioxidants against cataracts:** James M. Robertson, Allan P. Donner, and John R. Trevithick, "Vitamin E Intake and Risk of Cataracts in Humans," *Annals of the New York Academy of Sciences*, 1989; 570; 372–82.

Allen Taylor, "Role of Nutrients in Delaying Cataracts," *Annals of the New York Academy of Sciences*, 1992; 669; 111–23.

p. 162, **antioxidants stimulate immune functioning in patients with HIV and other infections:** G. O. Coodley et al., "Beta Carotene in HIV Infection," *Journal of Acquired Immune Deficiency Syndromes*, 1993; 6; 272–76.

M. Alexander, H. Newmark, and R. G. Miller, "Oral Beta Carotene Can Increase the Number of OKT4 Cells in Human Blood," *Immunology Letters*, 1985; 9; 221–24.

J. D. Kanofsky et al., "Is There a Role for Vitamin A or Beta Carotene in HIV Therapy?" (abstract) *Journal of the American College of Nutrition*, 1990; 9; 551.

p. 162, **beta carotene and lung cancer:** Regina G. Ziegler, "Vegetables, Fruits, and Carotenoids and the Risk of Cancer," *American Journal of Clinical Nutrition*, 1991; 53 (Suppl.); 251S–259S.

p. 162, **less favorable studies:** O. P. Heinonen, J. K. Huttunen, and D. Albanes, "The Effect of Vitamin E and Beta Carotene on the Incidence of Lung Cancer in Male Smokers," *New England Journal of Medicine*, 1994; 330(15); 1029–35.

E. Robert Greenberg et al., "A Clinical Trial of Antioxidant Vitamins to Prevent Colorectal Adenoma," *New England Journal of Medicine*, 1994; 331(3); 141–47.

p. 163, **British study on exacerbation of rheumatoid arthritis due to wheat and corn:** L. G. Darlington, "Dietary Therapy for Arthritis," *Rheumatic Disease Clinics of North America*, 1991; 17(2); 273–85.

p. 163, **trial in which hyperactive children reacted negatively to milk and chocolate:** J. Egger et al., "Controlled Trial of Oligoantigenic Diet Treatment in the Hyperkinetic Syndrome," *Lancet*, 1985; 1(8428); 540–45.

p. 163, **Egger's study on children with migraines:** J. Egger, "Is Migraine Food Allergy? A Double-Blind Controlled Trial of Oligoantigenic Diet Treatment," *Lancet,* 1983; 2; 865–69.

CHAPTER 12: *Other Medicines*

p. 166, **basic text of Chinese medicine:** Ilza Veith, trans., *The Yellow Emperor's Classic of Internal Medicine* (Berkeley: University of California Press, 1972).

p. 169, **history of osteopathic medicine:** Norman Gevitz, "Osteopathic Medicine: From Deviance to Difference," in Norman Gevitz, ed., *Other Healers: Unorthodox Medicine in America* (Baltimore: Johns Hopkins University Press, 1988).
Barbara Brennan and Anthony Rosner (cochairs) et al., "Manual Healing Methods," in *Alternative Medicine: Expanding Medical Horizons,* A Report to the National Institutes of Health on Alternative Medical Systems and Practices in the United States, NIH pub. no. 94-066 (Washington, D.C.: U.S. Government Printing Office, 1994).

p. 170, **history of chiropractic:** Walter I. Wardwell, "Chiropractors: Evolution to Acceptance," in Norman Gevitz, ed., *Other Healers: Unorthodox Medicine in America* (Baltimore: Johns Hopkins University Press, 1988).
Barbara Brennan and Anthony Rosner (cochairs) et al., "Manual Healing Methods," in *Alternative Medicine: Expanding Medical Horizons,* A Report to the National Institutes of Health on Alternative Medical Systems and Practices in the United States, NIH pub. no. 94-066 (Washington, D.C.: U.S. Government Printing Office, 1994).

p. 172, **AMA's "Committee on Quackery":** William Trever, *In the Public Interest* (Los Angeles: Scriptures Unlimited, 1972).

p. 172, **1991 court decision:** Chester A. Wilk et al *v.* AMA et al. Complaint no. 76C3777, decided September 25 in the U.S. District Court for the Northern District of Illinois, Eastern Division, Memorandum Opinion and Order. Susan Getzendanner, District Judge, 1987. Ruling upheld in 1991 by the U.S. Supreme Court.

p. 174, **as many as fifteen million people visit chiropractors:** Barbara Brennan and Anthony Rosner (cochairs) et al., "Manual Healing Methods," in *Alternative Medicine: Expanding Medical Horizons*, A Report to the National Institutes of Health on Alternative Medical Systems and Practices in the United States, NIH pub. no. 94-066 (Washington, D.C.: U.S. Government Printing Office, 1994).

p. 174, **osteopathic researchers have demonstrated subtle, rhythmic movements in the cranial bones of cats:** T. Adams et al., "Parietal Bone Mobility in the Anesthetized Cat," *Journal of the American Osteopathic Association,* 1992; 92; 599–622.
R. S. Heisey and T. Adams, "Role of Cranial Bone Mobility in Cranial Compliance," *Neurosurgery,* 1993; 33; 1–9.

p. 174, **chiropractors have shown decreases in nerve conduction in patients with subluxations:** Seth Sharpless, "Susceptibility of Spinal

Roots to Compression Block," in Murray Goldstein, ed., *The Research Status of Spinal Manipulative Therapy* (Washington, D.C.: U.S. Government Printing Office, 1975).

p. 174, **manipulation may relieve headaches:** G. B. Parker, H. Tupling, and D. S. Pryor, "A Controlled Trial of Cervical Manipulation for Migraine," *Australian and New Zealand Journal of Medicine,* 1978; 8; 589.
H. Vernon, "Manipulative Therapy in the Chiropractic Treatment of Headaches: A Retrospective and Prospective Study," *Journal of Manipulative Physiological Therapy,* 1982; 5; 109–12.

p. 174, **manipulation may diminish chronic pain:** M. E. Barker, "Manipulation in General Medical Practice for Thoracic Pain Syndromes," *British Osteopathic Journal,* 1983; 15; 95.

p. 174, **manipulation may transiently decrease high blood pressure:** A. P. Fichera and D. R. Celander, "Effect of Osteopathic Manipulative Therapy on Autonomic Tone as Evidenced by Blood Pressure Changes and Activity of the Fibrinolytic System," *Journal of the American Osteopathic Association,* 1969; 67; 1036–38.
J. P. Morgan et al., "A Controlled Trial of Spinal Manipulation in the Management of Hypertension," *Journal of the American Osteopathic Association,* 1985; 85; 308–13.
G. Plaugher and T. R. Bachman, "Chiropractic Management of a Hypertensic Patient," *Journal of Manipulative Physiological Therapy,* 1994; 16; 544–49.

p. 175, **effectiveness of manipulation in the treatment of lower back pain:** D. J. Brunarski, "Clinical Trials of Spinal Manipulation: A Critical Appraisal and Review of the Literature," *Journal of Manipulative Physiological Therapy,* 1985; 7; 243.
F. K. Hoehler, J. S. Tobis, and A. A. Buerger, "Spinal Manipulation for Low Back Pain," *Journal of the American Medical Association,* 1981; 245; 1835–39.

p. 175, **RAND Corporation literature review is cited in:** S. Haldeman, D. Chapman-Smith, and D. M. Peterson, *Guidelines for Chiropractic Quality Assurance and Practice Parameters* (Gaithersburg, Md.: Aspen Publishers, 1992).

U. S. Government Agency for Health Care Policy and Research literature review: Stanley J. Bigos (chair) et al., *Acute Low Back Problems in Adults.* AHCPR pub. no. 95-0642 (Rockville, Md.: Department of Health and Human Services, Public Health Service, Agency for Health Care Policy and Research, December 1994).

p. 179, **history of homeopathy:** Dana Ullman, *Discovering Homeopathy: Medicine for the 21st Century,* rev. ed. (Berkeley, Calif.: North Atlantic, 1991).

p. 182, **Harris Coulter's encyclopedic history of homeopathy:** Harris L. Coulter, *Divided Legacy: A History of the Schism in Medical Thought* (Berkeley, Calif.: North Atlantic, 1977).

p. 182, **Flexner report:** Abraham Flexner, *Medical Education in the United States and Canada* (New York: Carnegie Foundation for the Advancement of Teaching, 1910).

p. 184, **study on Rhus tox:** Peter Fisher et al., "Effect of Homeopathic Treatment on Fibrositis (Primary Fibromyalgia)," *British Medical Journal,* Aug. 5, 1989; 299; 365–66.

p. 184, **German work using homeopathy to treat varicose veins:** E. Ernst, T. Saradeth, and K. L. Resch, "Complementary Treatment of Varicose Veins—A Randomized, Placebo-Controlled, Double-Blind Trial," *Phlebology,* 1990; 157–63.

p. 184, **Oscillococcinum for treating flu:** J. P. Ferley et al., "A Controlled Evaluation of a Homeopathic Preparation in the Treatment of Influenza-Like Syndromes," *British Journal of Clinical Pharmacology,* 1989; 27; 329–35.

p. 184, **Arnica and Hypericum in decreasing postextraction dental pain:** Henri Albertini et al., "Homeopathic Treatment of Dental Neuralgia Using Arnica and Hypericum: A Summary of 60 Observations," *Journal of the American Institute of Homeopathy,* 1985; 78; 126–28.

p. 185, **microdoses of a combination of pollens in reducing hay fever:** D. T. Reilley et al., "Is Homeopathy a Placebo Response? Controlled trial of Homeopathic Potency, with Pollen in Hayfever as Model," *Lancet,* 1986; 2(8512); 881–86.

p. 185, **Arnica, Rhus tox, and Bryonia in diminishing the symptoms of rheumatoid arthritis:** R. G. Gibson et al., "Homeopathic Therapy in Rheumatoid Arthritis: Evaluation by Double-Blind Clinical Therapeutic Trial," *British Journal of Clinical Pharmacology,* May 9, 1980; 453–59.

p. 185, **various remedies to decrease severity of children's diarrhea:** J. Jacobs et al., "Treatment of Acute Childhood Diarrhea with Homeopathic Medicine: A Randomized Clinical Trial in Nicaragua," *Pediatrics,* 1994; 93(5); 719–25.

p. 185, **Caulophyllum to decrease rate of stillbirths in pigs:** C. Day, "Control of Stillbirths in Pigs Using Homeopathy," *Veterinary Record,* 1984; 114; 216.

p. 185, **homeopathic remedies can inhibit viral growth:** L. Singh and G. Gupta, "Antiviral Efficacy of Homeopathic Drugs Against Animal Viruses," *British Homeopathic Journal,* 1985; 74(3); 168.

p. 185, **homeopathic remedies can stimulate enzymatic and immune activity:** W. E. Boyd, "The Action of Microdoses of Mercuric Chloride on Diastase," *British Homeopathic Journal,* 1941; 31; 1–28; and 1942; 32; 106–11.

Elizabeth Davenas, Bernard Poitevin, and Jacques Benveniste, "Effect on Mouse Peritoneal Macrophages of Orally Administered Very High Dilutions of Silica," *European Journal of Pharmacology,* April 1987; 135; 313–19.

p. 187, **useful resources on Chinese medicine and acupuncture include:** Harriet Beinfield and Efrem Korngold, *Between Heaven and Earth: A Guide to Chinese Medicine.,* (New York: Ballantine Books, 1991). Leon Hammer, *Dragon Rises, Red Bird Flies: Psychology and Chinese Medicine* (Barrytown, N.Y.: Station Hill Press, 1990). Ted Kaptchuk, *The Web That Has No Weaver: Understanding Chinese Medicine* (Chicago: Contemporary Books, 1985).

p. 189, **James Reston article on acupuncture:** James Reston, "Now, About My Operation in Peking," *New York Times,* July 26, 1971, 1.

p. 197, **physiological characteristics of acupuncture points:** B. Pomeranz, "Scientific Basis of Acupuncture," in G. Stux and B. Pomeranz, eds., *Acupuncture: Textbook and Atlas* (Berlin: Springer-Verlag, 1986).

p. 198, **a number of mushrooms with immune-enhancing properties:** N. Ohno et al., "Structural Characterization and Antitumor Activity of the Extracts of the Matted Mycelium of Cultured *Grifola frondosa,*" *Chemical and Pharmacological Bulletin* (Tokyo), 1985; 33; 3395–401. I. Suzuki, "Antitumor and Immunomodulating Activities of a Beta-Glucan Obtained from Liquid-Cultured *Grifola frondosa.*" *Chemical and Pharmacological Bulletin* (Tokyo), 1989; 37; 410–13.

CHAPTER 13: *Helping One Another*

p. 206, **studies on people who have lost a husband or wife:** J. E. Dimsdale, "Emotional Causes of Sudden Death," *American Journal of Psychiatry,* 1977; 134; 1361–66.
G. L. Engel, "Sudden and Rapid Death During Psychological Stress: Folklore or Folk Wisdom?" *Annals of Internal Medicine,* 1971; 74; 771–82.
B. Lown et al., "Psychophysiological Factors in Sudden Cardiac Death," *American Journal of Psychiatry,* 1980; 137; 1325–35.
J. J. Lynch, *The Broken Heart: The Medical Consequences of Loneliness* (New York: Basic Books, 1977).
S. J. Schleifer et al., "Suppression of Lymphocyte Stimulation Following Bereavement," *Journal of the American Medical Association,* 1983; 250; 374–77.
J. B. Stoddard and J. P. Henry, "Affectional Bonding and the Impact of Bereavement," *Advances,* 1985, 2; 19–28.

p. 206, **surveys in Alameda County:** L. F. Berkman and S. L. Syme, "Social Networks, Host Resistance, and Mortality: A Nine-Year Follow-up Study of Alameda County Residents," *American Journal of Epidemiology,* 1979; 109; 186–204.

p. 206, **long-term surveys of patients:** J. S. House, C. Robbins, and H. M. Metzner, "The Association of Social Relationships and Activities with Mortality: Prospective Evidence from the Tecumseh Study," *American Journal of Epidemiology,* 1982; 116; 123–40.
J. House, K. R. Landis, and D. Umberson, "Social Relationships and Health," *Science,* 1988; 241; 540–45.

p. 207, **statistics on Alcoholics Anonymous:** Alcoholics Anonymous, personal communication.

p. 207, **National Alliance for the Mentally Ill (NAMI):** Lester Grinspoon, ed., "Self-Help Groups—Part II," *Harvard Mental Health Letter,* April 1993; 9(10); 1.

p. 207, **study of a thousand battered women:** Lester Grinspoon, ed., "Self-Help Groups—Part II," *Harvard Mental Health Letter,* April 1993; 9(10); 1.

p. 207, **Stanford's Arthritis Self-Help Course:** K. Lorig et al., "The Beneficial Outcomes of the Arthritis Self-Management Course Are Not Adequately Explained by Behavior Change," *Arthritis and Rheumatism,* 1989; 32; 91–95.

p. 208, **Jon Kabat-Zinn's chronic pain program:** Jon Kabat-Zinn, *Full Catastrophe Living: Using the Wisdom of Your Body and Mind to Face Stress, Pain, and Illness* (New York: Dell, 1990).

p. 208, **Herbert Benson's programs:** Herbert Benson and Miriam Klipper, *The Relaxation Response* (New York: Avon, 1976).
H. Benson, J. F. Beary, and M. P. Carol, "The Relaxation Response," *Psychiatry,* 1974; 37; 37–46.
A. D. Domar, M. M. Seibel, and H. Benson, "The Mind/Body Program for Infertility: A New Behavioral Treatment Approach for Women with Infertility," *Fertility and Sterility,* 1990; 53; 246–49.

p. 208, **David Spiegel's groups for women with breast cancer:** D. Spiegel et al., "Effect of Psychosocial Treatment on Survival of Patients with Metastatic Breast Cancer," *Lancet,* Oct. 14, 1989; 888–91.

p. 209, **Fawzy Fawzy's groups for people with malignant melanoma:** Fawzy I. Fawzy et al., "Malignant Melanoma: Effects of an Early Structured Psychiatric Intervention, Coping, and Affective State on Recurrence and Survival 6 Years Later," *Archives of General Psychiatry,* Sept. 1993; 50; 681–89.
Fawzy I. Fawzy et al., "A Structured Psychiatric Intervention for Cancer Patients: I. Changes Over Time in Methods of Coping and Affective Disturbance," *Archives of General Psychiatry,* Aug. 1990; 47; 720–25.
Fawzy I. Fawzy et al., "A Structured Psychiatric Intervention for Cancer Patients: II. Changes Over Time in Immunological Measures," *Archives of General Psychiatry,* Aug. 1990; 47; 729–35.

p. 210, **Dean Ornish's work at San Francisco's Preventive Medicine Research Institute:** D. Ornish et al., "Can Lifestyle Changes Reverse Coronary Heart Disease? The Lifestyle Heart Trial," *Lancet,* July 21, 1990; 336; 129–33.
"Multi-Center Lifestyle Heart Trial: Summary of Demonstration Project by the Preventive Medicine Research Institute," Sausalito, Calif., revised 5/19/95.

p. 210, **Michael Antoni's ten-week-long stress-management group:** M. H. Antoni et al., "Cognitive-Behavioral Stress Management Intervention Buffers Distress Responses and Immunologic Changes Following Notification of HIV-1 Seropositivity," *Journal of Consulting and Clinical Psychology,* 1991; 59; 906–15.

M. H. Antoni et al., "Psychosocial Stressors and Behavioral Interventions in Gay Men with HIV-1 Infection," *International Review of Psychiatry*, 1991; 3; 383–99.

p. 210, **George Solomon's research on long-term HIV survivors:** George F. Solomon and Lydia Temoshok, "A Psychoneuroimmunologic Perspective on AIDS Research: Questions, Preliminary Findings, and Suggestions," in L. Temoshok and A. Baum, eds., *Psychosocial Perspectives on AIDS* (Hillsdale, N.J.: Lawrence Erlbaum Associates, 1990).

Henry Dreher, "The Healthy Elderly and Long-Term Survivors of AIDS: Psychoimmune Connections. A Conversation with George F. Solomon, M.D.," *Advances*, 1988; 5(1); 6–14.

CHAPTER 14: *The Healing Path*

p. 220, **church attendance correlated with decreased rates of cancer, hypertension, strokes, and colitis and with lower overall rate of mortality:** G. W. Comstock and K. B. Partridge, "Church Attendance and Health," *Journal of Chronic Diseases*, 1972; 25; 665–72.

T. W. Graham et al., "Frequency of Church Attendance and Blood Pressure Elevation," *Journal of Behavioral Medicine*, 1978; 1(1); 37–43.

p. 220, **church attendance correlated with prevention of drug and alcohol abuse and adolescent suicide:** R. J. Watts et al., "Epidemiological Research on Blacks and Depression: A Sociocultural Perspective," paper presented at the annual meeting of the American Public Health Association, Washington, D.C., Nov. 1985.

p. 220, **we can make significant changes in the well-being of others:** Larry Dossey, *Healing Words: The Power of Prayer and the Practice of Medicine* (New York: HarperCollins, 1993).

p. 221, **research by Bernard Grad:** Bernard Grad, "Some Biological Effects of the 'Laying on of Hands': A Review of Experiments with Animals and Plants," *Journal of the American Society for Psychical Research*, Apr. 1975; 59(2); 95–126.

p. 221, **work of Dolores Krieger:** Dolores Krieger, "Therapeutic Touch: The Imprimatur of Nursing," *American Journal of Nursing*, May 1975; 75; 784–87.

p. 222, **work of William Braud and Marilyn Schlitz:** William G. Braud and Marilyn J. Schlitz, "Consciousness Interactions with Remote Biological Systems: Anomalous Intentionality Effects," *Subtle Energies*, 1992, 2(1); 1–46.

William Braud, "Psi and PNI: Exploring the Interface Between Parapsychology and Psychoneuroimmunology," *Parapsychology Review*, Jul.–Aug. 1986; 17(4); 1–4.

p. 222, **work of Randolph Byrd:** R. Byrd, "Positive Therapeutic Effects of Intercessory Prayer in a Coronary Care Unit Population," *Southern Medical Journal*, 1988; 81(7); 826–29.

p. 223, **books mentioned include:** Bernie Siegel, *Love, Medicine, and Miracles: Lessons Learned about Self-Healing from a Surgeon's Experience with Exceptional Patients* (New York: HarperCollins, 1986).

Deepak Chopra, *Quantum Healing: Exploring the Frontiers of Mind-Body Medicine* (New York: Bantam Books, 1989).

Deepak Chopra, *Ageless Body, Timeless Mind* (New York: Harmony Books, 1993).

Larry Dossey, *Healing Words: The Power of Prayer and the Practice of Medicine* (New York: HarperCollins, 1993).

p. 231, **a comprehensive, reasoned overview of alternative cancer treatments:** Michael Lerner, *Choices in Healing: Integrating the Best of Conventional and Complementary Approaches to Cancer* (Cambridge, Mass.: MIT Press, 1994).

p. 233, **resources on shamanism:** Roger N. Walsh, *Spirit of Shamanism* (Los Angeles: Jeremy P. Tarcher, 1990).

Mircea Eliade, *Shamanism: Archaic Techniques of Ecstasy* (Princeton, N.J.: Princeton University Press, 1964).

p. 233, **the power of the healing ordeal:** Caryle Hirshberg and Marc Ian Barasch, *Remarkable Recovery: What Extraordinary Healings Tell Us About Getting Well and Staying Well* (Riverhead/Putnam, 1995).

CHAPTER 15: *Creating the New Medicine*

p. 251, **visits by women to ERs that are related to physical abuse:** Teri Randall, "Domestic Violence Intervention Calls for More Than Treating Injuries," *Journal of the American Medical Association,* 1990; 264(8); 939–40.

Susan V. McLeer et al., "Education Is Not Enough: A Systems Failure in Protecting Battered Women," *Annals of Emergency Medicine,* 1989; 18(6); 651–53.

p. 252, **the Planetree Project:** Diane P. Martin et al., "The Planetree Model Hospital Project: An Example of the Patient as Partner," *Hospital and Health Services Administration,* 1990; 35(4); 591–601.

Rebecca Voelker, "New Trends Aimed at Healing by Design," *Journal of the American Medical Association,* 1994; 272(24); 1885–86.

p. 252, **brief psychotherapeutic intervention reduces hospitalization in hip fracture patients:** James J. Strain et al., "Cost Offset from a Psychiatric Consultation-Liaison Intervention with Elderly Hip Fracture Patients," *American Journal of Psychiatry,* 1991; 148; 1044–49.

p. 252, **relaxation and breathing techniques decrease anesthesia, postop medication, and complications:** L. D. Egbert et al., "Reduction of Postoperative Pain by Encouragement and Instruction of Patients," *New England Journal of Medicine,* 1964; 270; 825–27.

H. L. Bennett et al., "Preoperative Instructions for Decreased Bleeding During Spine Surgery," *Anesthesiology,* 1986; 65; A245.

M. Rogers and P. Reich, "Psychological Intervention with Surgical Patients: Evaluation Outcome," *Advances in Psychosomatic Medicine,* 1986; 15; 23–50.

E. Mumford et al., "The Effects of Psychological Intervention on Recovery from Surgery and Heart Attacks: An Analysis of the Literature," *American Journal of Public Health*, 1982; 72; 141–51.

p. 253, **childbirth has become a medical procedure:** Mindy A. Smith, Mack T. Ruffin, and Lee Green, "The Rational Management of Labor," *American Family Physician*, May 1, 1993; 47(6); 1471–81.

Mindy A. Smith et al., "A Critical Review of Labor and Birth Care," *Journal of Family Practice*, 1991; 33(3); 281–92.

p. 254, **self-hypnosis to reduce pain and anxiety of childbirth, contribute sense of confidence and control:** E. L. Rossi, *The Psychobiology of Mind-Body Healing: New Concepts of Therapeutic Hypnosis* (New York: W. W. Norton, 1986).

E. Fromm and S. Kahn, *Self-Hypnosis: The Chicago Paradigm* (New York: Guilford Press, 1990).

p. 254, **yoga to facilitate muscular strength and flexibility, encourage pelvic relaxation:** N. Fields, "Teaching the Gentle Way to Labour," *Nursing Times*, Feb. 8-14, 1995; 91(6); 44–45.

p. 254, **studies on *doulas*:** M. K. Klaus et al., "Maternal Assistance and Support in Labor: Father, Nurse, Midwife, or Doula?" *Clinical Consultations in Obstetrics and Gynecology*, 1992; 4(4); 211–17.

J. Kennell et al., "Continuous Emotional Support During Labor in a U.S. Hospital: A Randomized Controlled Trial," *Journal of the American Medical Association*, 1991; 265(17); 2197–237.

p. 254, **acupuncture stimulates labor gently, decreases pain, may reverse position of breech babies:** I. Skelton, "Acupuncture and Labour—A Summary of Results," *Midwives Chronicle*, May 1988; 134.

Wen Wei, "Correcting Abnormal Fetal Positions with Moxibustion," *Midwives Chronicle*, 1979; 103; 432.

S. Budd, "Traditional Chinese Medicine in Obstetrics," *Midwives Chronicle*, 1992; 105; 140.

S. Yelland, "Using Acupuncture in Midwifery Care," *Modern Midwife*, Jan. 1995; 5(1); 8–11.

p. 255, **worksite wellness programs:** Kenneth R. Pelletier, "A Review and Analysis of the Health and Cost-Effective Outcome Studies of Comprehensive Health Promotion and Disease Prevention Programs," *American Journal of Health Promotion*, Mar.–Apr. 1991; 5(4); 311–15.

p. 256, **Herbert Benson's relaxation techniques in schools:** Herbert Benson et al., "Increases in Positive Psychological Characteristics with a New Relaxation-Response Curriculum in High School Students," *Journal of Research and Development in Education*, 1994; 27; 224–31.

p. 257, **spending on "unconventional" medical care:** David M. Eisenberg et al., "Unconventional Medicine in the United States: Prevalence, Costs, and Patterns of Use," *New England Journal of Medicine*, Jan. 28, 1993; 328(4); 246–52.

p. 259, **workmen's compensation studies on chiropractic:** R. A. Martin, "A Study of Time Loss Back Claims: Workmen's Compensation Board," Medical director's report, state of Oregon, *Archives of the California Chiropractic Association,* 1975; 4(1).
First Research Corporation, *A Study and Analysis of the Treatment of Sprain and Strain Injuries in Industrial Cases* (Davenport, Iowa: International Chiropractic Association, 1960).
American Chiropractic Association, *Benefits of Chiropractic Inclusion in Your Health and Welfare Program* (Des Moines, Iowa, 1979).

p. 259, **worksite wellness and health promotion programs:** Kenneth R. Pelletier, "A Review and Analysis of the Health and Cost-Effective Outcome Studies of Comprehensive Health Promotion and Disease Prevention Programs," *American Journal of Health Promotion,* Mar./Apr. 1991; 5(4); 311–15.

p. 259, **work with people with chronic pain:** Margaret Caudill et al., "Decreased Clinic Use by Chronic Pain Patients: Response to Behavioral Medicine Intervention," *Clinical Journal of Pain,* 1991; 7; 305–10.

p. 259, **Stanford's Arthritis Self-Management Program:** K. Lorig et al., "Evidence Suggesting That Health Education for Self-Management in Patients with Chronic Arthritis Has Sustained Health Benefits While Reducing Health-Care Costs," *Arthritis and Rheumatism,* 1993; 36(4); 439–46.

p. 260, **massage for low-birth-weight babies:** T. M. Field et al., "Tactile/ Kinesthetic Stimulation Effects on Preterm Neonates," *Pediatrics,* 1986; 77(5); 654–58.

p. 260, **pairing every laboring mother with a *doula*:** M. K. Klaus et al., "Maternal Assistance and Support in Labor: Father, Nurse, Midwife, or Doula?" *Clinical Consultations in Obstetrics and Gynecology,* 1992; 4(4); 211–17.
J. Kennell et al., "Continuous Emotional Support During Labor in a U.S. Hospital: A Randomized Controlled Trial," *Journal of the American Medical Association,* 1991; 265(17); 2197–237.

p. 260, **cost-benefit analysis on Dean Ornish's Lifestyle Heart Trial:** D. Ornish et al., "Can Lifestyle Changes Reverse Coronary Heart Disease? The Lifestyle Heart Trial," *Lancet,* July 21, 1990; 336; 129–33. "Multi-Center Lifestyle Heart Trial: Summary of Demonstration Project by the Preventive Medicine Research Institute," Sausalito, Calif., revised 5/19/95.

p. 261, **single-payer plan:** Jim McDermott, "Evaluating Health System Reform: The Case for a Single-Payer Approach," *Journal of the American Medical Association,* Mar. 9, 1991; 271(10); 782–84.
Gordon D. Schiff et al., "A Better-Quality Alternative: Single-Payer National Health System Reform," *Journal of the American Medical Association,* Sept. 14, 1994; 272(10); 803–808.

Melvin Konner, *Dear America, A Concerned Doctor Wants You to Know the Truth About Health Reform* (Reading, Mass.: Addison Wesley, 1993).

p. 262, **currently 25 percent of our hospital costs:** Steffie Woolhandler, David U. Himmelstein, and James P. Lewontin, "Administrative Costs in U.S. Hospitals," *New England Journal of Medicine,* 1993; 329(6); 400–403.

p. 262, **levels of satisfaction higher for patients who see physicians who practice on their own:** Haya R. Rubin et al., "Patients' Ratings of Outpatient Visits in Different Practice Settings: Results from the Medical Outcomes Study," *Journal of the American Medical Association,* Aug. 18, 1993; 270(7); 835–40.

p. 263, **1991 GAO report:** U.S. General Accounting Office, *Canadian Health Insurance: Lessons for the United States,* Report to the Chairman, Committee on Government Operations, House of Representatives, pub. no. GAO/HRD-91-90 (Washington, D.C.: U.S. General Accounting Office, June 1991).

p. 266, **AMA study on defensive medicine:** Brian McCormick, "Study: Defensive Medicine Costs Nearly \$10 Billion," *American Medical News,* Feb. 15, 1993.

p. 268, **1991 study of 31,000 hospital records in New York state:** A. Russell Localio, et al., "Relation Between Malpractice Claims and Adverse Events Due to Negligence: Results of the Harvard Medical Practice Study," *New England Journal of Medicine,* July 25, 1991; 325(4); 245–50.

p. 269, **"no fault" malpractice system in New Zealand and Sweden:** Barry M. Manuel, "Professional Liability—A No-Fault Solution," *New England Journal of Medicine,* March 1, 1990; 322(9); 627–31.
Marilyn Rosenthal, *Dealing with Medical Malpractice: The British and Swedish Experience* (London and Durham, N.C.: Tavistock and Duke University Press, 1988).

p. 273, **1978 Office of Technology Assessment study:** U.S. Congress, Office of Technology Assessment, *Assessing the Efficacy and Safety of Medical Technologies,* stock no. 052-003-00593-0 (Washington, D.C.: U.S. Government Printing Office, September 1978).

p. 274, **report to the OAM:** *Alternative Medicine: Expanding Medical Horizons,* A Report to the National Institutes of Health on Alternative Medical Systems and Practices in the United States, (NIH pub. no. 94-066 (Washington, D.C.: U.S. Government Printing Office, 1994).

RESOURCES

Books ✍

Alternative Medicine: Expanding Medical Horizons. **(A Report to the National Institutes of Health on Alternative Medical Systems and Practices in the United States.) (NIH Publ. No. 94-066) Washington, DC: U.S. Government Printing Office, 1994.**
This book includes the work of over two hundred contributors and an editorial board. It is the most comprehensive and up-to-date compilation and evaluation of the research on a variety of alternative medical approaches. Dense and difficult going at times, but an invaluable reference work. The sections covering research on diet and nutrition, manipulative therapies, and mind-body approaches are particularly useful.

Benson, Herbert and E. Stuart. *The Wellness Book: The Comprehensive Guide to Maintaining Health and Treating Stress-Related Illness.* **Secaucus, NJ: Carol Publishing Group, 1992.**
An easy to read self-help guide. Each chapter focuses on a specific aspect of the mind-body approach, including exercise, nutrition, and stress management. It provides basic information and self-assessments and is full of illustrations and practical exercises.

Borysenko, Joan. *Minding the Body, Mending the Mind.* **Reading, MA: Addison-Wesley, 1987.**
A very good, readable, and practical introduction to the mind-body approach by a cell biologist and psychologist who's done laboratory research and clinical work. Joan Borysenko has a wonderful heart as well as an organized mind, and both are apparent here.

The Boston Women's Health Book Collective. *The New Our Bodies, Ourselves.* **New York: Simon & Schuster, 1984.**
Twenty years ago, this remarkable compilation of medical fact, personal experience, and political analysis provided a picture of the forces that shape the lives and health of women in the contemporary United States. This updated version provides clearly written and comprehensive information about pregnancy, menopause, sexuality, nutrition, lesbian relationships, and aging. It is one of the premier self-help books.

Chopra, Deepak. *Ageless Body, Timeless Mind.* **New York: Harmony Books, 1993.**
A practical and inspirational bestseller which suggests that attitude—as well as diet and exercise—can profoundly affect and slow down the aging process.

Chopra, Deepak. *Quantum Healing: Exploring the Frontiers of Mind/Body Medicine.* **New York: Bantam, 1990.**
A well-written and accessible essay on the power of the mind to affect the body. It makes an attempt to bring the discoveries of modern physics to bear on the mysteries of miraculous recoveries.

Dienstfrey, Harris. *Where the Mind Meets the Body.* **New York: HarperCollins, 1991.**
This is a good account of some of the pioneering work done in mind-body studies, including Herbert Benson's work on the relaxation response, Robert Ader's on psychoneuroimmunology, and Neal Miller's on biofeedback. It's clear, readable, and where appropriate, skeptical.

Ferguson, Tom (ed.) *Medical Self-Care: Access to Health Tools.* **New York: Summit Books, 1980.**
A classic compendium of information designed to help people to help themselves.

The Burton Goldberg Group. *Alternative Medicine: The Definitive Guide.* **Puyallup, WA: Future Medicine Publishing, 1993.**
An encyclopedic treatment of alternative therapies, including many that are highly controversial, and their uses for a variety of conditions. The information is presented through interviews with a variety of clinicians. It's extremely useful but neither as definitive nor as carefully documented as one would hope.

Goleman, Daniel and Joel Gurin (eds.) *Mind / Body Medicine: How to Use Your Mind for Better Health.* **Yonkers, NY: Consumer Reports Books, 1993.**
Some of America's leading physicians, psychologists, and medical researchers write about the connection between stress and illness, and a variety of mind-body approaches such as hypnosis, biofeedback, meditation, and psychotherapy.

Gordon, James S. *Holistic Medicine.* **New York: Chelsea House, 1988.**
A brief overview of the field and some of the techniques that are generally included in it.

Gordon, James S., Dennis T. Jaffe, and David E. Bresler (eds.) *Mind, Body, and Health: Toward an Integral Medicine.* **New York: Human Sciences Press, 1984.**
A compendium of articles on therapeutic approaches. The emphasis is on pioneering programs which have been developed to address specific

problems—chronic and acute pain, childbirth, aging, and others—rather than on specific modalities.

Hastings, Arthur C., James Fadiman, and James S. Gordon (eds.) *Health for the Whole Person: The Complete Guide to Holistic Medicine.* **Boulder, CO: Westview Press, 1980.**
For many years, this was the definitive book on the holistic approach and alternative therapeutic modalities. Each of the approximately thirty-five articles was written by an expert in the field. All have comprehensive and critically annotated bibliographies which, though no longer current, are still extremely useful.

Moyers, Bill. *Healing and the Mind.* **New York: Doubleday, 1993.**
A compilation of interviews on various aspects of the new medicine with participants in the television series of the same name. Moyers asks many of the questions that would naturally occur to viewers of this excellent series.

Northrup, Christiane. *Women's Bodies, Women's Wisdom.* **New York: Bantam, 1994.**
An overview of women's health by a gynecologist. It shows how psychological, social, and political factors and forces influence physical well being, and provides a good deal of practical information about health care and health promotion.

Pelletier, Kenneth. *Mind as Healer, Mind as Slayer: A Holistic Approach to Preventing Stress Disorders.* **New York: Delta, 1977.**
This pioneering book offers a clear, straightforward presentation of much of the research that has been done on the effects of stress on the human body. It is also a good summary of nonpharmacological techniques that have been used to alleviate the effects of stress, including meditation, autogenic training, and biofeedback.

Weil, Andrew. *Spontaneous Healing: How to Discover and Enhance Your Body's Natural Ability to Heal Itself.* **New York: Alfred A. Knopf, 1995.**
A clear, well-written discussion that emphasizes the power each of us has to mobilize our mind and body to heal ourselves. The book is particularly strong in explaining how the body heals itself and in presenting botanical treatments.

THE EVOLUTION OF MEDICINE

Carlson, Rick J. *The End of Medicine.* **New York: Wiley-Interscience, 1975.**
Carlson (a lawyer, health care consultant, and political organizer) crisply presents the case against a system of medical care that he describes as costly, dangerous, misguided, and ineffective.

Dubos, René. *Mirage of Health.* **New York: Harper and Row, 1959.**
In this remarkable volume Dubos, a Rockefeller Institute microbiologist, demonstrates the interrelationship between the health and disease of individuals and the biological and social environment in which people live. Dubos concludes that further improvements in the health of the peoples of developed nations will come not from new "magic bullets," but from improvements in our capacity to change and to adapt to our environment.

Garrison, F. H. *Contributions to the History of Medicine.* **New York and London: Hafner Publishing Co., 1966.**
The classic and still quite readable history of medicine.

Illich, Ivan. *Medical Nemesis: The Expropriation of Health.* **New York: Pantheon Books, 1982. (Originally published in 1976.)**
In this controversial book, Illich takes modern medicine to task. The heart of this densely written, meticulously documented polemic is that modern medicine has become a self-aggrandizing, imperialistic, and counterproductive enterprise that debilitates and demeans its patients as it gathers them into its domain.

Knowles, John H. (ed.) *Doing Better and Feeling Worse: Health in the United States.* **New York: Norton, 1977.**
This is a collection of essays by pillars of the American medical establishment on the problems and future directions of our health care system. John Knowles's message in particular is striking, because it stresses our individual responsibility for those attitudes and habits that affect our health.

Konner, Melvin. *Dear America, A Concerned Doctor Wants You to Know the Truth About Health Reform.* **Reading, MA: Addison-Wesley, 1993.**
This brief polemic makes an excellent case for the single-payer system of health care. It was written during the debate on President Clinton's proposal for health care reform, but its points are still relevant.

LaLonde, Marc. *A New Perspective on the Health of Canadians.* **Ottawa: Information Canada, 1975.**
This clear-thinking, elegantly written, brief (seventy-six pages) status report on the health of Canadians and what can be done to improve it, has been an inspiration to health-policy planners since its publication.

Lyons, Albert S. and R. Joseph Petrucelli. *Medicine: An Illustrated History.* **New York: Abradale Press, Harry N. Abrams, Inc., 1987.**
A lavishly illustrated, upbeat overview of the world's medical traditions. It is most useful on medicine prior to 1900.

McKeown, Thomas. *The Role of Medicine: Dream, Mirage, or Nemesis?* **London: Rock Carling Fellowship, Nuffield Provincial Hospitals Trust, 1976.**
Drawing on information derived from mortality and morbidity statistics in England and Wales in the last three centuries, McKeown demonstrates the central importance of changes in the environment, in nutrition, and in behavior for improving health.

Payer, Lynn. *Medicine and Culture.* **New York: Penguin, 1989.**
A survey which documents how much approaches to conventional medical practice can differ, even in Western countries. American medicine stands out as being particularly prone to using invasive technology.

PSYCHOLOGY

Erikson, Erik H. *Childhood and Society.* **New York: Norton, 1964.**
A wonderful—even illuminating book—about how we grow up and how that growing up is shaped by and in turn shapes society. Erikson is probably the most important psychoanalytic and psychological thinker and writer of the last 50 years. This really is *the* basic book for anyone who wants to understand the relationship between individual development and culture.

Frank, Jerome D. and Julia B. Frank. *Persuasion and Healing: A Comparative Study of Psychotherapy,* third edition. Baltimore: Johns Hopkins University Press, 1991.
This is an updated version of the classic examination of the universal elements in healing, by a professor emeritus of psychiatry at Johns Hopkins. Frank is particularly good on the role of belief and the importance of the interpersonal and cultural context in healing.

Justice, Blair. *Who Gets Sick: How Beliefs, Moods, and Thoughts Affect Your Health.* Los Angeles: Jeremy P. Tarcher, 1987.
An encyclopedic, readable compendium of "how beliefs, moods, and thoughts affect your health." Justice touches on nutrition as well as the psychosocial causes and concomitants of illness and health.

Laing, R. D. *The Politics of Experience.* New York: Ballantine Books, 1967.
An incandescent broadside against the conventional view of psychiatric disorders as diseases. Laing insists that much individual disturbance is a comprehensible response to a disturbed social and political environment.

Laing, R. D. *The Divided Self.* Baltimore, MD: Penguin Books, 1965. (Originally published in 1960.)
An elegantly written description of the way people deny their "true selves" in favor of a false, socially accommodating self. A useful means of understanding many of the ways we deny our needs and deform our being.

Minuchin, Salvador, Bernice Rosman, and Lester Baker. *Psychosomatic Families.* Cambridge, Mass.: Harvard University Press, 1978.
An extremely helpful discussion of the way family interactions shape and affect physical illness in children. The book is based on Minuchin and his colleagues' research at the Philadelphia Child Guidance Center.

RELAXATION, STRESS MANAGEMENT, AND BIOFEEDBACK

Davis, M., E. Eschelman, and M. Mathews. *The Relaxation and Stress Reduction Workbook.* Oakland, CA: New Harbinger Publications, Inc., 1988.
This is one of the most comprehensive and clearly written guides to stress reduction. Topics include imagery, assertiveness training, progressive muscle relaxation, self-hypnosis, meditation, autogenics, nutrition, biofeedback, coping skills, exercise, breathing, thought stopping, and time management.

Gordon, James S. *Stress Management.* New York: Chelsea House, 1990.
A good introduction to the causes, history, physiology, and effects of stress. It was written for "adolescents," so the clinical examples toward the end of the book rely primarily on the author's work with them.

Green, Elmer and Alyce Green. *Beyond Biofeedback.* Knoll, 1989.
The Greens, who for years worked at the Menninger Foundation, are pioneers in biofeedback. In this book, they discuss both its therapeutic uses and its implications for understanding the powers of the human imagination.

Jaffe, Dennis. *Healing from Within.* New York: Simon & Schuster, 1988.
A health psychologist's excellent guide to the use of the mind—through attitude change, relaxation, meditation, and imagery—in the treatment of physical and emotional disorders.

PSYCHONEUROIMMUNOLOGY

Dacher, Elliot S. *PNI: The New Mind-Body Healing Program.* **New York: Paragon, 1993.**
An internist's introduction to the science of psychoneuroimmunology, together with helpful exercises for using the mind to mobilize the immune system.

Dreher, Henry. *The Immune Power Personality: 7 Traits You Can Develop to Stay Healthy.* **New York: Dutton, 1995.**
A fine, comprehensive, well-written discussion of the ways attitude and emotion affect immune functioning. Dreher presents, in useful detail, the work of such researchers as George Solomon, who studied the effects of emotion on arthritis, and James Pennebaker, who explored the utility of self-expression through journal keeping.

Locke, S. and D. Colligan. *The Healer Within.* **New York: Dutton, 1985.**
A well-written and balanced evaluation of present research, theory, and clinical practice in the field of psychoneuroimmunology.

MEDITATION

Goleman, Daniel. *The Meditative Mind.* **Los Angles: J. P. Tarcher, 1988.**
A good overview of the world's meditative traditions, which mentions some of the scientific literature on meditation. Goleman is *The New York Times* psychology writer.

Kabat-Zinn, Jon. *Wherever You Go, There You Are.* **New York: Hyperion, 1994.**
A wise guide to bringing the practice of mindfulness into everyday life by the director of the Stress Management Clinic at the University of Massachusetts Medical Center.

LeShan, Lawrence. *How to Meditate.* **New York: Bantam, 1986. (Originally published in 1974.)**
A clear, concise introduction to meditative practice by one of the premier researchers in the psychology of healing.

Naranjo, Claudio. *How to Be.* **Los Angeles: J. P. Tarcher, 1991.**
A basic introduction to meditation which describes and differentiates three essential kinds—concentrative, awareness, and expressive. It was written twenty years ago by a Chilean psychiatrist and is now updated.

Nhat Hanh, Thich. *The Miracle of Mindfulness: A Manual on Meditation.* **Boston: Beacon Press, 1987. (Originally published in 1975.) Also,** *Peace Is Every Step: The Path of Mindfulness in Everyday Life.* **New York: Bantam, 1991.**
These are wonderful and wonderfully practical books by a Vietnamese Buddhist monk. They are a tonic for the soul.

HYPNOSIS AND IMAGERY

Achterberg, Jeanne. *Imagery in Healing: Shamanism and Modern Medicine.* **Boston: New Science Library Publisher, 1985.**
A research psychologist's thoughtful overview of how mind and culture influence the human body.

Cheek, David B. *Hypnosis: The Application of Ideomotor Techniques.*
Boston: Allyn, 1993.
David Cheek, an obstetrician and gynecologist, was one of the pioneers
in the use of hypnosis to treat physical disorders. This is an excellent intro-
duction to his methods and approach, and to the possibilities of hypnosis.
Epstein, Gerald. *Healing Visualizations: Creating Health with Imagery.*
New York: Bantam, 1989.
A guide, by a New York psychiatrist, to the use of imagery in healing.
Epstein is primarily a clinician rather than researcher, and this book pro-
vides many useful exercises to mobilize the mind to understand and assist
the body and itself.
Rossi, Ernest Lawrence. *The Psychobiology of Mind-Body Healing:
New Concepts of Therapeutic Hypnosis,* revised edition. New York:
W. W. Norton, 1993.
A very good, if sometimes dense introduction to the pathways
by which the mind affects the body. It is also an overview of some of
the hypnotic approaches developed by Milton Erickson. Rossi is a Jun-
gian psychologist who worked with Erickson for many years.

TOUCH, MOVEMENT, AND BREATHING

Downing, George. Illustrated by Ann Kent Rush. *The Massage Book.*
New York: Random House, 1972.
The classic introduction to massage therapy. The emphasis is on a relaxed,
meditative approach to touching others in a therapeutic way.
Feuerstein, Georg (ed.) and Stephan Bodian with the staff of Yoga
Journal. *Living Yoga: A Comprehensive Guide for Daily Life.* New York:
J. P. Tarcher / Putnam, 1993.
An introduction to the spirit and practice of yoga. This book contains a
number of essays with concrete information about yogic postures and
breathing techniques, as well as pieces on the spirit of yoga and its prac-
tice in daily life.
Gach, Michael R. and Carolyn Marco. *ACU-Yoga: Self-Help Tech-
niques to Relieve Tension.* New York: Japan Publications, 1981.
An interesting synthesis in which a common ground is found between
yogic postures and acupressure points. A very practical way to make
good use of both the Indian and Chinese healing approaches.
Hittleman, Richard. *Richard Hittleman's Yoga: 28-Day Exercise Plan.*
New York: Random House, 1995.
Yoga, like t'ai chi, is probably best learned in a class, but I've known peo-
ple who haven't had a class available who have used this book to very
good effect.
Huang, Chungliang Al. *T'ai Ji: Beginner's T'ai Ji Book.* Celestial Arts, 1995.
So far as I am concerned, the movements of t'ai chi must be learned in
the company of a teacher. This book, however, gives a nice sense of the
spirit of the practice.
Johnson, Don Hanlon. *Body, Spirit, and Democracy.* Berkeley, CA:
North Atlantic Books, 1993.
An excellent overview of and introduction to body-oriented therapies by
someone who has long practiced, deeply explored, and widely taught a
number of them.

Krieger, Dolores. *Accepting Your Power to Heal.* **Santa Fe, NM: Bear & Co., 1993.**
This book presents an introduction to the use of hands-on healing by the nurse-researcher who did some of the first studies on it. It is both readable and practical.

Lidell, Lucinda with Sara Thomas, et al. *The Book of Massage: The Complete Step-by-Step Guide to Eastern and Western Techniques.* **New York: Fireside/Gaia Books, 1984.**
A well-illustrated, easy to follow book that introduces the fundamentals of Swedish massage. Sections on touch, reflexology, and shiatsu are also included.

Lidell, Lucy et al. *The Sivananda Companion to Yoga.* **New York: Simon & Schuster, 1983.**
A well-illustrated introduction to hatha yoga postures as well as the philosophy on which yoga is based. There are also discussions of breathing techniques, diet, and meditation.

Loehr, James E. and Jeffrey Migdow. *Take a Deep Breath.* **New York: Random House, 1986.**
A clear, readable overview of the way breathing can be used to affect physical and psychological health. A number of different techniques are presented.

Montagu, Ashley. *Touching: The Human Significance of the Skin,* **third edition. New York: Harper & Row, 1986.**
A classic and highly readable work that covers scientific, interpersonal, and cross-cultural aspects of touch.

Murphy, Michael. *The Future of the Body: Explorations Into the Further Evolution of Human Nature.* **New York: Jeremy P. Tarcher/ Perigee, 1993.**
This book is the culmination of almost forty years of work by Michael Murphy, who cofounded The Esalen Institute. It is a massive compendium of information, some widely available, much little known, about the ways the mind and the body can affect one another. There are good overviews of Feldenkrais, Alexander work, Rolfing, and Reichian therapy, among other topics.

Reich, Wilhelm. *Selected Writings: An Introduction to Orgonomy.* **New York: Farrar, Straus, and Giroux, 1960.**
An excellent introduction to the work and thought of this psychoanalytic pioneer and maverick. Reich was the first to make explicit connections between political oppression, emotional illness, and disturbed biological functioning and was for years a leader in movements to alleviate all of them.

Swami Rama, Rudolph Ballentine, and Alan Hymes. *Science of Breath: A Practical Guide.* **Himalayan Publications, 1979.**
A good introduction to the physiology of breathing and the way meditative practice affects it.

FOOD AND NUTRITION

Balch, James F. and Phyllis A. Balch. *Prescription for Nutritional Healing.* **Garden City Park, NY: Avery, 1990.**
A self-help guide to nutritional supplements and their therapeutic use. Unfortunately not well-referenced.

Ballentine, Rudolph. *Transition to Vegetarianism: An Evolutionary Process.* Himalayan Press, 1987.
A good, sometimes frightening introduction to the importance of nutrition and to some of the ways we are polluting the planet and our own bodies and to some strategies for reversing the process. Ballentine was originally trained as a psychiatrist, and he spent many years in India studying nutrition, yoga, and meditation.

Carper, Jean. *Food—Your Miracle Medicine: How Food Can Prevent and Cure Over 100 Symptoms and Problems.* New York: Harper-Collins, 1993.
A terrific collection of information about the therapeutic use of foods and herbs for specific illnesses and disease states.

Crook, William G. Illustrated by Cynthia Crook. *Detecting Your Hidden Allergies.* Jackson, TN: Professional Books Future Health, 1988.
A good introduction to the causes and treatment of food allergies and their role in physical and behavioral problems, by a pediatrician who has also written about the prevalence and dangers of yeast infections.

Golan, Ralph. *Optimal Wellness.* New York: Bantam, 1995.
An excellent introduction to the use of natural therapies for health promotion and the treatment of illness. The book has very strong and practical sections on food allergy, hypoglycemia, nutritional deficiencies, and "dietary hazards and excesses."

Haas, Elson M. *Staying Healthy With Nutrition: The Complete Guide to Diet and Nutritional Medicine.* Berkeley, CA: Celestial Arts, 1992.
A fine overview of nutrition and of the use of nutritional therapies for specific illnesses.

McGee, Harold. *On Food and Cooking: The Science and Lore of the Kitchen.* New York: Collier Books, 1988. (Originally published in 1984.)
A wonderful reference book which tells you everything you might want to know about the hows and whys of preparing and cooking food. It contains an incredible amount of historical and scientific material presented in a clear and engaging way.

Robbins, John. *Diet for a New America.* Walpole, NH: Stillpoint, 1987.
A powerful statement about the ways we are destroying our food supply, and what we can do about it.

Shelton, Herbert. *The Science and Fine Art of Fasting.* Tampa, FL: Natural Hygiene Press, 1978.
The best of a small selection of books available on fasting. It is based on anecdotes only and therefore highlights the need for scientific investigation of this widely used modality.

The Surgeon General's Report on Nutrition. U. S. Government Printing Office, 1988.
This document presents the evidence that implicates our diet in our chronic illnesses. A good reference work—not a light read.

Williams, Roger John. *Biochemical Individuality.* Austin, TX: University of Texas Press, 1980.
A simple introduction to Williams's theory of biochemical individuality. Difficult to find, but worth reading.

HERBAL MEDICINE

Castleman, Michael. *The Healing Herbs: The Ultimate Guide to the Curative Power of Nature's Medicines.* New York: Bantam, 1995.
A concise, inexpensive, well-referenced guide to major western herbs.

Duke, James and S. Foster. *Peterson's Field Guide to Medicinal Plants.* Boston: Houghton-Mifflin, 1990.
A lavishly illustrated guide by one of the world's leading authorities on medicinal herbs.

Grieve, Maude. *A Modern Herbal.* New York: Dover, 1971. (Originally published in 1931.)
A classic herbal, rich with the lore of plant use.

Hoffman, D. *The Holistic Herbal.* Longmeade: Element Books Ltd., 1983.
A good introduction to the therapeutic use of a number of common herbs by a well-known teacher and practitioner.

THE OTHER MEDICINES

Beinfield, Harriet and Efrem Korngold. *Between Heaven and Earth: A Guide to Chinese Medicine.* Ballantine, 1992.
Probably the best and most complete introduction to the philosophy of Chinese medicine and acupuncture. It also gives a nice sense of how another culture views mind and body as inseparable and approaches illness in a more holistic way.

Bensky, Dan and Andrew Gamble. *Chinese Herbal Medicine: Materia Medica,* revised edition. Seattle: Eastland Press, 1993.
A comprehensive text that discusses the traditional uses of Chinese herbs and the modern scientific evidence that justifies these uses.

Coulter, Harris L. *Divided Legacy: A History of the Schism in Medical Thought.* Berkeley, CA: North Atlantic Press, 1977, 1977, 1981.
An encyclopedic treatment of the development of homeopathy and of the struggles that divided homeopaths from conventional physicians.

Cummings, Stephen and Dana Ullman. *Everybody's Guide to Homeopathic Medicines,* revised and expanded. New York: Jeremy P. Tarcher/Putnam, 1991.
A superior introduction to the use of homeopathic remedies. This is a book I recommend to my patients.

Eisenberg, David S. with Thomas Lee Wright. *Encounters With Qi: Exploring Chinese Medicine.* New York: Penguin Books, 1987.
An account of Chinese medicine and particularly of the communication of qi from healers to patients. The author is an American physician who studied and traveled widely in China.

Gevitz, Norman (ed.) *Other Healers: Unorthodox Medicine in America.* Baltimore: Johns Hopkins University Press, 1988.
The best single volume introduction to the history of the other medicines in the United States.

Grossinger, Richard. *Planet Medicine. Volume One: Origins; and Volume Two: Modalities.* Berkeley, CA: North Atlantic Books, 1995.
An extremely wide-ranging and often poetic look at the origins, purposes, and methods of healing in many cultures. Grossinger discusses shamanic theory and practice, classical Taoist healing, Ayurveda, Reichian therapy, and osteopathy, among other approaches.

Grossman, Richard. *The Other Medicine: An Invitation to Understanding and Using Them for Health and Healing*. Garden City, NY: Doubleday, 1985.
A nice, extremely readable, and practical introduction to such alternative approaches as homeopathy, herbalism, and Chinese medicine. It was written by an educator who has worked with several generations of New York City physicians-in-training.

Hammer, Leon. *Dragon Rises, Red Bird Flies: Psychology & Chinese Medicine*. Barrytown, NY: Station Hill Press, 1990.
A wise and comprehensive treatment of the five-element approach to Chinese medicine. The emphasis is on psychological issues and the utility of the five elements as a way of understanding and explaining behavior.

Kaptchuk, Ted. *The Web That Has No Weaver: Understanding Chinese Medicine*. Chicago: Contemporary Books, 1985.
An extremely useful introduction to the spirit and substance of traditional Chinese medicine by an American who studied in Macao.

Lonsdorf, Nancy, Veronica Butler, and Melanie Brown. *A Woman's Best Medicine: Health, Happiness, and Long Life Through Maharishi Ayur-Veda*. New York: Jeremy P. Tarcher / Putnam, 1995.
This is a readable introduction to the concepts and practices of Indian Ayurveda, as well as their relevance to women's health.

Redwood, Daniel. *A Time to Heal: How to Reap the Benefits of Holistic Health*. Virginia Beach, VA: A.R.E. Press, 1993.
A good introduction both to chiropractic and to one chiropractor's work. The section on chiropractic research presents a useful overview.

Reid, Daniel. *The Complete Book of Chinese Health and Healing*. Boston: Shambhala, 1995.
A good overview of the various aspects of Chinese medicine, this book is particularly strong in its discussion of qi gong.

Rose, Barry. *The Family Health Guide to Homeopathy*. Berkeley, CA: Celestial Arts, 1992.
A well-illustrated schematic guide to the treatment of a number of common illnesses and to frequently used homeopathic remedies. A good introduction to homeopathic symptom pictures and prescribing.

Sobel, David S. *Ways of Health: Holistic Approaches to Ancient and Contemporary Medicine*. New York: Harcourt Brace Jovanovich, 1979.
An extremely useful survey of other medical traditions. It includes some of the most telling critiques of Western medicine as well as snapshots from Hippocratic, Chinese, and American Indian sources.

Ullman, Dana. *Discovering Homeopathy: Medicine for the 21st Century,* revised edition. Berkeley, CA: North Atlantic Books, 1991.
A good introduction to the history and philosophy of homeopathy, with an excellent section on homeopathic research.

MIND-BODY APPROACH IN CLINICAL PRACTICE

Benjamin, Harold H. *The Wellness Community Guide to Fighting for Recovery from Cancer*. New York: Putnam, 1995.
This practical and reassuring book provides information on the emotional and social support that cancer patients need. Wellness communities around the country have provided guidance to more than 20,000 people with cancer.

Hirshberg, Caryle, and Marc Ian Barasch. *Remarkable Recovery: What Extraordinary Healings Tell Us about Getting Well and Staying Well.* New York: Riverhead/Putnam, 1995.
A wonderful and inspiring book based on case histories of people who recovered from apparently fatal illnesses. The book emphasizes the importance of attitude, faith, and human support in the face of overwhelming odds.

Kabat-Zinn, Jon. *Full Catastrophe Living: Using the Wisdom of Your Body and Mind to Face Stress, Pain, and Illness.* New York: Dell, 1990.
This book, by the director of a comprehensive program for the treatment of chronic illness at the University of Massachusetts Medical Center, gives a sense of the attitude that pervades that program—one of "mindfulness". It shows how yoga, meditation, and group support may be used in the treatment of chronic pain, anxiety disorders, and other conditions.

Lerner, Michael. *Choices in Healing: Integrating the Best of Conventional and Complementary Approaches to Cancer.* Cambridge, MA: MIT Press, 1994.
An extremely thoughtful and valuable overview of alternative cancer therapies. It is must reading for anyone with cancer.

Ornish, Dean. *Dr. Dean Ornish's Program for Reversing Heart Disease Without Drugs or Surgery.* New York: Ballantine, 1992.
Ornish's program for reversing heart disease offers a good perspective on the effective use of a comprehensive mind-body approach—including nutrition and exercise, relaxation techniques, yoga, and group support. This is a wonderful example of the way clinical work with the mind-body approach can not only provide enormous benefit to patients, but also yield persuasive research results.

Siegel, Bernie. *Love, Medicine, and Miracles: Lessons Learned about Self-Healing from a Surgeon's Experience with Exceptional Patients.* New York: HarperCollins, 1986.
A best seller by a Yale surgeon that has helped many people to realize that they can be "exceptions" to the grim statistics that often confront patients with cancer and other life-threatening illnesses.

Spiegel, David. *Living Beyond Limits: A Scientific Mind-Body Approach to Facing Life-Threatening Illness.* New York: Fawcett, 1994.
This is a popular account of Spiegel's work with women with metastatic breast cancer. The emphasis here is on the power of psychological support and self-expression to affect well-being and outcome.

SPIRITUALITY

Barasch, Marc Ian. *The Healing Path: A Soul Approach to Illness.* New York: Penguin, 1994.
A moving, well-written account of a what a journalist with thyroid cancer learned about himself and his illness as he worked to heal himself.

Borysenko, Joan. *Fire in the Soul: A New Psychology of Spiritual Optimism.* New York: Warner Books, 1994.
A wise and very personal guide to understanding life crises as part of a process of spiritual growth. This is a book I often recommend to my patients.

Dossey, Larry. *Healing Words: The Power of Prayer and the Practice of Medicine.* New York: HarperCollins, 1993.
A clear, well-written overview of the power of prayer to affect people physically and emotionally. The book is based on hundreds of published studies.

Institute of Noetic Sciences with William Poole. *The Heart of Healing.* Atlanta: Turner Publishing, 1993.
A nicely illustrated companion to the Institute of Noetic Sciences' series that appeared on Turner Broadcasting Systems. The emphasis of the book is on the power of the mind to affect our health, the therapeutic effect of spiritual practice, and intriguing but so-far inexplicable instances of remarkable recoveries.

Kornfield, Jack. *A Path With Heart: A Guide Through the Perils and Promises of Spiritual Life.* New York: Bantam, 1993.
A gentle, thoughtful approach to the meditative life by an American psychologist who spent years studying Buddhist practice in Southeast Asia.

Mitchell, Stephen. *The Enlightened Heart: An Anthology of Poetry.* New York: Harper, 1992.
An anthology of sacred poetry well chosen and well translated—from the Bible, Rumi, Lao Tzu, etc. Sample: "A good traveler has no fixed plans and is not intent upon arriving. A good artist lets his intuition lead him wherever it wants. A good scientist has freed himself of concepts and keeps his mind open to what is."—Lao Tzu.

Moore, Thomas. *Care of the Soul: A Guide for Cultivating Depth and Sacredness in Everyday Life.* HarperCollins, 1992.
A lovely and currently very popular book on the spiritual dimension of health and healing.

Suzuki, Shunryu and Trudy Dixon (ed.) *Zen Mind, Beginner's Mind.* New York: Weatherhill, 1970.
An elegant collection of talks by a great Zen teacher—very useful for those of us who spend too much time ruminating about the past or worrying about the future.

Walsh, Roger N. *The Spirit of Shamanism.* Los Angeles: Jeremy P. Tarcher, 1990.
A good overview of the historical, anthropological, and psychological literature on shamanic practices and states of mind. It was written by a California psychiatrist and philosopher.

Journals

Advances: The Journal of Mind-Body Health. Published by The Fetzer Institute, 9292 West KL Avenue, Kalamazoo, MI 49009. (616) 375-2000.

Alternative Therapies in Health and Medicine. Published by InnoVision Communications, a division of the American Association of Critical Care Nurses (AACN), 101 Columbia, Aliso Viejo, CA 92656. (800) 899-1712.

The Journal of Alternative and Complementary Medicine: Research on Paradigm, Practice, and Policy. Published by Mary Ann Liebert, Inc., 1651 Third Ave., New York, NY 10128. (212) 289-2300.

Organizations ∽

Center for Mind-Body Medicine
James S. Gordon, M.D., Director
5225 Connecticut Avenue, N.W.
Suite 414
Washington, DC 20015
(202) 966-7338
Fax (202) 966-2589

U.S. GOVERNMENT

Office of Alternative Medicine
9000 Rockville Pike
Building 31, Room 5B-37
Mailstop 2182
Bethesda, MD 20892
(301) 402-2466
Fax (301) 402-4741

MEDICAL AND NURSING

American Holistic Medical
  Association
4101 Lake Boone Trail
Suite 201
Raleigh, NC 27607
(919) 787-5181

American Holistic Nurses'
  Association
4101 Lake Boone Trail
Suite 201
Raleigh, NC 27607
(800) 278-AHNA
Fax (919) 787-4916

American Medical Student
  Association
1902 Association Drive
Reston, VA 22091
(703) 620-6600
Fax (703) 620-5873

Canadian Holistic Medical
  Association
491 Eglinton Avenue West, #407
Toronto, Ontario M5N 1A8
(416) 485-3071

FAMILY THERAPY

American Association for
  Marriage and Family Therapy
1133 15th Street, N.W., Suite 300
Washington, DC 20005
(202) 452-0109

Collaborative Family Health
  Care Coalition
40 West 12th Street
New York, NY 10011
(212) 675-2477

BIOFEEDBACK

Biofeedback Certification
  Institute of America
10200 West 44th Ave., Suite 304
Wheatridge, CO 80033
(303) 420-2902

MEDITATION

Insight Meditation Society
1230 Pleasant Street
Barre, MA 01005
(508) 355-4378

Kripalu Center for Yoga and Health
P.O. Box 793
Lenox, MA 01240
(413) 448-3400

San Francisco Zen Center
300 Page Street
San Francisco, CA 94102
(415) 431-3771

Washington Center for
  Meditation Studies
1834 Swann Street, N.W.
Washington, DC 20009
(202) 234-2866

HYPNOSIS

American Society of Clinical
  Hypnosis
2200 East Devon Avenue, Suite 291
Des Plaines, IL 60018
(708) 297-3317

Milton Erickson Foundation
3606 North 24th Street
Phoenix, AZ 85016
(602) 956-6196

IMAGERY

Academy for Guided Imagery
P.O. Box 2070
Mill Valley, CA 94942
(800) 726-2070

MASSAGE AND BODYWORK

American Massage Therapy
  Association
820 Davis Street, Suite 100
Evanston, IL 60201-4444
(708) 864-0123

North American Society of
  Teachers of the Alexander
  Technique
P.O. Box 517
Urbana, IL 61801
(800) 473-0620

The Feldenkrais Guild
706 Ellsworth Street, S.W.
P.O. Box 489
Albany, OR 97321
(800) 775-2118
(503) 926-0981
Fax (503) 926-0572

Rolf Institute
205 Canyon Boulevard
Boulder, CO 80302
(303) 449-5903
(800) 530-8875
Fax (303) 449-5978

NEO-REICHIAN THERAPY

Institute of Core Energetics
115 East 23rd Street
New York, NY 10010
(212) 982-9637

International Institute for
  Bioenergetic Analysis
144 East 36th Street, Suite 1A
New York, NY 10016
(212) 532-7742

THERAPEUTIC TOUCH

Nurse Healers Professional
  Associates, Inc.
175 Fifth Avenue
Suite 2755
New York, NY 10010
(212) 886-3776

YOGA

Yoga Journal
2054 University Avenue
Suite 600
Berkeley, CA 94704
(510) 841-9200

T'AI CHI

T'ai Chi Ch'uan Study Center
(correspondence address)
750 Miller Avenue
Great Falls VA 22066
(703) 759-9141

NUTRITION

American Dietetic Association
216 West Jackson
Suite 800
Chicago, IL 60606
(312) 899-0040

Center for Science in the Public
  Interest
1875 Connecticut Avenue, N.W.
Suite 300
Washington, DC 20009
(202) 332-9110
Fax (202) 265-4954

George Ohsawa Macrobiotic
Foundation
1999 Myers Street
Oroville, CA 95966-5340
(916) 533-7703

Physicians' Committee for
Responsible Medicine
P.O. Box 6322
Washington, DC 20015
(202) 686-2210

HERBAL MEDICINE

American Botanical Council
P.O. Box 201660
Austin, TX 78720
(512) 331-8868

American Herbalists' Guild
Box 1683
Soquel, CA 95073
(408) 464-2441

Herb Research Foundation
1007 Pearl Street, Suite 200
Boulder, CO 80302
(800) 748-2617
(303) 449-2265
NAPRALERT
(Natural Products Alert)
Program for Collaborative
Research in the
Pharmaceutical Sciences
M/C 877
College of Pharmacy - UIC
833 South Wood Street
Chicago, IL 60612
(312) 996-2246

ACUPUNCTURE AND CHINESE MEDICINE

American Academy of Medical
Acupuncture
5820 Wilshire Blvd., Suite 500
Los Angeles, CA 90036
(213) 937-5514

American Association of
Acupuncture and
Oriental Medicine
433 Front Street
Catasauqua, PA 18032-2506
(610) 266-1433

American Foundation of
Traditional Chinese Medicine
505 Beach Street
San Francisco, CA 94133
(415) 776-0502
Fax (415) 776-9053

AYURVEDA

The Ayurvedic Institute
P.O. Box 23445
Albuquerque, NM 87192
(505) 291-9698

College of Maharishi Ayurveda
at Maharishi International
University
1603 North Fourth Street
P.O. Box 282
Fairfield, IA 52557
(515) 472-8477

HOMEOPATHY

American Institute of
Homeopathy
1503 Glencoe
Denver, CO 80220
(303) 898-5477

Homeopathic Educational Services
2124 Kittredge Street
Berkeley, CA 94704
(510) 649-0294

National Center for Homeopathy
801 North Fairfax Street
Suite 306
Alexandria, VA 22314
(703) 548-7790
Fax (703) 548-7792

NATUROPATHY

American Association of
Naturopathic Physicians
P.O. Box 20386
Seattle, WA 98102
(206) 323-7610

Bastyr University of Natural
Health Sciences
144 N.E. 54th Street
Seattle, WA 98105
(206) 523-9585

CHIROPRACTIC

American Chiropractic Association
1701 Clarendon Boulevard
Arlington, VA 22209
(800) 986-4636
(703) 276-8800

International Chiropractors
Association
1110 North Glebe Road
Suite 1000
Arlington, VA 22201
(703) 528-5000

OSTEOPATHY

American Academy of
Osteopathy
3500 DePauw Blvd.
Suite 1080
Indianapolis, IN 46268
(317) 879-1881
Fax (317) 879-0563

American Osteopathic Association
142 East Ontario Street
Chicago, IL 60611
(312) 280-5800
Fax (312) 280-3860

CANCER PROGRAMS

CanHelp
3111 Paradise Bay Road
Port Ludlow, WA 98365-9771
(206) 437-2291
Fax (206) 437-2272

Commonweal Cancer
Help Program
P.O. Box 316
Bolinas, CA 94924
(415) 868-0970

Exceptional Cancer Patients
300 Plaza Middlesex
Middletown, CT 06457
(203) 343-5950
Fax (203) 343-5956

Healing Choices Report
Service/Equinox Press
144 St. John's Place
Brooklyn, NY 11217
(800) 929-WELL
(718) 636-4433
Fax (718) 636-0816

National Coalition for
Cancer Survivorship
1010 Wayne Avenue, Fifth floor
Silver Spring, MD 20910
(301) 505-2010

The Wellness Community
2200 Colorado Avenue
Santa Monica, CA 90404
(310) 453-2200

CLINICAL/EDUCATIONAL PROGRAMS

ARRIVE
(AIDS Risk Reduction for IV
Drug Users and Ex-Offenders)
151 West 26th Street
3rd Floor
New York, NY 10001
(212) 243-3434

Arthritis Self-Help Course
The Arthritis Foundation
P.O. Box 19000
Atlanta, GA 30326
(800) 283-7800

Mind/Body Medical Institute
Division of Behavioral Medicine
New England Deaconess Hospital
185 Pilgrim Road
Boston, MA 02215
(617) 732-9525
Fax (617) 738-7023

Preventive Medicine Research
Institute
900 Bridgeway, Suite One
Sausalito, CA 94965
(415) 332-2525
Fax (415) 332-5730

Stanford Arthritis Center
1000 Welch Road, Suite 204
Palo Alto, CA 94304
(415) 723-7935

Stress Reduction Clinic
University of Massachusetts
Medical Center
Worcester, MA 01655
(508) 856-1616

Upledger Institute
11211 Prosperity Farms Road
Palm Beach Gardens, FL 33410
(407) 622-4706
Fax (407) 622-4771

EDUCATIONAL PROGRAMS

American Holistic
Health Association
P.O. Box 17400
Anaheim, CA 92817-7400
(714) 779-6152

Esalen Institute
Big Sur, CA 93920
(408) 667-3000

Feathered Pipe Ranch
P.O. Box 1682
Helena, MT 59624
(406) 442-8196

Interface
55 Wheeler Street
Cambridge, MA 02138
(617) 876-4600

National Institute for the
Clinical Application of
Behavioral Medicine
P.O. Box 523
Mansfield Center, CT 06250
(203) 456-1153

New York Open Center
83 Spring Street
New York, NY 10012
(212) 219-2527

Oasis Center
7463 North Sheridan Road
Chicago, IL 60626
(312) 274-6777

Omega Institute for Holistic Studies
260 Lake Drive
Rhinebeck, NY 12572
(914) 266-4444
(800) 944-1001

Planetree Health Resource Center
2040 Webster Street
San Francisco, CA 94115
(415) 923-3680
Fax (415) 673-7650

FOUNDATIONS AND RESEARCH INSTITUTES

Fetzer Institute
9292 West KL Avenue
Kalamazoo, MI 49009-9398
(616) 375-2000

Institute of Noetic Sciences
P.O. Box 909
Sausalito, CA 94966
(415) 331-5650
Fax (415) 331-5673

Touch Research Institute
University of Miami School of
Medicine
P.O. Box 016820
Miami, FL 33101
(305) 547-6781

Index